Sample Sizes
for Clinical Trials

Steven A. Julious

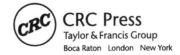

CRC Press
Taylor & Francis Group
Boca Raton   London   New York

CRC Press is an imprint of the
Taylor & Francis Group an **informa** business

A CHAPMAN & HALL BOOK

Chapman & Hall/CRC
Taylor & Francis Group
6000 Broken Sound Parkway NW, Suite 300
Boca Raton, FL 33487-2742

© 2010 by Taylor and Francis Group, LLC
Chapman & Hall/CRC is an imprint of Taylor & Francis Group, an Informa business

No claim to original U.S. Government works

Printed in the United States of America on acid-free paper
10 9 8 7 6 5 4 3 2 1

International Standard Book Number: 978-1-58488-739-3 (Hardback)

Library of Congress Cataloging-in-Publication Data

Julious, Steven A.
   Sample sizes for clinical trials / Steven A. Julious.
      p. ; cm.
   Includes bibliographical references and index.
   ISBN-13: 978-1-58488-739-3 (hardcover : alk. paper)
   ISBN-10: 1-58488-739-7 (hardcover : alk. paper)
   1. Clinical trials--Statistical methods. 2. Sampling (Statistics) I. Title.
   [DNLM: 1. Clinical Trials as Topic--methods. 2. Sample Size. QV 771 J94s 2009]

   R853.C55J85 2009
   615.5072'4--dc22   2008053599

Visit the Taylor & Francis Web site at
http://www.taylorandfrancis.com

and the CRC Press Web site at
http://www.crcpress.com

To my family

Contents

Preface

Probably the most common reason today for someone to come to see me for advice is for a sample size calculation, a calculation that, although relatively straightforward, is often left in the domain of a statistician.

Although the sample size calculated could easily be the end of matters, with time I have come to realise that the sample size of a trial is a process and not an end in itself.

Many years ago, when I was just starting out in my career, I was in dispute over a study being undertaken. An unscheduled interim analysis was requested, and I pushed back as the study had barely started; we had very little data, and I knew the request was more to do with politics—to have some results to present by year end—than science. I remember taking wise counsel from a sage statistician, who advised that sometimes you just have to let people fall on their face. On their face they royally fell.

Falling on my own face a number of times has provided salutary lessons. Trials that have been conducted that when done and reported failed to reject the null hypothesis less because the alternative was false but because the basic trial assumptions—around such aspects as trial variability and response rates—were optimistic or wrong.

I have always been uncomfortable calculating a sample size for a study, costing several million pounds, for which, for example, the variability used for the calculation was estimated through reading data from a graph in an article published in journal that was not very prestigious, and so with time I have come to the view that the imprecision of estimates in trials should be allowed for in calculations or at the very least investigated in the context of seeing how sensitive the study is to the assumptions being made.

The three most important factors in any study are design, design, design and a sample size calculation is a major component of the design. If you get your analysis wrong, it can be redone; however, if you get your design wrong—for example underestimating the sample size—you are scuppered. Good statistics cannot rescue bad designs; indeed there is an argument that if you have to do complicated statistics you have gotten your design wrong. I would further argue that you should spend as long designing a trial as analysing it. This is where the greatest leverage is and where you can make a bigger impact on a given study.

So you have calculated the sample size from estimates you yourself have obtained, you have investigated the sensitivity of the study to these estimates, you think the design is robust. But why stop there? When NASA launches a probe to Mars it does not point it in the general direction of the red planet, cross collected fingers and hope it hits the target; it reviews progress and tinkers and alters the trajectory. Clinical trials should be equally adaptive, and we should not wait with bated breath to the end of the study. Even though you are reasonably confident that the sample size is sound, it should not preclude sample size re-estimation during the course of the trial.

This is why I said that a sample size is a process, not an end unto itself. You first have to obtain estimated values to go into the sample size calculation. You then calculate your sample size, and you investigate how robust it is to the estimates. Finally, you implement sample size re-estimation as appropriate.

This book will be of relevance to researchers undertaking clinical research in the pharmaceutical and public sector. The focus of the book is on clinical trials, although it can be applied to other forms of prospective design. The book itself is based on a short course that has been presented a number of times, and the worked examples and problems are based on real-world issues.

Given the topic of the book, mentioning formulae is unavoidable. In addition the book is a little intentionally dry to enable the quick finding of an appropriate formula, application of a formula and a worked example. Given this, however, all results are presented within a practical context and with the addition of useful hints and tips to optimise sample size calculations.

Steven A. Julious

List of Figures

List of Tables

1

Introduction

This chapter describes the background of randomised controlled clinical trials and the main factors that should be considered in their design. The description of the issues associated with clinical trial design is made in the context of assessing innovative therapies. The different types of clinical trials, for different objectives, are then described in detail. It is highlighted how these different objectives have an impact on study design with respect to derivation of formulae for sample size calculations.

1.1 Background to Randomised Controlled Trials

Since the first reported 'modern' randomised clinical trial (Medical Research Council, 1948), clinical trials have become a central component in the assessment of new therapies. They have contributed to improvements in health care as measured by an increase in life expectancy by an average of 3 to 7 years and relief of poor quality of life related to chronic disease by an average of 5 years (Chalmers, 1998; Bunker, Frazier and Mosteller, 1994).

The primary objective of any clinical trial is to obtain an unbiased and reliable assessment of a given regimen response independent of any known or unknown prognostic factors; that is, clinical trials ensure that there is no systematic difference between treatments. Clinical trials are therefore designed to meet this primary objective (Julious and Zariffa, 2002). They do this first by ensuring, as much as possible, that the patients studied in the various regimen arms are objectively similar with reference to all predetermined relevant factors other than the regimens themselves (e.g. in terms of disease severity, demography, study procedures etc.). Second, they make sure that the assessment of the regimen response is independent of a given subject's regimen; finally, an appropriate control is included to quantify a given regimen response. To ensure the primary objective is met Julious and Zariffa (2002) described how the essential principles of clinical trial design can be summarised in terms of the ABCs of *Allocation* at random, *Blinded* assessment of outcome and *Control* with respect to a comparator group. These principles hold regardless of the type of trial.

1.2   Types of Clinical Trial

When planning a trial an essential step is the calculation of a sample size as studies that are either too small or too large may be judged unethical (Altman, 1980). For example, a study that is too large could have met the objectives of the trial before the actual study end had been reached, so some patients may have unnecessarily entered the trial and been exposed to a treatment with little or no benefit. A trial that is too small will have little chance of meeting the study objectives, and patients may be put through the potential trauma of a trial for no tangible benefit. This chapter, based on the work of Julious (2004d), discusses in detail the computation of sample sizes appropriate for

1. Superiority trials
2. Equivalence trials
3. Non-inferiority trials
4. As-good-as-or-better trials
5. Bioequivalence trials
6. Trials to a given precision

A distinction therefore is drawn to emphasise differences in trials designed to demonstrate 'superiority' and trials designed to demonstrate 'equivalence' or 'non-inferiority.' This is discussed with an emphasis on how differences in the null hypothesis can have an impact on calculations. The International Conference on Harmonisation of Technical Requirements for Registration of Pharmaceuticals for Human Use (ICH) guidelines ICH E3 (1996) and ICH E9 (1998) provide general guidance on selecting the sample size for a clinical trial. The ICH E9 (1998) guideline states that:

> The number of subjects in a clinical trial should always be large enough to provide a reliable answer to the questions addressed. This number is usually determined by the primary objective of the trial. ... The method by which the sample size is calculated should be given in the protocol together with any quantities used in the calculations (such as variances, mean values, response rates, event rates, differences to be detected).

This book is primarily written on the premise that just two treatments are to be compared in the clinical trial, and two study designs are discussed: parallel group and cross-over.

With a parallel group design subjects are assigned at random to the two treatments to form two treatment groups. It is hoped at the end of the trial that the two groups are the same in all respects other than the treatment received so that an unbiased assessment of treatment effect can be made.

With a cross-over trial all subjects receive both the treatments but the order that subjects receive the treatments is randomised. The big assumption here is that prior to starting the second treatment all subjects return to baseline, and that the order in which subjects receive treatment does not affect their response to treatment. Crossover trials cannot be used therefore in degenerative conditions in which subjects get worse over time. Also, they are more sensitive to bias than parallel group designs (Julious and Zariffa, 2002).

1.3 Assessing Evidence from Trials

Since it is rarely possible to collect information on an entire population, the aim of clinical trials (in the context of this book) is to use information from a sample to draw conclusions (or make inferences) about the population of interest. This inference is facilitated through making assumptions about the underlying distribution of the outcome of interest such that an appropriate theoretical model can be applied to describe outcome in the population as a whole from the clinical trial.

Note it is usual *a priori* to any analysis to make an assumption regarding the underlying distribution of your outcome measure for the trial. These assumptions are then to be investigated through various plots and figures for the observed data.

In the context of this book the *population* is a theoretical concept used for describing an entire group. One way of describing the distribution of a measurement in a population is by use of a suitable theoretical probability distribution.

1.3.1 The Normal Distribution

The Normal, or Gaussian, distribution (named in honour of C. F. Gauss, 1777–1855, a German mathematician) is the most important theoretical probability distribution in statistics. The distribution curve of data that are Normally distributed has a characteristic shape; it is bell shaped and symmetrical about a single peak (Figure 1.1). The Normal distribution is described completely by two parameters, the mean μ and the standard deviation σ. This means that for any Normally distributed variable, once the mean and variance σ^2 are known (or estimated), it is possible to calculate the probability distribution for observations in a population.

1.3.2 The Central Limit Theorem

The Central Limit Theorem (or the law of large numbers) states that given any series of independent, identically distributed random variables, their means

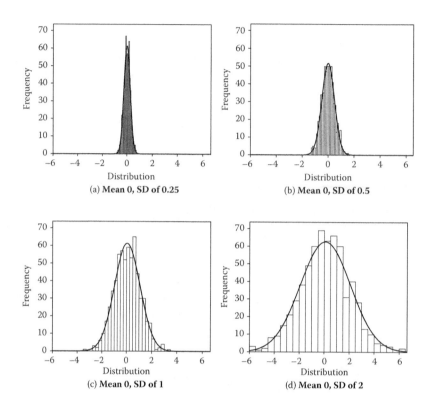

FIGURE 1.1 The Normal distribution (a) Mean 0, SD of 0.25; (b) Mean 0, SD of 0.5; (c) Mean 0, SD of 1; (d) Mean 0, SD of 2.

will tend to a Normal distribution as the number of variables increases. Put another way, the distribution of sample means drawn from a population will be Normally distributed whatever the distribution of the actual data in the population as long as the samples are large enough.

Each mean estimated from a sample is an unbiased estimate of the true population mean, and using the Central Limit Theorem we can infer that 95% of sample means will lie within 1.96 standard errors (of the mean) of the population mean. As we do not usually know the population mean the more important inference is that with the sample mean we are 95% confident that the population mean will fall within 1.96 standard errors of the sample mean.

The Normal distribution and the Central Limit Theorem are important as they underpin much of the subsequent statistical theory outlined in both this and subsequent chapters. This is because although only Chapters 3 through 8 discuss calculations for clinical trials in which the primary outcome is anticipated to take a Normal form, approximation to the Normal distribution

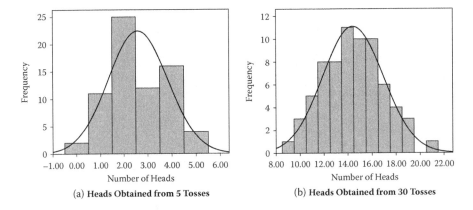

FIGURE 1.2 Coin-tossing experiment to illustrate the distribution of means from 60 samples with the number of heads obtained from (a) 5 and (b) 30 tosses of a coin.

(and what to do when Normal approximation is inappropriate) is important to subsequent chapters on binary and ordinal data.

To illustrate the Central Limit Theorem, consider the situation of tossing a coin. The distribution of the individual coin tosses would be uniform, half heads and half tails. That is, each outcome has an equal probability of being selected, and the shape of the probability density function of theoretical distribution is represented by a rectangle. According to the central limit theorem, if you were to select repeated random samples of the same size from this distribution and then calculate the means of these different samples, the distribution of the means would be approximately Normal, and this approximation would improve as the size of each sample increased. Figure 1.2 is taken from a recent practical with 60 students in a lecture. Figure 1.2a represents the distribution of the number of heads for 60 simulated samples of size 5. Even with such a small sample size the approximation to the Normal is remarkable, whilst repeating the experiment with samples of size 30 improves the fit to the Normal distribution (Figure 1.2b).

In reality, as we usually only take a single sample, we can use the Central Limit Theorem to construct an interval within which we are reasonably confident the true population mean will be included, that is, through calculation of a confidence interval.

1.3.3 Frequentist Approaches

Clinical trials are usually assessed through *a priori* declaring a null hypothesis, depending on the objective of the trial, and then formally testing this null hypothesis with empirical trial data.

An advantage of a sample size calculation for an applied medical statistician is that often it is the first time that formal consideration is given by a study team to some of the key aspects of the trial, such as primary objective, primary endpoint, and effect size of interest. Subsequent chapters discuss the sample size calculations for different objectives and endpoints. In this chapter we introduce the different types of clinical trial.

1.3.3.1 *Hypothesis Testing and Estimation*

Consider the hypothetical example of a trial designed to examine the effectiveness of two treatments for migraine. In the trial patients are to be randomly allocated to two groups corresponding to either treatment A or treatment B. Suppose the primary objective of the trial is to investigate whether there is a difference between the two groups with respect to a pain outcome; in this case we could carry out a significance test and calculate a *P*-value (a hypothesis test). The context here is that of a superiority trial. Other types of trial are discussed in this chapter and throughout the book.

1.3.3.2 *Hypothesis Testing: Superiority Trials*

In designing a clinical trial it is important to have a clear research question and to know the outcome variable to be compared. Once the research question has been stated, the null and alternative hypotheses can be formulated. For a superiority trial the null hypothesis H_0 is usually of the form of no difference in the outcome of interest between the study groups. The study or alternative hypothesis H_1 would then usually state that there is a difference between the study groups.

In lay terms the null hypothesis is what we are investigating, whilst the alternative is what we wish to show, that is:

H_0: We are investigating whether there is a difference between treatments.

H_1: We wish to show there is a difference between treatments.

Often when first writing H_0 and H_1 it is what the investigator wishes to show that is written as H_0. Hence, H_0 and H_1 can be confused. The confusion can arise as trials are usually named after the alternative hypothesis; for example, for an equivalence trial the H_0 is that two treatments differ, while the alternative is that they are equivalent. The same is true for non-inferiority and bioequivalence trials.

For the situation now, a superiority trial, we wish to compare a new migraine therapy against a control, and we are investigating the null hypothesis H_0 of no difference between treatments. We therefore wish to show that this null hypothesis is false and demonstrate that there is a difference at a given level of significance.

In general, the direction of the difference (e.g. that treatment A is better than treatment B) is not specified, and this is known as a *two-sided* (or two-tailed) test. By specifying no direction we investigate both the possibility that A is better than B and the possibility that B is better than A. If a direction is specified this is referred to as a *one-sided* (one-tailed) test, and we would be evaluating only whether A is better than B as the possibility of B being better than A is of no interest. There are further discussions of one-tailed and two-tailed tests when describing the different types of trial later in this chapter.

The study team began designing a trial with a research question. For the pain trial, the research question of interest was therefore

For patients with chronic pain which treatment for pain is the most effective?

There may be several outcomes for this study, such as mean pain score, alleviation of symptoms or time to alleviation. Assuming we are interested in reducing the mean pain score, then the null hypothesis H_0 for this research question would be:

There is no difference in the mean pain score between treatment A and treatment B groups.

The alternative hypothesis H_1 would be

There is a difference in the mean pain score between the two treatment groups.

Having *a priori* set the null and alternative hypotheses and subsequently performed the trial, collected the data and observed the outcomes, the next stage is to carry out a significance test. This is done by first calculating a test statistic using the study data. This test statistic is then compared to a theoretical value under the null hypothesis to obtain a *P*-value. The final and most crucial stage of hypothesis testing is to make a decision based on the *P*-value. To do this it is necessary to understand first what a *P*-value is and what it is not.

So, what does a *P*-value mean? A *P*-value is the probability of obtaining the study results (or results more extreme) if the null hypothesis is true. Common misinterpretations of the *P*-value are that it is either the probability of the data having arisen by chance or the probability that the observed effect is not a real one. The distinction between these incorrect definitions and the true definition is the absence of the phrase 'when the null hypothesis is true.' The omission of this phrase leads to the incorrect belief that it is possible to evaluate the probability of the observed effect being a real one. The observed effect in the sample is genuine, but what is true in the population is not known. All that can be known with a *P*-value is, if there truly is no difference

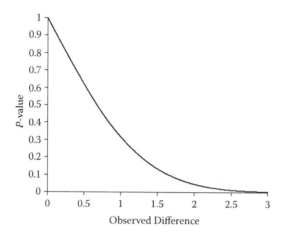

FIGURE 1.3 The relationship between the observed difference and the *P*-value under the null hypothesis.

in the population, how likely is the result obtained (from the sample). Thus a small *P*-value indicates that the difference obtained is unlikely if there genuinely was no difference in the population.

In practice, what happens in a trial is that the null hypothesis that two treatments are the same is stated, that is, $\mu_A = \mu_B$ or $\mu_A = \mu_B = 0$. The trial is then conducted, and a particular difference d is observed where $\bar{x}_A - \bar{x}_B = d$. Due to pure randomness even if the two treatments are truly the same we would seldom actually observe $\bar{x}_A - \bar{x}_B = 0$ but some random difference. Now if d is small (say a 1 mm mean difference in VAS pain score), then the probability of seeing this difference under the null hypothesis could be very high, say $P = 0.995$. If a larger difference is observed, then the probability of seeing this difference by chance is reduced; with a mean difference of 5 mm, the *P*-value could be $P = 0.562$. As the difference increases, the *P*-value falls such that a difference of 20 mm may equate to $P = 0.021$. In this relationship (illustrated in Figure 1.3) as d increases the *P*-value (under the null hypothesis) falls.

It is important to remember that a *P*-value is a probability and its value can vary between 0 and 1. A 'small' *P*-value, say close to zero, indicates that the results obtained are unlikely when the null hypothesis is true, and the null hypothesis is rejected. Alternatively, if the *P*-value is 'large,' then the results obtained are likely when the null hypothesis is true, and the null hypothesis is not rejected. But how small is small? Conventionally the cut-off value or two-sided significance level for declaring that a particular result is statistically significant is set at 0.05 (or 5%). Thus if the *P*-value is less than this value the null hypothesis (of no difference) is rejected, and the result is said to be statistically significant at the 5% or 0.05 level (Table 1.1). For the pain example, if the *P*-value associated with the mean difference in the VAS pain score was 0.01, then as this is less than the cut-off value of 0.05

TABLE 1.1

Statistical Significance

	$P < 0.05$	$P \geq 0.05$
Result is	Statistically significant	Not statistically significant
Decision	Sufficient evidence to reject the null hypothesis	Insufficient evidence to reject the null hypothesis

we would say that there was a statistically significant difference in the pain score between the two groups at the 5% level.

The choice of 5% is somewhat arbitrary, and though it is commonly used as a standard level for statistical significance its use is not universal. Even where it is, one study that is statistically significant at the 5% level is not usually enough to change practice; replication is usually required (i.e. at least one more study with statistically significant results). For example, to get a regulatory license for a new drug usually two statistically significant studies are required at the 5% level, which equates to a single study at the 0.00125 significance level. It is for this reason that larger 'super studies' are conducted to get significance levels that would change practice (i.e. a lot less than 5% and maybe nearer to 0.1%).

The origin of setting the level of statistical significance at 5% is not really known. Much of what we refer to as statistical inference is based on the work of R. A. Fisher (1890–1962), who first used 5% as a level of statistical significance acceptable to reject the null hypothesis. One theory is that 5% was used because Fisher published some statistical tables with different levels of statistical significance, and 5% was the middle column (another is that five is the number of toes on Fisher's foot, which maybe is just as plausible).

An exercise to do, for instance with students, to demonstrate empirically that 5% is a reasonable level for statistical significance is to toss a coin and tell the students whether a head or a tail has been observed, but keep saying heads. After around six tosses ask the students when they stopped believing the toss indication was the truth. Usually about half would say after four tosses and half after five. The probability of getting four heads in a row is 0.063, and the probability of getting five heads in a row is 0.031, hence 5% is a figure about which most people would intuitively start to disbelieve a hypothesis.

The significance level of 5% has to a degree become a tablet of stone, which could be considered strange given that it may well be based on a gut feeling. However, it is such a tablet of stone that it is not unknown for a P-value to be presented as $P = 0.049999993$ as P must be less than 0.05 to be significant, and written to two decimal places $P = 0.05$ is considered to present far less evidence for rejection of the null hypothesis than $P = 0.049999993$.

Although the decision to reject or not reject the null hypothesis may seem clear-cut, it is possible that a mistake may be made, as can be seen from the shaded cells of Table 1.2. For example a 5% significance level means that we

TABLE 1.2

Making a Decision

| | The Null Hypothesis Is Actually | |
Decide to	False	True
Reject the null hypothesis	The power	Type I error
Reject the null hypothesis	Type II error	Correct decision

would only expect to see the observed difference (or one greater) 5% of the time under the null hypothesis. Alternatively we can rephrase this to state that even if the two treatments are the same 5% of the time we will conclude that they are not, and we will make an error. This error is known as a Type I error. Therefore, whatever is decided, the decision may correctly reflect what is true in the population: the null hypothesis is rejected when in fact it is false, or the null hypothesis is not rejected when in fact it is true. Alternatively, it may not reflect what is true in the population: the null hypothesis may be rejected when it is in fact true, which would lead us to a false positive and a Type I error, or the null hypothesis may not be rejected when in fact it is false. This would lead to a false negative and a Type II error. Acceptable levels of the Type I and Type II error rates are set before the study is conducted. As mentioned the usual level for declaring a result to be statistically significant is set at a two-sided level of 0.05 prior to an analysis (i.e. the Type I error rate is set at 0.05 or 5%). In doing this we are stating that the maximum acceptable probability of rejecting the null when it is in fact true (committing a Type I error, α error rate) is 0.05. The P-value that is then obtained from our analysis of the data gives us the probability of committing a Type I error (making a false-positive error).

The concepts of Type I and Type II errors as well as study power (1 – Type II error) are dealt with further in this chapter and throughout the book as these are important components of sample size calculation. Here, however, it must be highlighted that they are set *a priori* when considering the null and alternative hypotheses.

1.3.3.3 *Statistical and Clinical Significance or Importance*

Discussion so far has dealt with hypothesis testing. However, in addition to statistical significance, it is useful to consider the concept of clinical significance or importance. Whilst a result may be statistically significant, it may not be clinically important; conversely an estimated difference that is clinically important may not be statistically significant. For example, consider a large study comparing two treatments for high blood pressure; the results suggest that there is a statistically significant difference ($P = 0.023$) in the amount by which blood pressure is lowered. This P-value relates to a difference of 3 mmHg between the two treatments.

Whilst the difference is statistically significant, it could be argued that a difference of 3 mmHg is not clinically important. Hence, although there is a statistically significant difference this difference may not be sufficiently large enough to convince anyone that there is a truly important clinical difference.

This is not a trivial point. Often *P*-values alone are quoted, and inferences about differences between groups are made based on this one statistic. Statistically significant *P*-values may be masking differences that have little clinical importance. Conversely it may be possible to have a *P*-value greater than the magic 5% but for there to be a genuine difference between groups: Absence of evidence does not equate to evidence of absence.

The issue of clinical significance is particularly important for non-inferiority and equivalence trials, discussed separately in this chapter, for which margins are set that confidence intervals must preclude. *P*-values are seldom quoted here. These margins are interpreted in terms of clinically meaningful differences.

1.4 Superiority Trials

As discussed, in a superiority trial the objective is to determine whether there is evidence of a statistical difference in the comparison of interest between the regimens with reference to the null hypothesis that the regimens are the same. The null (H_0) and alternative (H_1) hypotheses may take the form

H$_0$: The two treatments have equal effect with respect to the mean response ($\mu_A = \mu_B$).

H$_1$: The two treatments are different with respect to the mean response ($\mu_A \neq \mu_B$).

In the definition of the null and alternative hypotheses μ_A and μ_B refer to the population mean response on regimens A and B, respectively. In testing the null hypothesis there are two errors we can make:

I. Rejecting H$_0$ when it is actually true.

II. Retaining H$_0$ when it is actually false.

As described, these errors are usually referred to as Type I and Type II errors, respectively (Neyman and Pearson, 1928, 1933a,b, 1936a,b, 1938). The aim of the sample size calculation is to find the minimum sample size for a fixed probability of Type I error to achieve a value of the probability of a Type II error. The two errors are commonly referred to as the regulator's (Type I) and investigator's (Type II) risks, and by convention are fixed at rates of 0.05 (Type I) and 0.10 or 0.20 (Type II). The Type I and Type II risks carry different weights as they reflect the impact of the errors. With a Type I error medical practice may switch to the investigative therapy with resultant costs, whilst with a Type II error medical practice would remain unaltered.

In general, we usually think not in terms of the Type II error but in terms of the power of a trial (1 – probability of a Type II error), which is the probability of rejecting H_0 when it is in fact false. Key trials should be designed to have adequate power for statistical assessment of the primary parameters. The Type I error rate that is usually taken as standard for a superiority trial is 5%. It is recommended that the power to consider as standard to be 90%, with the minimum to be considered to be 80%. However, it is debatable regarding which level of power we should use, although it should be noted that, compared to a study with 90% power, with just 80% power we are doubling Type II error for only a 25% saving in sample size.

Neyman and Pearson introduced the concept of the two types of error, Types I and II, in the 1930s. The labelling of these two types of error was arbitrary though as the authors simply listed the two types of error that could be made as sub-bullets that were numbered with the prefixes of I and II. Subsequently the authors then referred to the errors as errors of Type I and errors of Type II. If these sub-bullets had different labelling, of A and B say, then statisticians would have a different nomenclature.

The purpose of the sample size calculation is hence to provide sufficient power to reject H_0 when in fact some alternative hypothesis is true. For the calculation we must have a prespecified value, for difference in the means, for the alternative hypothesis d (Campbell, Julious and Altman, 1995). The amount d is chosen as a clinically important difference or effect size and is the main factor in determining a sample size. Reducing the effect size by half will quadruple the required sample size (Fayers and Machin, 1995). Usually the effect size is taken from clinical judgement or is based on previous empirical experience in the population to be examined in the current trial. This is discussed in greater detail in Chapter 2.

Formally the aim is to calculate a sample size suitable for making inferences about a certain function of given model parameter μ, $f(\mu)$ say. For data that take a Normal form $f(\mu)$ will be $\mu_A - \mu_B$, that is, the difference in means of two populations A and B. Now let S be a sample estimate of $f(\mu)$. Thus S is defined as the difference in the sample means. As we are assuming that the data from the clinical trial are sampled from a Normal population, then, using standard notation, $S \sim N(f(\mu), Var(S))$, giving

$$\frac{S - f(\mu)}{\sqrt{Var(S)}} \sim N(0,1).$$

A basic equation can now be developed in general terms from which a sample size can be estimated. Let α be the overall Type I error level, with $\alpha/2$ of this Type I error equally assigned to each tail of the two-tailed test and let $Z_{1-\alpha/2}$ denote the $(1 - \alpha/2)$ 100% of a standard Normal distribution.

Thus, an upper two-tailed, α-level critical region for a test of $f(\mu) = 0$ is

$$|S| > Z_{1-\alpha/2}\sqrt{Var(S)},$$

where $||$ means take the absolute value of S ignoring the sign. For this critical region against an alternative that $f(\mu) = d$, for some chosen d, to have power $(1 - \beta)\%$ we require

$$d - Z_{1-\beta}\sqrt{Var(S)} = Z_{1-\alpha/2}\sqrt{Var(S)}, \tag{1.1}$$

where β is the overall Type II error level, and $Z_{1-\beta}$ is the $100(1 - \beta)\%$ point of the standard Normal distribution. Thus, in general terms for a two-tailed, α-level test we require

$$Var(S) = \frac{d^2}{(Z_{1-\beta} + Z_{1-\alpha/2})^2}, \tag{1.2}$$

where $Var(S)$ will be unknown and depends on the sample size. Once $Var(S)$ is written in terms of sample size, these expressions can be solved to give the sample size.

Chapters 3 and 4 for parallel group and cross-over trials, respectively, detail the calculations for trials in which the data are expected to take a Normal form, while Chapter 9 (for parallel group) and Chapter 10 (for cross-over) describe the calculations for binary data. The calculations for ordinal and survival data are given in Chapters 14 and 15, respectively.

1.5 Equivalence Trials

In certain cases the objective is not to demonstrate superiority but to demonstrate that two treatments have no clinically meaningful difference, that is, they are equivalent. The null (H_0) and alternative (H_1) hypotheses may take the form

H_0: The two treatment differences are different with respect to the mean response ($\mu_A \neq \mu_B$).

H_1: The two treatments have equal effect with respect to the mean response ($\mu_A = \mu_B$).

Usually these hypotheses are written in terms of a clinical difference d and become

H_0: $\mu_A - \mu_B \leq -d$ or $\mu_A - \mu_B \geq +d$.
H_1: $-d < \mu_A - \mu_B < +d$.

The statistical tests of the null hypotheses are an example of an intersection-union test (IUT), in which the null hypothesis is expressed as a union and the alternative as an intersection. To conclude equivalence, we need to reject each component of the null hypothesis.

Note that in an IUT each component is tested at level α giving a composite test, which is also of level α (Berger and Hsu, 1996).

A common approach with equivalence trials is to test each component of the null hypothesis, called the two one-sided test (TOST) procedure. In practice, this is operationally the same as constructing a $(1 - 2\alpha)100\%$ confidence interval for $f(\mu)$ where equivalence is concluded provided that each end of the confidence interval falls completely within the interval $(-d, +d)$ (Jones et al., 1996). Here, $(-d, +d)$ represents the range within which equivalence will be accepted.

Note as each test is carried out at the α level of significance then, under the two null hypotheses, the overall chance of committing a Type I error is less than α (Senn, 1997, 2001b). Hence, the TOST and $(1 - 2\alpha)100\%$ confidence interval approaches are conservative. There are enhancements that can be applied, but they are of no practical importance for formally powered clinical trials (Senn, 1997, 2001b). As a consequence the TOST approach is only discussed for equivalence trials (and bioequivalence trials in a separate discussion).

Figure 1.4 shows how confidence intervals are used to test the different hypotheses in superiority, non-inferiority and equivalence trials. The special case of bioequivalence is covered elsewhere in the chapter.

Here, δ represents the standardised equivalence and non-inferiority limits ($\Delta = d/\sigma$), and the solid line shows the confidence interval for the treatment difference.

In ICH E10 (2000) some detail in the description of equivalence trials and the related non-inferiority trials (discussed elsewhere in the chapter) is provided, whilst ICH E9 (1998) and ICH E3 (1996) discuss the appropriate analysis of such trials.

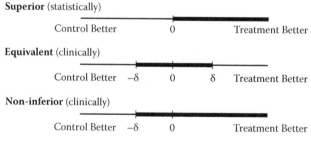

* Δ is variable

FIGURE 1.4 The difference among equivalence, non-inferiority and superiority.

In this section the sample size formulae are initially derived:

i. For the general case of inequality between treatments (i.e., $f(\mu) = \Delta$)

ii. Adopting the same notation and assumptions as superiority trials

iii. Under the assumption that the equivalence bounds $-d$ and d are symmetric about zero

This section then moves on to the special case of no treatment difference, replacing (i) with

i. For the special case of no mean difference (i.e. $f(\mu) = 0$).

1.5.1   General Case

As with superiority trials we require

$$\frac{S - f(\mu)}{\sqrt{Var(S)}} \sim N(0,1).$$

Hence, the $(1 - 2\alpha)$ 100% confidence limits for a non-zero mean difference would be

$$S - \Delta \pm Z_{1-\alpha} \sqrt{Var\ S}.$$

To declare equivalence the lower and upper confidence limits should be within $\pm d$

$$S - \Delta - Z_{1-\alpha} \sqrt{Var(S)} > -d \quad \text{and} \quad S - \Delta + Z_{1-\alpha} \sqrt{Var(S)} < d. \qquad (1.3)$$

Thus, for the TOST with this critical region there are two opportunities under the alternative hypothesis to have a Type II error for some chosen d and power $(1 - \beta)$:

$$\Delta + d - Z_{1-\beta_1} \sqrt{Var(S)} = Z_{1-\alpha} \sqrt{Var(S)} \text{ and } \Delta - d - Z_{1-\beta_2} \sqrt{Var(S)} = -Z_{1-\alpha} \sqrt{Var(S)}$$

$$(1.4)$$

where β_1 and β_2 are the probability of a Type II error associated with each one-sided test from the TOST procedure, and $\beta = \beta_1 + \beta_2$. Hence, we require

$$Z_{1-\beta_1} = \frac{\Delta + d}{\sqrt{Var(S)}} + Z_{1-\alpha} \quad \text{and} \quad Z_{1-\beta_2} = \frac{\Delta - d}{\sqrt{Var(S)}} - Z_{1-\alpha}. \qquad (1.5)$$

Alternatively, Senn (1997) considered the calculation of the Type II error in terms of the power and hence had a slightly different nomenclature. However, they are equivalent.

1.5.2   Special Case of No Treatment Difference

With symmetric equivalence bounds we require

$$S \pm Z_{1-\alpha}\sqrt{Var\ S},$$

Thus, to declare equivalence we should have

$$S - Z_{1-\alpha}\sqrt{Var(S)} > -d \quad \text{and} \quad S + Z_{1-\alpha}\sqrt{Var(S)} < d.$$

With the TOST procedure the Type II error for some chosen d and power $(1 - \beta)$ will come from

$$d - Z_{1-\beta}\sqrt{Var(S)} = Z_{1-\alpha}\sqrt{Var(S)} \quad \text{and} \quad -d - Z_{1-\beta}\sqrt{Var(S)} = -Z_{1-\alpha}\sqrt{Var(S)}.$$

Hence,

$$Z_{1-\beta/2} = \frac{d}{\sqrt{Var(S)}} - Z_{1-\alpha},$$

giving

$$Var(S) = \frac{d^2}{(Z_{1-\alpha} + Z_{1-\beta/2})^2}. \tag{1.6}$$

Chapter 5 describes the calculations for which the data are expected to take a Normal form. The more complex calculations for binary data are discussed in Chapter 12. The calculations for ordinal and survival data are given in Chapters 14 and 15, respectively.

1.6   Non-inferiority Trials

In certain cases the objective of a trial is not to demonstrate that two treatments are different or that they are equivalent but rather to demonstrate that a given treatment is not clinically inferior compared to another, that is, that a treatment is non-inferior to another. The null (H_0) and alternative (H_1) hypotheses may take the form

H_0: A given treatment is inferior with respect to the mean response.

H_1: The given treatment is non-inferior with respect to the mean response.

As with equivalence trials these hypotheses are written in terms of a clinical difference d, which again equates to the largest difference that is clinically acceptable (Committee for Proprietary Medicinal Products [CPMP], 2000; Committee for Medicinal Products for Human Use [CHMP], 2005):

H_0: $\mu_A - \mu_B \leq -d$.
H_1: $\mu_A - \mu_B > -d$.

Detail is given in ICH E3 (1996) and ICH E9 (1998) on the analysis of non-inferiority trials, whilst ICH E10 (2000) goes into detail regarding the definition of d.

To conclude non-inferiority, we need to reject the null hypothesis. In terms of the equivalence hypotheses mentioned this is the same as testing just one of the two components of the TOST procedure and reduces to a simple one-sided hypothesis test. In practice, this is operationally the same as constructing a $(1 - 2\alpha)100\%$ confidence interval and concluding non-inferiority provided that the lower end of this confidence interval is above $-d$. Figure 1.4 shows how confidence intervals are used to test the different hypotheses in superiority, equivalence and non-inferiority trials.

Adopting the same notation and under the same assumptions as for superiority trials but with $f(\mu) = -\Delta$ and the additional assumption that the non-inferiority bound is $-d$, the lower $(1 - 2\alpha)100\%$ confidence limit is

$$S - \Delta - Z_{1-\alpha} \sqrt{Var\ S}. \tag{1.7}$$

To declare non-inferiority the lower end of the confidence interval should lie above $-d$:

$$S - \Delta - Z_{1-\alpha} \sqrt{Var(S)} > -d. \tag{1.8}$$

For this critical region we therefore require a $(1 - \beta)100\%$ chance that the lower limit lies above $-d$. Hence,

$$Z_{1-\beta} = \frac{-d + \Delta}{\sqrt{Var(S)}} - Z_{1-\alpha'} \tag{1.9}$$

giving

$$Var(S) = \frac{(d - \Delta)^2}{(Z_{1-\alpha} + Z_{1-\beta})^2}. \tag{1.10}$$

Depending on the type of data Chapters 6 (for Normal), 11 (for binary), 14 (for ordinal) and 15 (for survival) describe the calculations.

1.7 As-Good-as-or-Better Trials

For certain clinical trials the objective is to demonstrate either that a given treatment is not clinically inferior or that it is clinically superior when compared to the control, that is, that the treatment is "as good as or better" than the control. Therefore two null and alternative hypotheses are investigated in such trials. First the non-inferiority null and alternative hypotheses

> H_0: A given treatment is inferior with respect to the mean response $(\mu_A \leq \mu_B)$.
>
> H_1: The given treatment is non-inferior with respect to the mean response $(\mu_A > \mu_B)$.

If this null hypothesis is rejected, then a second null hypothesis is investigated:

> H_0: The two treatments have equal effect with respect to the mean response $(\mu_A = \mu_B)$.
>
> H_1: The two treatments are different with respect to the mean response $(\mu_A \neq \mu_B)$.

Practically these two null hypotheses are investigated through the construction of a 95% confidence interval to investigate where the lower (or upper, as appropriate) bound lies. Figure 1.4 highlights how the two separate hypotheses for superiority and non-inferiority are investigated.

The as-good-as-or-better trials are really a subcategory of either superiority or non-inferiority trials. However, in this book this class of trials is put in a separate section to highlight how these trials combine the null hypotheses of superiority and non-inferiority trials into one closed testing procedure whilst maintaining the overall Type I error (Morikawa and Yoshida, 1995; Bauer and Kieser, 1996; Julious, 2004d).

To introduce the closed testing procedure this section first describes the situation in which a one-sided test of non-inferiority is followed by a one-sided test of superiority. The more general case in which a one-sided test of non-inferiority is followed by a two-sided test of superiority is then described.

In describing as-good-as-or-better trials this book draws heavily on the work of Morikawa and Yoshida (1995). The CPMP (2000) recently issued a points to consider document.

1.7.1 A Test of Non-inferiority and One-Sided Test of Superiority

The null ($H1_0$) and alternative ($H1_1$) hypotheses for a non-inferiority trial can be written as

> $H1_0: \mu_A - \mu_B \leq -d.$
> $H1_1: \mu_A - \mu_B > -d.$

which alternatively can be written as

$H1_0$: $\mu_A - \mu_B \leq 0$.
$H1_1$: $\mu_A - \mu_B > 0$.

The corresponding null ($H2_0$) and alternative ($H2_1$) hypotheses for a superiority trial can be written as

$H2_0$: $\mu_A - \mu_B \leq 0$.
$H2_1$: $\mu_A - \mu_B > 0$.

What is clear from the definitions of these hypotheses is that if $H2_0$ is rejected at the α level, then $H1_0$ would also be rejected. Also, if $H1_0$ is not rejected at the α level, then $H2_0$ would also not be rejected. This is because $\mu_A - \mu_B + d \geq \mu_A - \mu_B$. Hence, both $H1_0$ and $H2_0$ are rejected if they are both statistically significant; neither $H1_0$ nor $H2_0$ is rejected if $H1_0$ is not significant; only $H1_0$ is rejected if only $H1_0$ is significant.

Based on these properties a closed test procedure can be applied to investigate both non-inferiority and superiority whilst maintaining the overall Type I error rate without α adjustment. To do this the intersection hypothesis $H2_0 \cap H1_0$ is first investigated; if rejected, this is followed by a test of $H1_0$ and $H2_0$. In this instance $H2_0 \cap H1_0 = H1_0$, so both non-inferiority and superiority can be investigated through the following two steps (Morikawa and Yoshida, 1995): First investigate the non-inferiority through the hypothesis $H1_0$. If $H1_0$ is rejected, then $H2_0$ can be tested. If $H1_0$ is not rejected, then the investigative treatment is inferior to the control treatment. If $H2_0$ is rejected in the next step, then we can conclude that the investigative treatment is superior to the control. Else if $H2_0$ is not rejected, then non-inferiority should be concluded.

1.7.2 A Test of Non-inferiority and Two-Sided Test of Superiority

The null ($H3_0$) and alternative ($H3_1$) hypotheses for a two-sided test of superiority can be written as:

$H3_0$: $\mu_A = \mu_B$.
$H3_1$: $\mu_A < \mu_B$ or $\mu_A > \mu_B$.

These are equivalent to TOSTs at the $\alpha/2$ level of significance—summing to give an overall Type I error of α—with the investigation of $H2_0$ against the alternative of $H2_1$ and the following hypotheses:

$H4_0$: $\mu_A \geq \mu_B$.
$H4_1$: $\mu_A < \mu_B$.

In applying the closed test procedure in this instance it is apparent that the intersection hypothesis $H1_0 \cap H3_0$ is always rejected as it is empty, so both

$H1_0$ and $H3_0$ can be tested. Because there is no intersection the following steps can be applied (Morikawa and Yoshida, 1995):

1. If the observed treatment difference is greater than zero and $H3_0$ is rejected, then $H1_0$ is also rejected, and we can conclude that the investigative treatment is superior to control.

2. If the observed treatment difference is less than zero and $H3_0$ is rejected and $H1_0$ is not, then the control is statistically superior to the investigative treatment. If $H1_0$ is also rejected, then the investigative drug is worse than the control but is not inferior (practically although this may be difficult to claim).

3. If $H3_0$ is not rejected but $H1_0$ is, then the investigative drug is non-inferior compared to the control.

4. If neither $H1_0$ nor $H3_0$ is rejected, then we must conclude that the investigative treatment is inferior to the control.

Note that when investigating the $H1_0$ and $H3_0$ hypotheses using the procedure described, $H3_0$ will be tested at a two-sided α level of significance whilst $H1_0$ will be tested at a one-sided $\alpha/2$ level of significance. Thus, the overall level of significance is maintained at α.

1.8   Assessment of Bioequivalence

In this chapter, trials were described in which we wished to demonstrate that the two therapies were clinically equivalent. In equivalence trials the comparators may be completely different in terms of route of administration or even actual drug therapies, but what we wish to determine is whether they are clinically the same. However, in bioequivalence trials the comparators are ostensibly the same; we may have simply moved manufacturing sites or had a formulation changed for marketing purposes. Bioequivalence studies are therefore conducted to show these two formulations of the drug have similar *bioavailability*—the amount of drug in the bloodstream. The assumption in bioequivalence trials is that if the two formulations have equivalent bioavailability, then we can infer that they have equivalent therapeutic effect for both efficacy and safety. The pharmacokinetic bioavailability is therefore a surrogate for the clinical endpoints. As such we would expect the concentration-time profiles for the test and reference formulations to be superimposable (see Figure 1.5 for an example) and the two formulations to be clinically equivalent for safety and efficacy.

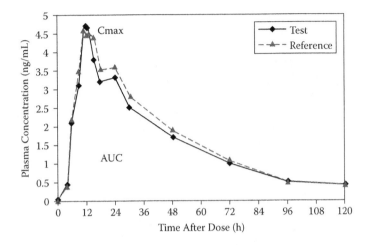

FIGURE 1.5 An example of pharmacokinetic profiles for test and reference formulations.

In bioequivalence studies, therefore, we can determine whether *in vivo* the two formulations are bioequivalent by assessing whether the concentration-time profiles for the test and reference formulations are superimposable (Senn, 1998). Assessing if the rate and extent of absorption are the same usually does this. The pharmacokinetic parameter AUC (area under the concentration curve) is used to assess the extent of absorption, and the parameter C_{max} (maximum concentration) is used to assess the rate of absorption. Figure 1.5 gives a pictorial representation of these parameters. If the two formulations are bioequivalent, then they can be switched without reference to further clinical investigation and can be considered interchangeable.

The null and alternative hypotheses are similar to those for equivalence studies:

H_0: The test and reference formulations give different drug exposures ($\mu_T \neq \mu_R$).

H_1: The test and reference formulations give equivalent drug exposure ($\mu_T - \mu_R$).

Similar to other types of trials the objective of a bioequivalence study is to test the null hypothesis to see if the alternative is true. The 'standard' bioequivalence criteria demonstrate that average drug exposure on the test is within 20% of the reference on the log scale (FDA, 2000, 2001; CPMP, 1998). Thus, the null and alternative hypotheses can be rewritten as

H_0: $\mu_T/\mu_R \leq 0.80$ or $\mu_T/\mu_R \geq 1.25$.
H_1: $0.80 < \mu_T/\mu_R < 1.25$.

We can declare two comparator formulations to be bioequivalent if we can demonstrate that the mean ratio is wholly contained within 0.80 to 1.25. To test the null hypothesis we undertake TOSTs at the 5% level to determine whether $\mu_T/\mu_R \le 0.80$ or $\mu_T/\mu_R \ge 1.25$. If neither of these tests hold, then we can accept the alternative hypothesis of $0.80 < \mu_T/\mu_R < 1.25$. As we are performing two simultaneous tests on the null hypothesis, both of which must be rejected to accept the alternative hypothesis, the Type I error is maintained at 5%. Similar to equivalence trials discussed in this chapter the convention is to represent the TOSTs as a 90% confidence interval around the mean ratio of μ_T/μ_R, which summarises the results of two one-tailed tests.

In summary, a test formulation of a drug is said to be bioequivalent to its reference formulation if the 90% confidence interval for the ratio test:reference is wholly contained within the range 0.80 to 1.25 for both AUC and C_{max}. As both AUC and C_{max} must be equivalent to declare bioequivalence there is no need to allow for multiple comparisons.

Note that this example raises the issue of loss of power when we have multiple endpoints. Here both AUC and C_{max} needed to hold to declare bioequivalence, so the Type I error is not inflated. However, such "and" comparisons may affect the Type II error, depending on the correlation between the endpoints, as there is twice the chance to make a Type II error, which can have an impact on the power (Koch and Gansky, 1996; CPMP, 2002). The most extreme situation would be for two independent "and" comparisons in which the Type II error is doubled. However, here AUC and C_{max} are highly correlated, and as we select the highest variance from the two to calculate the sample size this means that any increase in the Type II error could be offset by the fact that for either AUC or C_{max} the power is greater than 90% for the calculated sample size.

For compounds with certain indications other parameters, such as C_{min} (defined as the minimum concentration over a given period) or T_{mic} (defined as time above a minimum inhibitory concentration over a given period), may also need to be assessed.

Note that the criteria for acceptance of bioequivalence may vary depending on factors such as which regulatory authority's guidelines are followed and the therapeutic window of the compound formulated, so the 'standard' criteria may not always be appropriate.

The methodology described in this section can also be applied to other types of in vivo assessment such as the assessment of a food (FDA, 1997), drug interaction (CPMP, 1997; FDA, 1999b) or special populations (FDA, 1998, 1999a). The criteria for acceptance for other types of *in vivo* assessment may vary depending on the guidelines (FDA 1999a) or *a priori* clinical assessment (CPMP, 1997; FDA, 1997, 1999b).

It may be worth noting the statistical difference between testing for equivalence and bioequivalence with reference to investigating the null hypothesis. In equivalence trials the convention is to undertake TOSTs at the 2.5% level, which in turn are represented by a 95% confidence interval;

in a bioequivalence trial TOSTs at the 5% level are undertaken that are represented by a 90% confidence interval. Thus, in bioequivalence trials the overall Type I error is 5%—twice that of equivalence trials, in which the overall Type I error is 2.5%. Chapter 6 details the actual sample size calculations.

1.8.1 Justification for Log Transformation

The concentration-time profile for a one-compartment intravenous dose can be represented by the following equation:

$$c(t) = Ae^{-\lambda t},$$

where t is time, A is the concentration at $t = 0$ and λ is the elimination rate constant (Julious and Debarnot, 2000). It is evident from this equation that drug concentration in the body falls exponentially at a constant rate λ. A test and reference formulation are superimposable, therefore, only when $c_L(t) = c_R(t)$. On the log scale this is equivalent to $\log(A_T) - \lambda_T = \log(A_R) - \lambda_R$, which for $\lambda_T = \lambda_R$ (which *a priori* we would expect) becomes $\log(A_T) = \log(A_R)$. Thus, on the log scale the difference between two curves can be summarised on an additive scale. It is on this scale that such pharmacokinetic parameters as the rate constant λ and the half-life are derived (Julious and Debarnot, 2000). This simple rationale also follows through for statistics used to measure exposure (AUC) and absorption (C_{max}) as well as the pharmacokinetic variance estimates (Lacey et al., 1997; Julious and Debarnot, 2000). Hence, unless there is evidence to indicate otherwise, the data are assumed to follow a log Normal distribution; hence the default is to analyse $\log_e$ AUC and $\log_e C_{max}$. The differences on the $\log_e$ scale (test-reference) are then back-transformed to obtain a ratio. It is the back-transformed ratio and its corresponding 90% confidence interval that are used to assess bioequivalence.

1.8.2 Rationale for Using Coefficients of Variation

All statistical inference for bioequivalence trials is undertaken on the log scale and back-transformed to the original scale for interpretation. Thus, the within-subject estimate of variability on the log scale is used for both inference and sample size estimation. With the interpretation of the mean effect on the original scale it is good also to have a measure of variability also on the original scale. This measure of variability is usually the coefficient of variability (CV) as for log-Normally distributed data the following exact relationship between the CV on the arithmetic scale and the standard deviation σ on the log scale holds (Diletti, Hauschke and Steimijans, 1991; Julious and Debarnot, 2000):

$$CV = \sqrt{(e^{\sigma^2} - 1)}.$$

For small estimates of σ^2 ($\sigma < 0.30$) the CV can be approximated by

$$CV = \sigma.$$

1.8.3   Individual and Population Bioequivalence

The assessment of bioequivalence as defined in this chapter is based on average bioequivalence in which only the formulation means are required to be equivalent. Paradigms for bioequivalence based on population and individual bioequivalence have also been proposed (Schall and Williams, 1996; Hauck and Anderson, 1992) for which there are regulatory guidelines (FDA, 2001). These alternative approaches also involve formulation variabilities as well as their means in the assessment bioequivalence. To calculate a sample size recommendations have been made based on simulations (FDA, 2001).

The merits of the concepts of individual and population bioequivalence are debatable, and some authors have questioned the concepts (Senn, 2001b). There are a number of reasons for this. The first is that for two formulations A and B in a study it could be possible to declare A to have individual or population bioequivalence with B while the converse is not true.

The second reason is that there is no hierarchy to the assessments. If in a study individual bioequivalence was declared between two formulations it is not then possible to automatically be able to conclude population bioequivalence and average bioequivalence. In fact it is possible to be able to conclude individual bioequivalence and yet have a point estimate outside the standard average bioequivalence bounds of (0.80, 1.25).

The final reason is turning the arguments for individual and population bioequivalence assessment around. The justification for their use is that they allow for an assessment of switchability and prescribability of two formulations that have greater clinical meaning. This may apply if the study conducted is in a patient population with clinical endpoints. However, bioequivalence studies are conducted in healthy volunteers using surrogate endpoints (pharmacokinetics), so the argument pertaining to "switchability" and "prescribability" fails.

1.9   Estimation to a Given Precision

In the previous sections of the chapter calculations were discussed with reference to some clinical objectives, such as the demonstration of equivalence. However, often a preliminary or pilot investigation is conducted in which the objective is to provide evidence of what the potential range of values is with a view to doing a later definitive study (Wood and Lambert, 1999; Day, 1988; Julious and Patterson, 2004; Julious, 2004d). Such studies may also have sample sizes based more on feasibility than formal consideration (Julious, 2005b).

In a given drug's development, it may be the case that reasonably reliable estimates of between-subject and within-subject variation for the endpoint of interest in the reference population are available, but the desired magnitude in the treatment difference of interest will be unknown. This may be the case, for example, when considering the impact of an experimental treatment on biomarkers (Biomarkers Definitions Working Group, 2001) or other measures not known to be directly indicative of clinical outcome but potentially indicative of pharmacological mechanism of action. In this situation, drug and biomarker development will be in such an early stage that no prespecified treatment difference is known. In such exploratory or 'learning' studies (Sheiner, 1997), what is proposed in this book is that the sample size be selected to provide a given level of precision in the study findings, not to power in the traditional fashion for a (in truth unknown) desirable and prespecified difference of interest.

For such studies, rather than testing a hypothesis, it is more informative to give an interval estimate or confidence interval for the unknown $f(\mu)$.

Recall that $(1 - \alpha)$ 100% confidence interval for $f(\mu)$ has half-width

$$w = Z_{\alpha/2}\sqrt{Var(S)}. \tag{1.11}$$

Hence, if you are able to specify a requirement for w and write $Var(S)$ in terms of n, then the expression can be solved for n. It should be noted though that if the sample size is based on precision calculations, then the protocol should clearly state this as the basis for the size of the study.

A similar situation occurs when the sample size is determined primarily by practical considerations. In this case you may quote the precision of the estimates obtained based on the half-width of the confidence interval and provide this information in the discussion of the sample size. Again it must be clearly stated in the protocol that the size of the study was determined based on practical, and not formal, considerations.

The estimation approach also could be useful if you wish to quantify a possible effect across several doses or not only to power on a primary endpoint overall but also to have sufficient precision in given subgroup comparisons. The former of these may be a neglected consideration for clinical trials even though there is some regulatory encouragement as the CPMP (2002) Points to Consider on Multiplicity Issues in Clinical Trials stated:

> Sometimes a study is not powered sufficiently for the aim to identify a single effective and safe dose but is successful only at demonstrating an overall positive correlation of the clinical effect with increasing dose. This is already a valuable achievement. Estimates and confidence intervals are then used in an exploratory manner for the planning of future studies.

Indeed in an early phase or pilot trial instead of powering a single dose against a placebo we could undertake a well-designed study based on the precision approach with several doses estimated against the placebo. As the CPMP document acknowledged this could be a very informative trial.

Sample size calculations for precision-based trials are discussed in Chapters 8, 13, 14 and 15 for Normal, binary, ordinal and survival data, respectively.

 Key Messages

- When undertaking a clinical trial we are looking to make inference about true population responses.
- When making this inference we can make false-positive (Type I) or false-negative (Type II) errors.
- The setting and definition of these errors depend on the objective of the individual trial.

2

Seven Key Steps to Cook Up a Sample Size

2.1 Introduction

In many ways the actual calculation of a sample size is the final step in an iterative calculation process. This chapter describes some of these steps, from defining the trial objective to selection of an appropriate endpoint. There is also a description of how each interacts to have an impact on the sample size.

2.2 Step 1: Deciding on the Trial Objective

The first decision is to decide on the primary objective for the trial (as described in Chapter 1). This then has an impact on the definition of the statistical null and alternative hypotheses. Chapter 1 described the main trial objectives that could be assessed:

- Superiority
- Non-inferiority
- Equivalence
- Bioequivalence
- Precision

Even within an individual trial there may be an assessment of a number of objectives (e.g. in an as-good-as-or-better trial where there is an assessment of both non-inferiority and superiority within one hierarchical approach).

With several treatment arms there may also be an assessment of different objectives depending on the investigative arm comparison. For example with a three-arm trial with a new investigative treatment compared to both placebo and an active control, the investigative treatment may be compared to placebo to assess superiority or against the active control to make a non-inferiority assessment. Here a decision should be made regarding the primary objective of the trial. The sample size for the study will be based on this primary objective.

2.3   Step 2: Deciding on the Endpoint

The next step is deciding on the endpoint to be assessed in the trial. The primary endpoint should enable an assessment of the primary objective of the trial. It is beyond the scope of this book to go into the detail on endpoint selection as this depends on many things, such as the objective of the trial.

With respect to the actual mechanics of a sample size calculation the calculation would depend on the form of the endpoint and whether it is

- Normal
- Binary
- Ordinal
- Survival (time to event)

The sample size calculations for different endpoints for different objectives are described in subsequent chapters.

2.4   Step 3: Determining the Effect Size (or Margin)

Steps 1 and 2 can be relatively easy steps to climb. What may be difficult could be deciding on what effect size (or margin) to base the sample size since the purpose of the sample size calculation is to provide sufficient power to reject the null hypothesis when in fact some alternative hypothesis is true.

In terms of a superiority trial we might have a null hypothesis that the two means are equal versus an alternative that they differ by an amount d. The amount d is chosen as a clinically important difference or effect size and is the main factor in determining a sample size. Reducing the effect size by half will quadruple the required sample size (Fayers and Machin, 1995).

To some degree the determination of what is an appropriate effect size (or margin) does have a qualitative component. However, if possible it is best to base the calculation on some form of quantitative assessment, especially if the endpoint chosen is established already in the investigated population.

2.4.1   Obtaining an Estimate of the Treatment Effects

If we have several clinical investigations, then we need to obtain an overall estimate of the treatment effect. To do this we could follow meta-analysis methodologies (Whitehead and Whitehead, 1991). To obtain an overall estimate across several studies we could use

$$d_s = \frac{\sum_{i=1}^{k} w_i d_i}{\sum_{i=1}^{k} w_i},$$

(2.1)

where d_s is an estimate of the overall response across all the studies, d_i is an estimate of the response from study i, w_i is the reciprocal of the variance from study i ($w_i = 1/\operatorname{var}(d_i)$) and k is the number of studies. Hence, define

$$d_i \sim N\left(d_s, w_i^{-1}\right), \tag{2.2}$$

and thus

$$\sum_{i=1}^{k} w_i d_i \sim N\left(d_s \sum_{i=1}^{k} w_i, \sum_{i=1}^{k} w_i\right). \tag{2.3}$$

Hence overall we can define

$$d_s = \frac{\Sigma_{i=1}^{k} w_i d_i}{\Sigma_{i=1}^{k} w_i} \sim N(\mu, \sigma). \tag{2.4}$$

where σ is the population variance and μ is the population mean. The variance for d_s is defined as $s_s = 1/\Sigma_{i=1}^{k} w_i$; consequently a 95% confidence interval for the overall estimate can be obtained from

$$d_s \pm Z_{1-\alpha/2} \sqrt{\frac{1}{\Sigma_{i=1}^{k} w_i}}. \tag{2.5}$$

Note that the methodology applied here is that of fixed-effects meta-analysis. Random trial-to-trial variability in the "true" control group rate has not been investigated. The approaches described in this section can allow us to undertake this investigation.

We could apply a random effects approach by replacing w_i with w_i^* where w_i^* comes from (Whitehead and Whitehead, 1991)

$$w_i^* = \left(w_i^{-1} + \tau^2\right)^{-1} \tag{2.6}$$

where τ is defined as

$$\tau^2 = \frac{\Sigma_{i=1}^{k} w_i (d_i - d_s)^2 - (k-1)}{\Sigma_{i=1}^{k} w_i - \left(\Sigma_{i=1}^{k} w_i^2 / \Sigma_{i=1}^{k} w_i\right)}. \tag{2.7}$$

Simply, τ can crudely be thought of as

$$\tau^2 = \frac{\text{Variation in the treatment difference between groups}}{\text{Variation in the variation between groups}}. \tag{2.8}$$

If $\tau^2 = 0$ then the weighting for the fixed-effect analysis is used.

The corresponding (random effects) confidence interval would be given by

$$d_s \pm Z_{1-\alpha/2}\sqrt{\frac{1}{\Sigma_{i=1}^{k} w_i^*}}. \tag{2.9}$$

The relative merits of fixed- versus random-effects meta-analysis is not discussed here. In this chapter the methodology applied is that of fixed-effects meta-analysis.

One thing to highlight is that it is not so much random-effects analysis but random effects planning that is of importance. The fundamental assumption when considering retrospective data in planning a trial is that the true response rates are the same from trial to trial and observed rate responses only vary according to sampling error. What this touches on, in fact, is the heterogeneity of trials, especially trials conducted sequentially over time or in different regions for instance. This is discussed in greater detail in an example in Section 2.5.2.

2.4.1.1   *Worked Example with a Binary Endpoint*

Suppose we are planning a study in a rheumatoid arthritis population in which the binary responder endpoint ACR20 is taken as the primary endpoint. For now it does not matter what ACR20 is per se, but it is a scale from the American College of Rheumatology (ACR) on which a *responder* is defined as someone who improves by 20%. The primary endpoint therefore is the proportion of people who have this response. Figure 2.1 gives a graphical summary for the absolute difference in response (active versus placebo). The bottom two lines (fixed and random) give estimates of the overall responses using fixed- and random-effects meta-analyses. Fixed meta-analysis was taken to give the overall estimates for this worked example.

These results could be used to consider an effect size for the study currently planned. From this analysis the overall response rate on placebo was 32%, while that for active was 50%; these were estimated from separate meta-analyses not presented here. The overall estimate of the difference (given in Figure 2.1) between active and placebo is 18% while the minimum observed difference was 12%.

Such analyses could form the basis for discussions with a study team regarding which treatment effect to use in the planned study.

2.4.1.2   *Worked Example with Normal Endpoint*

In the same program as the one described for rheumatoid arthritis suppose we are planning a second study in an osteoarthritis population. An endpoint to be used in the planned trial is Western Ontario and McMaster University Osteoarthritis Index (WOMAC) physical function which is measured on a visual analogue scale (VAS).

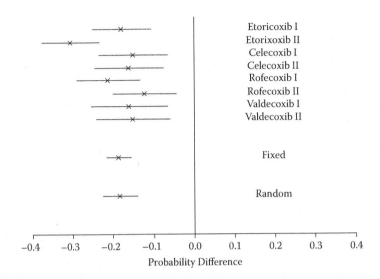

FIGURE 2.1 Meta-analysis of active against placebo in a rheumatoid arthritis population for absolute difference for ARC20.

An issue that became apparent was that different studies used different VASs. This can be resolved by instead using the mean difference $\bar{x}_A - \bar{x}_B$ via the scale-independent standardised estimate of effect $(\bar{x}_A - \bar{x}_B)/s$ and doing a meta-analysis with these standardised differences (Whitehead and Whitehead, 1991). Figure 2.2 gives a graphical summary of the meta-analysis.

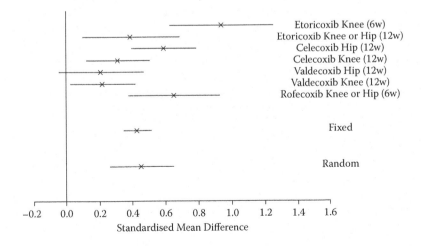

FIGURE 2.2 Meta-analysis for WOMAC physical function for a standardised mean difference in an osteoarthritis population.

With a standard meta-analysis this can be an issue as $(\bar{x}_A - \bar{x}_B)/s$ could be considered harder to interpret than $\bar{x}_A - \bar{x}_B$. However, in terms of interpretation the use of standardised effects is more straightforward (discussed in Chapter 3). These are used in sample size calculations and in construction of tables.

For this analysis the overall standardised effect was 0.46, which with standard deviation assumed to be 22 mm would equate to a difference of 10 mm since $0.46 = 10/22$ (actually $0.46 = 10.12/22$ as there is a small rounding error). In addition the minimum effect observed was 0.22 (equating to a difference of 4.5 mm).

2.4.2   Point Estimate

We have discussed thus far the challenges in quantifying an effect size through empirical use of data particularly across several studies. Suppose, however, we only have a single trial on which to base an effect size.

To consider this problem we first need to consider the following situation: we have designed a study with the standard deviation assumed to be s about an effect size d. We calculate a sample size n with 90% power and two-sided significance level of 5%.

The trial is run, and you see exactly the same effect d and the same standard deviation s as you designed. So what is your two-sided P-value? It is not 5% but actually $P = 0.002$, much less than the significance level designed around. This is because of the distribution under the alternative hypothesis.

Suppose the alternative hypothesis is true; the response would be distributed centrally about d as highlighted in Figure 2.3. If the alternative hypothesis is correct, there is only a 50% chance to see an effect greater than d, and there is even a chance of seeing zero or an effect where $P > 0.05$, which is why we have Type II errors (the chance of declaring no difference when a difference actually exists).

In fact to have a statistically significant result of $P < 0.05$, if the data are distributed around a true effect d on which the study is powered then we would only need to see an effect that is 0.65 of d.

The consequence of what we have discussed is that care needs to be exercised if an observed effect from a single study is to be used as the effect size to design a future study. To be confident of having the desired power the observed P-value would need to be nearer 0.002 than 0.05.

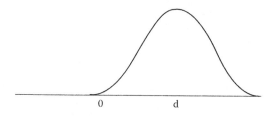

0   d

FIGURE 2.3 Treatment response under the alternative hypothesis.

2.4.3 Choice of Equivalence or Non-inferiority Limit

The choice of the Type I error in the setting of the non-inferiority/equivalence limit is a controversial issue. The limit is defined as the largest difference that is clinically acceptable such that a larger difference than this would matter in clinical practice (Committee for Proprietary Medicinal Products [CPMP], 2000). This difference also cannot be (International Conference on Harmonisation of Technical Requirements for Registration of Pharmaceuticals for Human Use [ICH] E10, 2000)

> ...greater than the smallest effect size that the active (control) drug would be reliably expected to have compared with placebo in the setting of the planned trial.

However, beyond this there is not much formal guidance. Jones et al. (1996) recommended that the choice of limit be set at half the expected clinically mean-ingful difference between the active control and placebo. There is no hard regu-latory guidance, although the CPMP (1999) in a concept paper originally stated that for non-mortality studies it might be acceptable to have an equivalence limit "of one half or one third of the established superiority of the comparator to placebo, especially if the new agent has safety or compliance advantages".

In the draft notes for guidance that followed the CHMP (2005) moved away from such firm guidance and stated the following

> It is not appropriate to define the non-inferiority margin as a propor-tion of the difference between active comparator and placebo. Such ideas were formulated with the aim of ensuring that the test product was superior to (a putative) placebo; however they may not achieve this purpose. If the reference product has a large advantage over placebo this does not mean that large differences are unimportant, it just means that the reference product is very efficacious.

The CHMP now talk of having a margin that ensures that there is "no important loss of efficacy" caused through switching from reference to test and that the margin could be defined from a "survey of practitioners on the range of differences that they consider to be unimportant".

Generally, the definition of the acceptable level of equivalence or non-inferiority is made with reference to some retrospective superiority com-parison to placebo (Hung et al., 2003; D'Agostino, Massaro and Sullivan, 2003; Wiens, 2002). Methodologies for indirect comparisons to placebo have been discussed in detail by Hasselblad and Kong (2001). In this context the definition of the non-inferiority and equivalence limits should address the following (Wiens, 2002; D'Agostino, Massaro and Sullivan, 2003; Julious, 2004d):

1. There must be confidence that the active control would have been different from placebo had one been employed.

2. There should be a determination that there is no clinically meaningful difference between investigative treatment and the control.

3. Through comparing the investigative treatment to control there should be an ability indirectly to be able to determine that it is superior to placebo.

Points 1 and 3 are important as there is a view that non-inferiority and equivalence trials reward "failed" studies; that is, if we conducted a poor trial in which it would not have been possible to demonstrate the active control to be superior to placebo, then a poor investigative therapy may slip through via comparison to this control. However, Julious and Zariffa (2002) pointed out that this may not be the case as poor studies are poor for most objectives.

We can therefore infer that the clinical difference used for the limits of equivalence and non-inferiority will be smaller than the difference used for placebo-controlled superiority trials. There also is no generic definition for its setting; its definition will need to be defined on a study-by-study or indication-by-indication basis with consultation with the appropriate agencies and experts.

2.5   Step 4: Assessing the Population Variability

One of the most important components in sample size calculation is the variance estimate used. This variance estimate is usually made from retrospective data, sometimes from a number of studies. To adjudicate on the relative quality of the variance Julious (2004d) recommended considering the following aspects of the trials from which the variance is obtained:

1. Design: Is the study design ostensibly similar to the one you are designing? On the basic level are the data from a randomised controlled trial? Observational or other data may have greater variability. If you are undertaking a multicentre trial is the variance also estimated from a similarly designed trial? Were the endpoints similar to those you plan to use? Not just the actual endpoints, but were the times relative to treatment of both the outcome of interest and the baseline similar to your own?

2. Population: Is the study population similar to your own? The most obvious consideration is to ask whether the demographics were the same, but if the trial conducted was a multicentre one, was it conducted in similar countries? Different countries may have different types of care (e.g. different concomitant medication) and so may have different trial populations. Was the same type of patient enrolled the same (same number of mild, moderate and severe cases)? Was the

study conducted during the same seasons (relevant for conditions such as asthma)?

3. Analysis: Was the same statistical analysis undertaken? This means not just the question of whether the same procedure was used for the analysis but whether the same covariates were fitted to the model. Were the same summary statistics used?

The accuracy of the variance will obviously influence the sensitivity of a trial to the assumptions made about the variance and will obviously influence the strategy of an individual clinical trial. Depending on the quality of the variance estimate (or even if we have a good variance estimate) it may be advisable, as discussed in this chapter, to have some form of variance re-estimation during the trial.

We now highlight how the points raised need to be considered through two case studies. In each of these examples we make the assumption that the effect size of interest is known but what what must be ascertained is the control response rate (for binary data) or the population variability (for continuous Normal data).

2.5.1 Binary Data

For binary data the assumptions about the control response rate critically influence the sample size. This is because in determining an investigative treatment response rate it may be the control response p_A and a fixed effect size d that may be used to conjecture regarding the investigative response ($p_B = p_A + d$). We highlight the issues through a worked example.

2.5.1.1 *Worked Example of a Variable Control Response with Binary Data*

Table 2.1 gives the data from eight different studies for the control response rate (Stampfer et al., 1982). The e_i here are the number of events (myocardial infarctions) observed in each study. As you can see, the response rates vary between 8% and 27% across the different studies. The rightmost two columns give the workings for calculations for w_i and $w_i p_i$ and hence the calculations for the overall estimates.

The response from each study and the overall response estimate are given in Figure 2.4. From this we can estimate the overall response from a fixed-effects meta-analysis (the fixed line in the figure) to be 14.3% with standard error 0.0086. Hence, the 95% confidence interval around the overall estimate is 0.126 to 0.160.

There may be some evidence of heterogeneity across the studies used in this example. This may be because certain trials were sampled from "different" populations. It could raise the question of whether an overall response should be used or whether to use only trials, for example, from the same geographic region. In Section 2.5.2 we discuss in greater detail

TABLE 2.1

Control Data by Individual Study

Trial	Control e_i	Total	P_i	w_i	$p_i w_i$
1	15	84	0.179	572.66	102.26
2	94	357	0.263	1,840.44	484.60
3	17	207	0.082	2,746.05	225.52
4	18	157	0.115	1,546.72	177.33
5	29	104	0.279	517.18	144.21
6	23	253	0.091	3,061.30	278.30
7	44	293	0.150	2,295.89	344.78
8	30	159	0.189	1,038.68	195.98
Total	270	1,614		13,618.91	1,952.97

how regional and demographic differences may have an impact on calculation for Normal data.

2.5.2 Normal Data

Even if we have a good estimate of the variance, what guarantee is there that the trial population from which the population is taken will be the same as the one from which the prospective trial will be drawn? We could perform two apparently identical trials (same design, same objectives, same centres), but this would not be a guarantee that each trial would be drawn from the

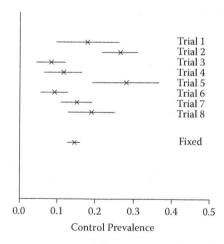

FIGURE 2.4 Plot of point estimates and confidence intervals for individual studies and overall.

same population. For example, if the trials were done at different times (e.g., years), then the concomitant medicines used in the trials may change over time, which could change the populations. Likewise with respect to time the technologies associated with the trials may change: from technologies associated with study conduct to the technology used to actually assess subjects. Again we highlight the issues through a worked example.

2.5.2.1 *Worked Example of Assessing Population Differences with Normal Data*

In designing a clinical trial for depression, variability data were collated from a number of trials. The primary endpoint for the prospective trial was the Hamilton Depression Scale (HAMD) (Hamilton, 1960). An appropriate estimate of the variance was thus required to use in the design of the prospective study.

The placebo data from 20 randomised controlled trials were collated for the primary endpoint of the HAMD 17-item scale. The data sets were based on the intent-to-treat data set as this would be the primary analysis population in the future trial.

A summary of the top-level baseline demographic data for each trial is given in Table 2.2. The data span 18 years, from 1983 to 2001. The studies were conducted in the two regions of Europe and North America in a number of populations. The duration of the studies varied from 4 to 12 weeks.

As discussed in Chapter 3, to get an overall estimate of the variance across several studies we can use the following result:

$$s_p^2 = \frac{\sum_{i=1}^{k} df_i s_i^2}{\sum_{i=1}^{k} df_i}, \tag{2.10}$$

where k is the number of studies, s_i^2 is the variance estimate from study i (estimated with df_i degrees of freedom) and s_p^2 is the minimum variance unbiased estimate of the population variance. This result therefore weights the individual variances to get an overall estimate such that the larger studies have greater weight in the variance estimate than smaller studies.

Using (2.10) the pooled estimate of the variance is 55.03, which is estimated with 1,543 degrees of freedom. However, there does seem to be some heterogeneity in the sample variances in the different subpopulations, given in Table 2.3, with the variability overall in the paediatric population 46.09 (on 85 degrees of freedom) and in the adult population 58.59 (on 312 degrees of freedom). Also, albeit on smaller populations in Europe, there seems to be a difference between the two regions of North America and Europe. These differences are not trivial, with differences in variances of 20% knocking on to a consequent 20% difference in the sample size estimate.

Note though that this investigation of the heterogeneity ignores factors like HAMD entry criteria at baseline and study duration, which may also

TABLE 2.2

Trial Information and Variances from 20 Randomised Controlled Trials' Placebo Data

Study	HAMD Entry Criteria	Number of Centres	Duration	Year	Population	Region	Phase	Sample Size	Degrees of Freedom	Variance
1	18	1	6	1984	Adult	North America	II	25	22	41.59
2	18	1	6	1985	Adult/geriatric	North America	II	169	160	59.72
3	18	6	6	1985	Adult/geriatric	North America	III	240	232	57.11
4	21	3	6	1986	Adult/geriatric	North America	III	12	9	62.97
5	18	10	6	1985	Adult/geriatric	North America	III	51	49	58.32
6	18	28	12	1991	Adult/geriatric	North America	III	117	109	42.51
7	18	23	12	1991	Adult/geriatric	North America	III	140	133	68.98
8	18	12	8	1992	Adult/geriatric	North America	III	129	121	51.81
9	18	1	6	1982	Adult	Europe	III	21	19	62.44
10	15	1	6	1983	Adult/geriatric	Europe	III	10	8	44.71
11	15	12	12	1994	Adult/geriatric	North America	III	85	80	38.81
12	13–18	12	8	1994	Paediatric	North America	III	87	85	46.09
13	15	18	10	1994	Adult	North America	IV	43	41	60.01
14	15	20	12	1996	Adult	North America	III	101	99	61.42
15	20	20	12	1996	Adult	North America	III	110	108	61.65
16	18	29	12	1996	Geriatric	North America	III	109	105	45.54
17	20	40	8	2001	Adult/geriatric	North America	III	146	140	58.36
18	18	1	4	1983	Adult	Europe	III	23	20	43.64
19	18	1	4	1983	Adult	Europe	III	3	1	19.32
20	18	1	4	1989	Adult	Europe	II	4	2	43.9

TABLE 2.3

Baseline Demographics and Variances from 20 Randomised Controlled Trials' Placebo Data

Population	Overall s_p^2	Overall df	Europe s_p^2	Europe df	North America s_p^2	North America df
All	55.03	1,543	50.48	50	55.19	1,493
Adult	58.59	312	51.58	42	59.70	430
Adult/geriatric	55.66	1,041	44.71	8	55.74	1,033
Paediatric	46.09	85	.	.	46.09	85
Geriatric	45.54	105	.	.	45.54	105

have an impact on the heterogeneity of the studies. There is no evidence of any trends by time.

We could do a statistical test to assess heterogeneity between the study variances through Bartlett's test, which can be applied and compared to the chi-squared distribution (Bartlett, 1937; Armitage and Berry, 1987):

$$M/C \sim \chi^2_{k-1} \tag{2.11}$$

where

$$M = \left(\sum_{i=1}^{k} df_i \right) \log\left(s_p^2\right) - \sum_{i=1}^{k} df_i \log\left(s_i^2\right)$$

$$C = 1 + \frac{1}{3(k-1)} \left[\sum_{i=1}^{k} \left(\frac{1}{df_i} \right) - \frac{1}{\Sigma_{i=1}^{k} df_i} \right]$$

Armitage and Berry (1987) recommended using C in the test statistic only in marginal cases as it is usually close to 1.

For an overall test of heterogeneity the Bartlett test returns a P-value of 0.561 (excluding C in the calculation) and 0.519 (including C). Thus, although there seems to be some evidence of differences in the different demographic populations the Bartlett test statistic infers that the individual studies themselves are drawn from the same population (and thus the demographic differences may be down to chance).

The variance data can also be examined pictorially. Data taken from a chi-squared distribution can be approximated to a Normal distribution with mean $\sqrt{2df - 1}$ and variance 1. This result only technically holds for large n (and there are some small sample sizes in the case study). However, most of the studies are reasonably large. Hence, by taking away $\sqrt{2df_i - 1}$ from each study (and dividing by 1) we can convert each of the variances to a scale that approximates to the standard Normal. From these amended variances a Normal probability plot can be constructed.

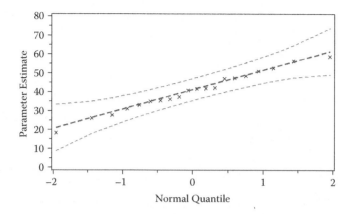

FIGURE 2.5 Normal probability plot of the observed variances across the 20 studies in the heteroskedasticity case study.

Figure 2.5 gives the Normal probability plot for the data. The bounds around the line are confidence bounds calculated using the methodologies of Friendly (1991). Thus, this figure pictorially supports the result from the Bartlett test.

This case study is good in that at first, with 20 studies, it seems that we have ample data on which to estimate a variance for a sample size calculation. However, by definition the reason why there were so many studies was to interrogate the treatment response in different populations. Once we drilled down into the data to optimise calculations for the prospective trial (same population; same study design and same region), there were less data to rely on.

When assessing the data at a global level, however, there seemed to be no heteroskedasticity between the studies. The evidence seems to suggest that the assumption that each study was drawn from the same population holds, and that a global, pooled estimate of the variance should be sufficient to power the prospective study.

2.6   Step 5: Type I Error

The results of any study are subject to the possibility of error; the purpose of the sample size calculation is to reduce the risk of errors due to chance to a level we will accept.

Figure 2.6 pictures the response anticipated under the null hypothesis with a superiority trial. Even if the null hypothesis is true there is still a chance that an extreme value would be observed such that it is rejected.

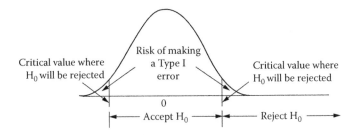

FIGURE 2.6 Illustration of a Type I error.

Type I error therefore is the chance of rejecting the null hypothesis when it is true. We can reduce the risk of making a Type I error by increasing the level of "statistical significance" we demand—the level at which a result is declared significant is also known as the Type I error rate. For example, in Figure 2.6 we could move the tails further and further away from 0 before we will accept a difference as statistically significant (i.e. reduce the significance level).

To a degree, the setting of the Type I error level is determined by precedent and is dictated by the objective of the study. It is often termed *society's risk* as medical practice may change depending on the results, so falsely significant results have a consequence.

2.6.1 Superiority Trials

For a superiority trial in which a two-sided significance test will be undertaken the convention is to set the Type I error at 5%. For a one-sided test the convention is to set the significance level at half of this (i.e. 2.5%) (ICH E9, 1998). However, these are conventions; although to a degree they could be considered the 'norm' there may be instances for superiority trials in which the Type I error rate is set higher depending on the therapeutic area and phase of development or lower.

An example for which the error rate may be set lower could be when instead of undertaking two clinical trials for a drug submission one is undertaken. Here the Type I error rate may be set at 0.125% as this is equivalent in terms of statistical evidence to two trials set at 5%.

2.6.2 Non-Inferiority and Equivalence Trials

The convention for non-inferiority and equivalence trials is to set the Type I error rate at half of that employed for a two-sided test used in a superiority trial (i.e. one-tailed significance level of $\alpha = 0.025$). However, setting the Type I error rate for non-inferiority and equivalence trials at half that for superiority trials could be considered consistent with superiority trials. This is because although in a superiority trial we have a two-sided 5% significance level in practice for most trials in effect what we have is a one-sided investigation with a 2.5% level of significance. The reason for this is that you usually have an investigative therapy and a control therapy, and it is only statistical superiority of the investigative therapy that is of interest.

Throughout the rest of the book when equivalence and non-inferiority trials are discussed the assumption is that $\alpha = 0.025$ and that 95% confidence intervals are used in the final statistical analysis.

Bioequivalence studies, described in Chapter 6, are different with respect to their Type I errors as two simultaneous tests at 5% and 90% confidence intervals are used.

2.7   Step 6: Type II Error

A Type II error is what you make when you do not reject a null hypothesis when it is false (and the alternative hypothesis is true). Figure 2.7 gives an illustration of the Type II error. From this you can see that under the alternative hypothesis there is a distribution of responses if the alternative is true centred around a difference d. From this figure you can see that under the alternative hypothesis there is still a chance a difference will be observed that will provide insufficient evidence to reject the null hypothesis.

The aim of the sample size calculation therefore is to find the minimum sample size for a fixed probability of Type I error to achieve a value of the probability of a Type II error. The Type II error is often termed the investigator's risks and by convention is fixed at rates of 0.10 to 0.20. The Type I error (usually set at 5% as discussed) and Type II risks carry different weights as they reflect the impact of the errors. As stated, with a Type I error medical practice

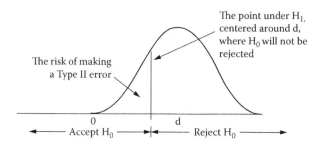

FIGURE 2.7 Illustration of a Type II error.

may switch to the investigative therapy with resultant costs, whilst with a Type II error medical practice would remain unaltered.

In general, we usually think not in terms of the Type II error but in terms of the power of a trial (1 – probability of a Type II error), which is the probability of rejecting the H_0 when it is in fact false. Pivotal trials should be designed to have adequate power for statistical assessment of the primary parameters. The Type I error rate of 5% is usually taken as standard for a superiority trial. He is recommended that the power to be consider to be standard be 90% with 80% the minimum considered. It is debatable regarding which level of power we should use, although it should be noted that, compared to a study with 90% power, with just 80% power we are doubling Type II error for only a 25% saving in sample size.

2.8   Step 7: Other Factors

The sample size is actually the evaluable number of subjects required for analysis. The final step in the calculation is to ask what the required total sample size is to ensure the evaluable number of subjects for analysis. For example, although you may enrol and randomise a certain number of subjects you may then find that 10–20% may drop out before an evaluation is made. Certain protocols specify that there must be at least one evaluable post-dose observation to be included in a statistical analysis. ICH E9 (1998) refers to the data set used as the analysis data set. Therefore, to account for having a proportion of subjects with no post-randomisation information we should recruit a sufficient number of subjects to ensure the evaluable sample size.

In addition, for trials such as those to assess non-inferiority, the per protocol data set would either be a primary or co-primary data set, so here the evaluable sample size would equate to the per protocol population.

As with obtaining a quantification of treatment effect or a variance discussed in Section 2.5 the number of dropouts or subjects in the per protocol data set could be assessed from retrospective studies and maybe pooled through methods such as meta-analysis. An example of the type of analysis is given in Figure 2.8, which provides the results of an analysis to quantify trial completion rates, which are used to assess the number of subjects in a completer data set as well as to assess how to analyse the data for the primary endpoint. There is a large amount of variability in the completion rates of the trials in this example, and although we do not go into detail of this here, an investigation would need to be made regarding which of these studies would be the most appropriate for the study planned.

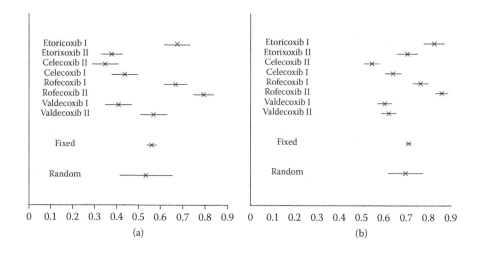

FIGURE 2.8 Trial completion rates: (a) placebo and (b) active.

  Key Messages

- Obtaining an estimate of the variance is an essential step in the sample size calculation.
- An effect size for calculating the study could be obtained through evaluating effects seen in previous studies.
- Caution needs to be exercised if the effect is estimated from just a single study.
- An estimated sample size is actually an evaluable sample size, and additional sample size calculations may be required to ensure a trial is of sufficient size to achieve the evaluable sample size.

3

Sample Sizes for Parallel Group Superiority Trials with Normal Data

3.1 Introduction

This chapter describes the calculations for clinical trials in which the expectation is that the data will take a plausibly Normal form and discusses the standard sample size calculations for trials in which the objective is to determine superiority. The chapter then describes how to undertake sensitivity analyses around the sample size calculations when designing a trial.

3.2 Sample Sizes Estimated Assuming the Population Variance to Be Known

As discussed in Chapter 1, in general terms for a two-tailed, α-level test we require

$$Var(S) = \frac{d^2}{(Z_{1-\beta} + Z_{1-\alpha/2})^2}, \tag{3.1}$$

$$Var(S) = \frac{\sigma^2}{n_A} + \frac{\sigma^2}{n_B} = \frac{r+1}{r} \cdot \frac{\sigma^2}{n_A}, \tag{3.2}$$

where σ^2 is the population variance estimate, and $n_B = rn_A$. Note (3.2) is minimised when $r = 1$ for fixed n. Substituting (3.2) into (3.1) gives (Brush, 1988; Lemeshow et al., 1990)

$$n_A = \frac{(r+1)(Z_{1-\beta} + Z_{1-\alpha/2})^2 \sigma^2}{rd^2}. \tag{3.3}$$

Note that in this section, and throughout the chapter for parallel group trials with Normal data, the assumption is made that the variances in each group are equal, that is, that $\sigma_A^2 = \sigma_B^2 = \sigma^2$. This assumption is referred to as *homoskedasticity*. There are alternative formulae for the case of unequal variances (Schouten, 1999; Singer, 2001), and Julious (2005d) described how the assumptions of homogeneity have an impact on statistical analysis. However, in the context of clinical trials under the null hypothesis the assumption is that the populations are the same, which would infer equal variances (as well as equal means).

When the clinical trial has been conducted and the data have been collected and cleaned for analysis it is usually the case that for the analysis the population variance σ^2 is considered unknown, and a sample variance estimate s^2 is used. As a consequence of this a *t*-statistic as opposed to a *Z*-statistic is used for inference. This fact should be represented in the sample size calculation, rewriting (3.3) so that *t* as opposed to *Z*-values are used. Hence, if the population variance is considered unknown for the statistical analysis (which is usually the case) the following could be used:

$$n_A \geq \frac{(r+1)(Z_{1-\beta} + t_{1-\alpha/2,\, n_A(r+1)-2})^2 \sigma^2}{rd^2}. \tag{3.4}$$

Unlike (3.3) this result does not give a direct estimate of the sample size as n_A appears on both the left and right sides of (3.4). It is best to rewrite the equation in terms of power and then use an iterative procedure to solve for n_A:

$$1 - \beta = \Phi\left(\sqrt{\frac{rn_A d^2}{(r+1)\sigma^2}} - t_{1-\alpha/2, n_A(r+1)-2} \right), \tag{3.5}$$

where $\Phi(\bullet)$ is defined as the cumulative density function of $N(0,1)$. However, it is not just a simple case of replacing *Z*-values with *t*-values when a sample variance is used in the analysis. In this situation the power should be estimated from a cumulative *t*-distribution as opposed to a cumulative Normal distribution (Senn, 1993; Brush, 1988; Chow, Shao and Wang, 2002; Julious, 2004d). The reason for this is that by replacing σ^2 with s^2 (3.5) becomes

$$1 - \beta = P\left(\sqrt{\frac{rn_A d^2}{(r+1)s^2}} - t_{1-\alpha/2, n_A(r+1)-2} \right), \tag{3.6}$$

where $P(\bullet)$ denotes a cumulative distribution defined from 3.6. This equation can in turn be rewritten as

$$1 - \beta = P\left(\frac{\sqrt{rn_A}\, d / \sqrt{(r+1)}\,\sigma}{\sqrt{s^2/\sigma^2}} - t_{1-\alpha/2, n_A(r+1)-2} \right), \tag{3.7}$$

by dividing top and bottom by σ^2. Thus, we have a Normal distribution over a square root of a chi-squared distribution, which by definition is a *t*-distribution. More specifically, in fact as the power is estimated under the alternative hypothesis, and under this hypothesis $d \neq 0$, the power should hence be estimated from a non-central *t*-distribution with degrees of freedom $n_A(r+1) - 2$ and non-centrality parameter $\sqrt{rn_A/(r+1)\sigma^2}$ (Senn, 1993; Brush, 1988; Chow, Shao and Wang, 2002; Kupper and Hafner, 1989; Julious, 2004d). Thus, (3.5) can be rewritten as

$$1 - \beta = \text{probt}\left(t_{1-\alpha/2, n_A(r+1)-2}, \; n_A(r+1)-2, \; \sqrt{\frac{rn_A d^2}{(r+1)\sigma^2}} \right), \qquad (3.8)$$

where $\text{probt}(\bullet, \; n_A(r+1)-2, \; \sqrt{rn_A d^2/(r+1)\sigma^2})$ denotes the cumulative distribution function of a Student's non-central *t*-distribution with $n_A(r+1)-2$ degrees of freedom and non-centrality parameter $\sqrt{rn_A d^2/(r+1)\sigma^2}$. Note here that the notation $\text{probt}(\bullet, \; n_A(r+1)-2, \; \sqrt{rn_A d^2/(r+1)\sigma^2})$ is the same as that used in the statistical package SAS notation. Note also that when $d = 0$ then we have a standard (central) *t*-distribution.

The differences between a non-central *t*-distribution and a Normal distribution could be considered trivial for all practical purposes as illustrated by Figure 3.1, which plots the distributions together for different effect sizes. The fact that the two lines are mainly superimposable is telling. Note that when there is no difference between treatments (Figure 3.1a) the slightly fatter distribution is the *t*-distribution. For each figure the fatter of the two distributions is the *t*-distribution. At the most "extreme" (Figure 3.1d) we can see that the *t*-distribution is slightly skewed compared to the Normal distribution, but the difference between the distributions is small.

Practically we could use (3.3) for the initial sample size calculation and then calculate the power for this sample size using (3.8), iterating as necessary until the required power is reached. To further aid in these calculations a correction factor of $Z^2_{1-\alpha/2}/4$ can be added to (3.3) to allow for the Normal approximation (Guenther, 1981; Campbell, Julious and Altman, 1995; Julious, 2004d)

$$n_A = \frac{(r+1)(Z_{1-\beta} + Z_{1-\alpha/2})^2 \sigma^2}{rd^2} + \frac{Z^2_{1-\alpha/2}}{4}. \qquad (3.9)$$

For quick calculations the following formula to calculate sample sizes, with 90% power and a two-sided 5% Type I error rate, can be used:

$$n_A = \frac{10.5\sigma^2}{d^2} \frac{(r+1)}{r}, \qquad (3.10)$$

or for $r = 1$

$$n_A = \frac{21\sigma^2}{d^2}. \qquad (3.11)$$

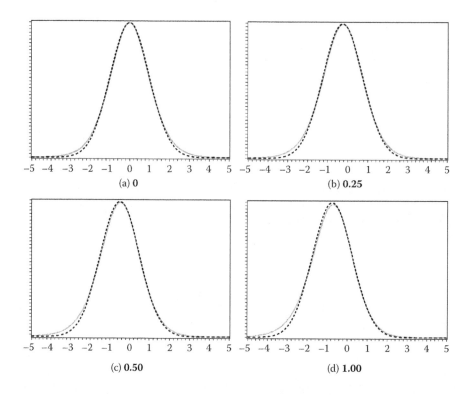

FIGURE 3.1 The Normal (dotted line) and *t*-distribution (solid line) estimated with 10 degrees of freedom for different effect sizes: (a) 0.0, (b) 0.25, (c) 0.50, (d) 1.00.

The result of (3.10) comes from putting a 10% Type II error rate and a two-sided Type I error of 5% into (3.3). Table 3.1 gives the actual calculated value from which (3.3) is derived.

Equations (3.11) and (3.10) are close approximations to (3.8), giving sample size estimates only one or two lower and thus providing quite good initial

TABLE 3.1

Calculated Values for $2(Z_{1-\beta} + Z_{1-\alpha/2})^2$ for a Two-Sided Type I Error Rate of 5% and Various Type II Error Rates

α	β	$2(Z_{1-\beta} + Z_{1-\alpha/2})^2$
0.05	0.20	15.70
0.05	0.15	17.96
0.05	0.10	21.01
0.05	0.05	25.99

TABLE 3.2

Sample Sizes for One Group, n_A ($n_B = n_A$), in a
Parallel Group Study for Different Standardised
Differences and Allocation Ratios for 90% Power
and a Two-Sided Type I Error of 5%

	Allocation Ratios			
δ	1	2	3	4
0.05	8,407	6,306	5,605	5,255
0.10	2,103	1,577	1,402	1,314
0.15	935	702	624	585
0.20	527	395	351	329
0.25	338	253	225	211
0.30	235	176	157	147
0.35	173	130	115	108
0.40	133	100	89	83
0.45	105	79	70	66
0.50	86	64	57	53
0.55	71	53	47	44
0.60	60	45	40	37
0.65	51	38	34	32
0.70	44	33	30	28
0.75	39	29	26	24
0.80	34	26	23	21
0.85	31	23	20	19
0.90	27	21	18	17
0.95	25	19	17	15
1.00	23	17	15	14

estimates. Equation (3.5) is closer to (3.8), mainly giving the same result and occasionally underestimating by just 1. Although the difference in sample size estimates is small using the non-central *t*-distribution relative to the complexity added to the calculations the results are easy to program and hence tabulate for ease of calculation. As such, Table 3.2 gives sample sizes using (3.8) for various standardised differences ($\delta = d/\sigma$).

3.3   Worked Example 3.1

The worked example described here is based on real calculations done day to day by applied medical researchers designing clinical trials. The first calculation undertaken in the worked example includes a common mistake when undertaking sample size calculations; this is followed by the correct calculations.

TABLE 3.3

Baseline Characteristics Mean (and standard deviation) Unless Presented as a Count (%)

	Intervention Group	
	Vestibular Rehabilitation	Usual Medical Care
Sample size	83	87
Age	62.93 (15.21)	61.01 (14.42)
Duration of dizziness (months)	98.00 (141.48)	101.01 (135.25)
Number (%) of participants		
Female	59 (71%)	62 (71%)
Whose occupation		
Managerial/professional	39 (36%)	33 (22%)
Intermediate	18 (23%)	23 (28%)
Routine/semiroutine	21 (27%)	26 (32%)
Taking medication for dizziness	44 (53%)	43 (49%)
Who had previously undertaken balance retraining	3 (4%)	2 (2%)
Vertigo Symptom Scale	16.57 (11.28)	14.70 (9.21)
Movement-provoked dizziness	27.28 (5.72)	26.56 (7.64)
Postural stability eyes open	586.49 (249.27)	561.38 (278.66)
Postural stability eyes closed	897.99 (459.94)	820.27 (422.45)
Dizziness Handicap Inventory	**40.98 (22.52)**	**37.89 (19.74)**
SF-36–Physical Functioning	65.67 (30.30)	69.37 (27.28)
HADS–Anxiety	7.37 (4.60)	7.24 (4.66)
HADS–Depression	3.77 (3.10)	3.48 (2.67)

The calculations were based on the results taken from Yardley et al. (2004) in a trial of vestibular rehabilitation for chronic dizziness. In this trial the intervention arm was compared to usual care in a single-blind manner. The trial was not chosen because it had anything wrong with it but more because it was a well-analysed study that provided all the requisite information for calculations.

3.3.1　Initial Wrong Calculation

Suppose now you wished to repeat the trial of Yardley et al. (2004) but with a single primary endpoint of "Dizziness Handicap Inventory" assuming an effect size of 5 to be of importance. It is decided to do the calculations with a two-tailed Type I error of 5% and 90% power.

The data for the variability are to be taken from Yardley et al. (2004), given in Table 3.3.

As there are two variance estimates an overall estimate of the population variance is obtained from the following:

$$s_p^2 = \frac{\sum_{i=1}^{k} df_i s_i^2}{\sum_{i=1}^{k} df_i}. \tag{3.12}$$

The degrees of freedom can be taken as the sample size minus one. Hence, the pooled estimate of the variance is

$$s_p^2 = \frac{82 \times 22.52^2 + 86 \times 19.74^2}{82 + 86} = 447.01,$$

$$(3.13)$$

giving a standard deviation of 21.14.

In truth (3.12) is a somewhat artificial calculation here in that we have only two variances from which to obtain an overall estimate. However, the result (3.13) can be generalised to many variances.

With an effect size of 5 the estimate of the sample size is 375.77 or 376 evaluable subjects per arm using (3.3); the quick calculation of (3.10) provides the same sample size estimate. The result (3.8) that allows for the fact that a sample variance will be used in the analysis also estimates the sample size to be 376 evaluable subjects per arm.

3.3.2   Correct Calculations

The calculations now are repeated. Instead of using the table of baseline characteristics from Yardley et al. (2004), the variances taken from the statistical analysis (given in Table 3.4) are now used. Here the mean differences are quoted with corresponding confidence interval. These were taken were from an analysis of covariance (ANCOVA) including the term for baseline in the analysis. For the confidence interval a pooled estimate of the standard deviation was used (s_p).

TABLE 3.4

Statistical Analysis

Measure	N (Missing)	Vestibular Rehabilitation Mean (SE)	Usual Medical Care Mean (SE)	Difference between Groups	P-Value
Vertigo Symptom Scale	170 (13)	9.88 (0.76)	13.67 (0.74)	−3.48 (−5.59 to −1.38)	0.001
Movement-provoked dizziness	169 (17)	14.55 (1.19)	20.69 (1.14)	−6.15 (−9.40 to −2.90)	0.001
Postural stability eyes open	168 (20)	528.71 (19.68)	593.71 (18.98)	−65.00 (−119.01 to −11.00)	0.019
Postural stability eyes closed	160 (20)	731.95 (32.05)	854.25 (30.48)	−122.29 (−209.85 to −34.74)	0.006
Dizziness Handicap Inventory	170 (18)	31.09 (1.52)	35.88 (1.48)	−4.78 (−8.98 to −0.59)	0.026

As a result a pooled estimate of the standard deviation can be estimated because the confidence interval can be estimated from

$$\bar{x}_A - \bar{x}_B \pm Z_{1-\alpha/2} s_p \sqrt{1/n_A + 1/n_B}. \tag{3.14}$$

Hence

$$s_p = \frac{\text{Upper CI bound} - \text{Lower CI bound}}{2Z_{1-\alpha/2}\sqrt{1/n_A + 1/n_B}}, \tag{3.15}$$

and an estimate of the standard deviation is

$$s_p = \frac{8.98 - 0.59}{2 \times 1.96\sqrt{1/83 + 1/87}} = 13.95. \tag{3.16}$$

Note that we have used Z-values here but we could also use *t*-values and *t* tables for this calculation.

Using the same effect size of 5 the sample size estimate is now 163.63 or 164 evaluable subjects per arm using (3.3), the same as the quick result (3.10). The sample size estimate from (3.8) is 165 subjects, which we use in the following worked examples.

This sample size estimate is less than half the estimate from the previous calculation. This is because Table 3.3 used a variance estimated from summary statistics, while Table 3.4 used a variance estimated from an ANCOVA. This second variance is considerably smaller.

This point is not a trivial one. A consequence is that if you are planning to undertake an ANCOVA with baseline fitted as a covariate as your final analysis, then the calculations described here that use a variance from an ANCOVA would be the correct approach. Failure to allow for baseline in sample size calculations when baseline will be accounted for in the final analysis could lead to a substantial overestimation of the sample size. Section 3.5 revisits this problem.

3.3.3   Accounting for Dropout

Suppose there was an anticipation of 15% dropouts in the planned study. The estimated sample sizes so far were evaluable subjects. What is therefore required is an estimate of the total sample size to get the requisite evaluable sample size.

Taking 165 as the evaluable sample size the total sample size would therefore be

$$165/0.85 = 194.12$$

or 195 subjects per arm.

If possible the evaluable sample size could still be used for recruitment with the number of subjects enrolled until 165 evaluable subjects have completed the trial. In such instances the total sample size calculations would still be of value as they could be used for budgetary or planning purposes.

Note a very common mistake when calculating the total sample size is to multiply the evaluable sample size by 1.15 and not divide by 0.85. Here this would erroneously return a sample size of 189.75 or 190 subjects.

3.4   Worked Example 3.2

It has been highlighted how important it is to use a variance estimate from an ANCOVA if such an analysis is to be undertaken in the planned study. However, often articles do not give confidence intervals but simply a mean difference and *P*-value. Suppose Table 3.4 presented the results in such a way then for the same effect size (5), power (90%) and Type I error rate (5%) the following calculations could be undertaken: We know that the *P*-value is calculated from

$$\frac{\bar{x}_A - \bar{x}_B}{s_p \sqrt{1/n_A + 1/n_B}}. \tag{3.17}$$

We also know what the *P*-value is, so the standard deviation can be estimated from

$$s_p = \frac{(\bar{x}_A - \bar{x}_B)}{Z_{P-value} \sqrt{1/n_A + 1/n_B}}. \tag{3.18}$$

If we use Normal distribution tables, then the Z-value to give a *P*-value of 0.026 is 2.226. Hence the pooled estimate for the standard deviation is

$$s_p = \frac{(35.88 - 31.09)}{2.226 \times \sqrt{1/87 + 1/83}} = 13.995. \tag{3.19}$$

Note that, as with the confidence intervals discussed, we could also use *t*-values and *t* tables for this calculation.

The sample size estimate would hence be estimated from (3.8) as 166 evaluable subjects per arm.

3.5   Design Considerations

3.5.1   Inclusion of Baselines or Covariates

In the analysis of the results of a clinical trial, the effects of treatment on the response of interest are often adjusted for predictive factors, such as demographic (like gender and age) or clinical covariates (such as baseline response), by fitting them concurrently with treatment. This section concentrates on the case when baseline is the predictive covariate of interest (although the results are generalisable to other factors), the design is a parallel group design and an ANCOVA, allowing for the baseline, is to be the final analysis. The Committee for Proprietary Medicinal Products (CPMP) issued notes for guidance on the design and analysis of studies with covariates (CPMP, 2003).

Frison and Pocock (1992) gave a variance formula for various numbers of baseline measures:

$$\text{Variance} = \sigma^2 \left(1 - \frac{p\rho^2}{1+(p-1)\rho} \right). \tag{3.20}$$

Here, ρ is the Pearson correlation coefficient between observations—assuming compound symmetry—and p is the number of baseline or measures taken per individual. From this equation a series of correction factors can be calculated (Machin et al., 1997) that give the variance reduction and consequent sample size reduction for different correlations and numbers of baselines. The assumption here is that there is balance between treatments and the baseline (or covariate) of interest. Any imbalance will increase the variance from (3.20) and consequent sample size (Senn, 1997). With randomisation the imbalance should be minimised, however.

From (3.20) it is clear that for fixed numbers of baseline measures the higher the correlation is, the greater the reduction in variance and consequent sample size will be. For example, if three baseline measures were to be taken and the expected correlation between baseline and outcome is 0.5, the effect would be to reduce the variance to $0.6250 \times \sigma^2$. However, for the same number of baseline measures if the expected correlation between baseline and outcome is 0.7 then the effect would be to reduce the variance to $0.3875 \times \sigma^2$.

Another result from (3.20) is that for fixed correlation it seems that although there is incremental benefit with increasing numbers of baselines this incremental benefit asymptotes at three baselines for all practical purposes. The results in Table 3.5 demonstrate this, giving the correction factors for a fixed

TABLE 3.5

Effect of Number of Baselines on the Variance

Number of Baselines	Variance
1	0.7500
2	0.6667
3	0.6250
4	0.6000
5	0.5833
6	0.5714

correlation between baseline and outcome of 0.50 and difference numbers of baseline measures.

The results of Frison and Pocock (1992) are a little simplistic; for example, they assume that the within-subject errors are independent (Senn, Stevens and Chaturvedi, 2000). However, they do highlight the advantages of taking baselines in clinical trials.

The results in this section demonstrate the importance, when estimating the sample size, to take the variance estimate from the full model in which all covariates are present. They also highlight how, if we ignore baseline and covariate information when doing sample size calculations, we could potentially be overestimating the sample size, which was demonstrated also in Worked Example 3.1. The variance taken from an analysis that allows for covariates should always be used in the sample size calculations if ANCOVA is to be the planned analysis.

3.5.2   Post-dose Measures Summarised by Summary Statistics

Often in parallel group clinical trials, patients are followed up at multiple time points. Making use of all of the information obtained on a patient has the desirable property of increasing the precision for estimating the effects of treatment. Naturally, as the precision is increased the variability is decreased, and we consequently need to study fewer patients to achieve a given power. Suppose we are interested in looking at the difference in the average of all of the post-dose measures:

$$H_0 : \bar{\mu}_A = \bar{\mu}_B \text{ versus } H_1 : \bar{\mu}_A \neq \bar{\mu}_B,$$

where $\bar{\mu}_A$ and $\bar{\mu}_B$ represent the means of the average of the post-dose measures in the two treatment populations. It should be noted that often in clinical trials when data are measured longitudinally it is the rate of change of a particular endpoint that is of interest. For example, in respiratory trials of chronic lung disease the hypothesis may focus on whether a treatment changes the annual decline in lung function. However, the simplest approach of taking the summary measure as the simple average of the post-dose assessments for each subject and taking the average of these averages across treatments to obtain $\bar{\mu}_A$ and $\bar{\mu}_B$ is assumed to be the summary statistic used.

Assuming we have r post-dose measures and that the correlation between those measures is ρ the variance can be calculated as

$$\text{Variance} = \frac{\sigma^2[1+(r-1)\rho]}{r}, \tag{3.21}$$

where σ^2 represents the variance of a given individual post-dose measurement.

When looking at (3.21) it seems that as the correlation between post-dose measures increases the variance increases, as does the total sample size required. This is because, although it may seem counterintuitive, the advantage of taking additional measurements decreases as the correlation increases.

This fact is due to how the total variance σ^2 is constructed (Julious, 2000):

$$\sigma^2 = \sigma_b^2 + \sigma_w^2, \tag{3.22}$$

where σ_w^2 is the within-subject component of variation (as in cross-over trials), and σ_b^2 is the between-subject component of variation.

It is important here to distinguish between the within- (intra-) subject and the between- (inter-) subject components of variation. The within-subject component of variation quantifies the expected variation among repeated measurements on the same individual. It is a compound of true variation in the individual (and is discussed again in Chapter 4). The between-subject component of variation quantifies the expected variation of single measurements from different individuals. If only one measurement is made per individual it is impossible to estimate σ_w^2 and σ_b^2; consequently, only the total variation, given in (3.22), can be estimated.

If we know the between-subject variance and the correlation between the measures the within-subject variance can be derived from

$$\sigma_w^2 = \left(\frac{1-\rho}{\rho}\right)\sigma_b^2. \tag{3.23}$$

Therefore, for known variance components of σ^2 and correlation between measures, the variance that takes account of the number of post-dose measures is defined as

$$\text{Variance} = \sigma_b^2 + \frac{\sigma_w^2}{r}. \tag{3.24}$$

Thus, formula (3.21) is actually quite intuitive. As for constant r the higher the correlation, from (3.23), the lower the within-subject variance is and, from (3.24), the lower the total variance and consequent sample size are. However, as ρ increases and σ_w^2 falls, the effect of taking repeated measures diminishes as σ_w^2 already constitutes a small part of the overall variance.

Equation (3.21) also gives the incremental benefit of taking additional post-dose measures for fixed correlation. Like with the number of baselines it seems that although there is incremental benefit with increasing numbers of post-dose measures, the incremental benefit asymptotes at four post-dose measures for all practical purposes. The results in Table 3.6 demonstrate this, giving the correction factors for a fixed correlation between post-dose measures of 0.50 and difference numbers of post-dose measures.

3.5.3 Inclusion of Baseline or Covariates as Well as Post-dose Measures Summarised by Summary Statistics

As noted further savings in sample size can be achieved by accounting for baseline as a covariate. Frison and Pocock (1992) defined an additional

TABLE 3.6

Effect of Number of Post-dose Measures on the Variance

Number of Post-Dose Measures	Variance
1	1.0000
2	0.7500
3	0.6667
4	0.6250
5	0.6000
6	0.5833

variance measure to account for the baseline (or multiple baselines) as a covariate and difference numbers of post-dose measures. Assuming there are p baseline visits and r post-dose visits the variance is defined as

$$\text{Variance} = \sigma^2 \left[\frac{1+(r-1)\rho}{r} - \frac{p\rho^2}{1+(p-1)\rho} \right]. \qquad (3.25)$$

3.6 Revisiting Worked Example 3.1

In Chapter 2 it was highlighted how assessing the variance used in the sample size calculations was important. What is an issue with the Yardley et al. (2004) paper used in the calculations in Worked Example 3.1 is that the primary analysis was a last observation carried forward (LOCF) analysis that included baseline (i.e. if there were no post-measurements then baseline was used to impute the outcome).

If you are not planning to undertake such an imputation, then there is an issue with using the variance from this study as the variance in your study would be larger. It is easy to demonstrate why.

Suppose we are designing a study with a single baseline and we have the variance from an ANCOVA defined as σ_c^2. Thus, if we are using baseline in an LOCF, then fitting baseline as a covariate will produce an extraspecial prediction of post-dose assessment. Formally, the correlation between baseline and post-dose assessment can be shown to be (Julious and Mullee, 2008)

$$\rho_{BLOCF} = \lambda + \rho(1-\lambda), \qquad (3.26)$$

where λ is the proportion of subjects for whom baseline is being carried forward. It can be seen from visual inspection of (3.20) and (3.26) that the greater the λ, the greater the ρ_{BLOCF} is and the smaller the variance. Obviously if $\lambda = 1$ then $\rho_{BLOCF} = 1$.

TABLE 3.7

Increases in Correlation Due to Baseline Carried Forward for
Different Actual Correlations between Baseline and Post-dose
Assessment and Different Proportion of Missing Data

	Proportion of Subjects Missing Data (λ)			
ρ	0.050	0.100	0.150	0.200
0.90	0.905	0.910	0.915	0.920
0.80	0.810	0.820	0.830	0.840
0.70	0.715	0.730	0.745	0.760
0.60	0.620	0.640	0.660	0.680
0.50	0.525	0.550	0.575	0.600

For the illustrative example taken from Yardley et al. (2004) we have
$\rho = 0.67$ and $\lambda = 0.12$. Hence, from (3.26) we have $\rho_{BLOCF} = 0.71$. In practice the
correlation between baseline and post-dose assessments would be expected
to be lower than for correlations between just post-dose assessments.

The objective of this little exercise is to reinforce the importance of investigating how a study is to be analysed. If the planned analysis is different from
the study from which the variance estimate was taken, then this may have
an impact on the sample size.

An investigation of (3.20) and (3.26) is made in Table 3.7 for plausible values
of λ and ρ. The leftmost column gives the actual correlation between baseline and post-dose assessment (assuming no data missing). The subsequent
columns give the correlations between baseline and post-dose assessment
for different proportions of missing data (assuming baseline is carried forward in a LOCF through a BLOCF).

3.6.1   Reinvestigating the Type II Error

Often when calculating a sample size the estimate produced for the effect
size of interest could be smaller than that anticipated originally leading to
sample sizes which may not be feasible. One solution to this problem would
be to reduce the power of the study to 80%, say, for which for the same effect
size (5) and standard deviation (13.95) the evaluable sample size would need
to be 124 subjects per arm compared to 164 subjects per arm for 90% power.

Hence, 25% fewer subjects are required for an 80% powered study compared to a 90% powered study (or 33% more subjects are required for a 90%
powered study compared to an 80% powered study). However, within an
individual study it should be highlighted that you are doubling the Type II
error for this sample size saving.

In truth a sample size calculation is in many ways a negotiation. Another
common situation is when the sample size is fixed and we wish to determine
the effect size that can be detected for this sample size. This is fine as far as it

goes, but it depends on how the calculation is then written. If the text in the protocol appeared as

> For 90% power and a two-tailed Type I error rate of 5% with an estimate of the population standard deviation of 13.95 and an effect size of 5.742 the sample size is estimated as 125 evaluable subjects per arm.

This would be inappropriate as the sample size came first and was not calculated. It is far better to say what the actual power is and if nothing else to flag the risks being taken for budgetary concerns. More appropriate wording would be of the form

> The sample size is 125 evaluable subjects per arm. This sample size is based on feasibility. However, with 90% power and a two-tailed Type I error rate of 5% with an estimate of the population standard deviation of 13.95 this sample size could detect an effect size of 5.742.

3.7   Sensitivity Analysis

One potential issue with conventional calculations is that they usually rely on retrospective data to quantify the variance to be used in the calculations. If this variance is therefore estimated imprecisely, then it would have an impact on the calculations.

A main assumption in the calculations therefore is that the variance used in the calculations is the population variance when in fact we have estimated it from a previous study. What therefore needs to be assessed *a priori* is the sensitivity of the study design to the assumption around the variance. On the issue of sensitivity the International Conference on Harmonisation of Technical Requirements for Registration of Pharmaceuticals for Human Use (ICH) E9 (1998) makes the following comment, with the emphasis that of the author:

> The method by which the sample size is calculated should be given in the protocol, together with the estimates of any quantities used in the calculations (such as variances, mean values, response rates, event rates, difference to be detected). ... It is important to investigate the **sensitivity** of the sample size estimate to a variety of deviations from these assumptions.

The sensitivity of the trial design to the variance is relatively straightforward to investigate and can be done using the degrees of freedom of the variance estimate used in the calculations. This concept was described by Julious (2004a). Firstly, we need to calculate the sample size conventionally using an appropriate variance estimate. Next, using the degrees of freedom for this variance and the chi-squared distribution, we can calculate the upper one-tailed 95th percentile, say, for the variance using

$$s_p^2(95) < \frac{df}{\chi_{0.05,df}^2} s_p^2.$$

(3.27)

Here, s_p^2 is taken from (3.12), which is estimated with the degrees of freedom

$$df_p = \sum_{s=1}^{n} df_i.$$

(3.28)

Then this upper estimate of the variance can be used in (3.8) to investigate the power. This would give an assessment of the sensitivity of the study to deviations from the variability assumptions by investigating a study's power to an extreme plausible value that the variance could take.

3.7.1   Worked Example 3.3

For Worked Example 3.1 we had a pooled estimate of the standard deviation of 13.95 and we wished to detect a difference of 5 with 90% power and two-sided significance level of 5%. The variance was estimated from 170 subjects, which would correspond to around 168 degrees of freedom.

We have $\chi_{0.05,168}^2 = 138.03$; hence from (3.26) we have

$$s_p^2(95) < \frac{168}{138.03} \times 13.95^2 = 235.15.$$

Therefore a highly plausible value for s_p is 15.33. If the true standard deviation was nearer to 15.33 than the 13.95 used in the calculations, then we would actually have 84% power. We could hence conclude that that study is reasonably robust to the assumptions about the variance.

Suppose, however, the sample variance estimate was only estimated with 25 degrees of freedom. We would then have $\chi_{0.05,25}^2 = 14.61$; hence we would have that

$$s_p^2(95) < \frac{25}{14.61} \times 13.95^2 = 194.60.$$

We thus have a highly plausible value for s_p as 18.25. If the true standard deviation was nearer to 18.25 than the 13.95 used in the calculations, then we would actually have 70% power. This is not too alarming, but consideration may need to be given to accounting for this imprecision somehow. We could do a sample size re-estimation (discussed separately in this chapter), or else it may be expedient to highlight to the team the sensitivity of the study design to the assumptions being made in the sample size calculation.

3.8 Calculations Taking Account of the Imprecision of the Variance Used in the Sample Size Calculations

We have highlighted thus far how when designing a trial typically σ^2 would be unknown, but the choice of sample size, which depends crucially on σ^2, has to be decided before any observations in the prospective trial have been made. The simplest approach is just to assume that σ^2 is known and take an 'assumed value,' which is the basis for traditional sample size formulae discussed in this chapter. In reality the assumed value is obtained from an estimate s^2 of σ^2 from previous similarly designed studies using the same endpoint.

To account for the fact that we are using s^2 and not σ^2 the following result can be used to estimate the power (Julious, 2002; Julious and Owen, 2006):

$$probt\left(\sqrt{\frac{rn_A d^2}{(r+1)s^2}}, m, t_{1-\alpha/2, n_A(r+1)-2}\right) \geq 1-\beta, \tag{3.29}$$

where m here is the degrees of freedom about s^2, the estimated variance. When (3.29) is rewritten in terms of the sample size it becomes

$$n_A \geq \frac{(r+1)s^2[tinv(1-\beta, m, t_{1-\alpha/2, n_A(r+1)-2})]^2}{rd^2}, \tag{3.30}$$

which if we replace the t-statistic with the Z-statistic becomes

$$n_A = \frac{(r+1)s^2[tinv(1-\beta, m, Z_{1-\alpha/2})]^2}{rd^2} \tag{3.31}$$

This last result, (3.31), may be thought of as a version of (3.3) that has been adjusted for uncertainty about the unknown true sampling standard deviation σ.

As relationships (3.20) and (3.30) both have to be solved by iteration for a given power (3.31) can be used to provide initial values to start the iteration. From simple empirical observation it seems that an expected power of at least $1 - \beta$ is ensured through adding 1 to the sample size obtained from (3.31).

It is worth noting when considering the approximate formula for n_A of (3.3) and (3.31) that the ratio of these depends on α, β and m but not on r, s or d. Hence a ratio of (3.3) and (3.31) would give you an inflation factor (IF) to account for the imprecision in the sample variance.

$$\text{Inflation Factor (IF)} = \frac{(r+1)s^2[tinv(1-\beta, m, Z_{1-\alpha/2})]^2}{[Z_{1-\beta}+Z_{1-\alpha/2}]^2} \tag{3.32}$$

TABLE 3.8

Multiplication Factors for Different Levels of Two-Sided
Significance, Type II Error and Degrees of Freedom

		Two Significance Level (α)			
m	β	0.010	0.025	0.050	0.100
5	0.05	2.232	2.145	2.068	1.980
	0.10	1.819	1.761	1.711	1.652
	0.15	1.614	1.571	1.533	1.489
	0.20	1.482	1.449	1.419	1.385
	0.50	1.122	1.120	1.117	1.114
10	0.05	1.488	1.454	1.425	1.392
	0.10	1.346	1.322	1.301	1.276
	0.15	1.268	1.249	1.233	1.214
	0.20	1.215	1.200	1.187	1.172
	0.50	1.056	1.055	1.054	1.053
25	0.05	1.172	1.160	1.150	1.139
	0.10	1.126	1.117	1.109	1.101
	0.15	1.100	1.092	1.086	1.079
	0.20	1.081	1.075	1.070	1.065
	0.50	1.021	1.021	1.021	1.021
50	0.05	1.083	1.077	1.072	1.067
	0.10	1.061	1.057	1.053	1.049
	0.15	1.049	1.045	1.042	1.039
	0.20	1.040	1.037	1.034	1.032
	0.50	1.010	1.010	1.010	1.010
75	0.05	1.054	1.051	1.047	1.044
	0.10	1.040	1.037	1.035	1.032
	0.15	1.032	1.030	1.028	1.026
	0.20	1.026	1.024	1.023	1.021
	0.50	1.007	1.007	1.007	1.007
100	0.05	1.040	1.038	1.035	1.033
	0.10	1.030	1.028	1.026	1.024
	0.15	1.024	1.022	1.021	1.019
	0.20	1.020	1.018	1.017	1.016
	0.50	1.005	1.005	1.005	1.005

Some values for (3.32) are given in Table 3.8. This table could be used to provide multiplication factors when standard formulae are used to calculate the
sample size, such as (3.3), (3.4) or (3.8), to account for the imprecision in the
variance.

Note the sample sizes from (3.31) converge to (3.4) as n_A becomes large.
In this chapter, using (3.8), the sample sizes were also derived from a non-
central t-distribution. However, as (3.31) converges to (3.4) there will be
instances for large m for which (3.31) gives a sample size one smaller than
(3.8). For the IFs, because $Z_{1-\alpha/2}$ not $t_{1-\alpha/2,n_A(r+1)-2}$ is used, (3.8) becomes (3.3).

Hence, the IFs hold regardless of the original sample size calculation as they are large sample results.

3.8.1 Worked Example 3.4

We revisit Worked Example 3.3 in which it was imagined that the variances were estimated with 25 degrees of freedom. Previously the sample size, assuming the variance in the calculations to be a population variance, was estimated using (3.8) at 165 patients in each arm of the trial. From Table 3.8 we can see that to account for the imprecision in the sample variance we would need to increase the sample size estimated by 11% to 184 (rounded from 183.15) patients per arm. An inversion of this argument would be to say that by assuming that the standard deviation was a population estimate the sample size could be considered to be underestimated by 10%.

It may seem an unrealistic scenario to undertake a large study in which the calculations are based on such few degrees around the variance. However, it is not an unknown occurrence to design a study based on a few degrees of freedom, particularly early in drug development. For all trials, therefore, particularly those in which the design is sensitive to assumptions, it is strongly recommended to have some form of adaptive component to the design.

3.9 Interim Analyses and Sample Size Re-estimation

When NASA (National Aeronautics and Space Administration) launches a rocket to Mars it does not point the rocket in the general direction of its target and launch it with a vain hope that in 2 years it will hit the red planet. It continuously monitors the course of the rocket, tinkering and modifying its route to optimise the chances of success. Analogously in clinical trials why should we set up the study and then hope that the assumptions on which the trial was designed were correct?

Throughout this chapter the trial design assumptions we have investigated have been about the trial's variability. One approach to the problem of having an uncertain estimate of the variability is to be adaptive. The advantage of being adaptive is that it allows you to alter or stop the course of a study during its actual conduct such that unexpected occurrences are not encountered for the first time when the study has been completed and the final analysis undertaken. There are three approaches that we can adopt for adaptive designs (Julious, 2004a):

1. Group sequential design: The sample size in each group is fixed, but interim analyses are undertaken to test the null hypothesis with a decision made at each analysis to stop the trial for success or failure or to enrol another cohort.

2. Fixed interim analyses: The parameters used in the estimation of the sample size are re-estimated, such as the variance for Normal data, and the sample size is adjusted accordingly. The null hypothesis is not tested.

3. A combination of approaches 1 and 2: At the interim analyses both the null hypothesis is investigated and the sample size is re-estimated—conditional on whether the trial is stopped for success or failure.

The first two approaches are relatively straightforward, but the third is more complex as the sample size re-estimation depends on a decision on the null hypothesis. This section concentrates on the first two designs but only in the context of the effect on the sample size.

3.9.1   Interim Analyses

There are methodological considerations when deciding whether to undertake an interim analysis. However, an initial consideration may well be budgetary, and a main consideration here could be the possible increase in the sample size as the sample size has an impact on the cost of the study.

The impact of the interim analysis on the sample size is determined by why we are undertaking the interim analysis. We need to maintain the overall Type I error rate at the nominal level set *a priori* (usually 5%) and having interim analyses has the potential to increase the Type I error. Therefore to maintain the overall Type I error at or below the nominal level we need to make an appropriate adjustment. Adjusting the Type I error will in turn have an impact on the sample size. The effects of the different adjustments are now discussed in detail.

3.9.1.1   *Worked Example 3.5*

For Worked Example 3.1 it was calculated that 165 subjects per arm were required. Suppose for the study three equally placed interim analyses are planned. The purpose of these interim analyses is primarily to assess safety; however, efficacy will also be examined, although the study will only stop for efficacy for "wonder" effects (i.e. very highly significant results).

O'Brien and Fleming (1979) stopping rules were hence proposed for the study as these set stopping boundaries that are very hard to cross at the difference interim analyses. Table 3.9 gives the stopping boundaries for the different interim analyses. For example, at the very first interim analysis the critical value for the Z-statistic is 4.084, which would equate to a P-value of 0.000044.

There is a penalty for these interim looks: At the end of the study the Z- value is 2.042, and the nominal P-value is 0.044003. As the nominal P-value has been reduced at the end there is a penalty in the form of the sample size

TABLE 3.9

O'Brien–Fleming Stopping Boundaries and *P*-values for Different Interim Analyses

	Proportion of Information			
	0.25	0.50	0.75	1.00
Critical value	4.084	2.888	2.358	2.042
Nominal *P* value	0.000044	0.003878	0.018375	0.041146

although as only a small proportion of the alpha has been spent early, so the sample size has been increased by 9 to 174. Hence the cost in terms of sample size is quite small.

Suppose there is a desire to stop the study early. For this, the trial is run as a sequential trial with a request that the alpha is spent equally at each interim analysis. Pocock (1983) stopping rules can be used.

Table 3.10 gives the stopping boundaries for the different interim analyses. For example at the very first interim analysis the critical value for the Z-statistic is 2.368, which would equate to a *P*-value of 0.017869. The penalty for the interim looks is now greater, such that if the trial went to the final analysis without stopping the final *P*-value would be 0.017869. As more alpha has been spent at the interim analyses there is a greater penalty in terms of the sample size, with it having to increase to 209 subjects per arm to account for the interim analysis.

A more generic solution for the O'Brien–Fleming method can be found using Table 3.11 and Table 3.12. The final row for each column for Table 3.11 is taken from O'Brien and Fleming (1979). The subsequent rows are taken by multiplying this value by

$$\sqrt{\frac{J}{i}}, \tag{3.33}$$

where J is the total number of interim analyses, and i is the interim analysis number.

The nominal significance levels for the boundary values are given in Table 3.12. Hence, to calculate a sample size when five analyses are to be undertaken use a

TABLE 3.10

Pocock Stopping Boundaries and *P*-values for Different Interim Analyses

	Proportion of Information			
	0.25	0.50	0.75	1.00
Critical value	2.368	2.368	2.368	2.368
Nominal *P*-value	0.017869	0.017869	0.017869	0.017869

TABLE 3.11

Critical Values for O'Brien–Fleming Method for Different Interim
Analyses Schedules

Interim Number	Number of Interim Analyses			
	2	3	4	5
1	2.802856	3.438023	4.084116	4.554668
2	**1.966977**	2.431049	2.887906	3.220637
3		**1.984943**	2.357965	2.629639
4			**2.042058**	2.277334
5				**2.036909**

conventional result—such as (3.3), (3.4) and (3.8)—but use the significance level
of 0.041659 taken from Table 3.12 to calculate the sample size.

Pocock's method is a little more straightforward; calculate the nominal
level of significance for each interim as

$$\alpha \ln(1 + (e - 1)/J), \tag{3.34}$$

from which the critical values are calculated. This nominal level of significance, given in Table 3.13, is then used to calculate the sample size using (3.3),
(3.4) or (3.8).

Note the methodology for calculating sample sizes allowing for interims described here is a little conservative as it only uses the significance
levels at the final analysis to calculate the sample size. In the actual
trial the study planned could also have declared a significant result at
each of the interims that is not being accounted for in the sample size
calculations.

In summary, therefore, how you spend your P affects the impact of the
interim analysis. If you have small P's at the interim analysis then you will
have a big P at the end. However, if you have bigger P's at the interim, then
you will have a smaller P at the end.

TABLE 3.12

Nominal P-values for O'Brien–Fleming Method for Different Interim
Analyses Schedules

Interim Number	Number of Interim Analyses			
	2	3	4	5
1	0.005065	0.000586	0.000044	0.000005
2	0.049186	0.015055	0.003878	0.001279
3		0.047151	0.018375	0.008548
4			0.041146	0.022766
5				0.041659

TABLE 3.13

Critical Values and Nominal Significance Levels for Pocock Method for Different Interim Analyses Schedules

	Number of Interim Analyses			
	2.000000	**3.000000**	**4.000000**	**5.000000**
Nominal significance level	0.031006	0.022642	0.017869	0.014770
Critical value	2.156999	2.279428	2.368328	2.437977

3.9.2   Sample Size Re-estimation

If the variance estimates are imprecisely estimated prior to the start of the trial, a sample size re-assessment could be made at some point during the study.

A simple solution would be to have an independent third party analyse the data in an unblinded manner and provide a new estimate of the variance. There may be strictly no methodological issues with this approach; however, there could be a concern if there are just two arms in the trial as the total variation would be known or easily estimated.

Source of Variation	DF	SS	MS
Between Treatment Group	XX	XX	XX
Within Group	XX	XX	XX
Total	XX	XX	

If the third party uses with the within-group variation for sample size re-assessment, then the within-group variation may become known.

Source of Variation	DF	SS	MS
Between Treatment Group	XX	XX	XX
Within Group	XX	XX	XX
Total	XX	XX	

Then through knowing the within-group variation and the total variation we would be able to estimate the between-group effect.

Source of Variation	DF	SS	MS
Between Treatment Group	XX	XX	XX
Within Group	XX	XX	XX
Total	XX	XX	

With more than two treatment arms this issue may be less of a concern.

The convention when undertaking a sample size re-assessment is to have some form of restricted sample size re-estimation with the following procedure applied:

1. Take an initial estimate of the same size n (say).
2. After a proportion of subjects has been enrolled (say $n/2$) re-calculate the sample size n_1 using the same sample size criteria Type I error, power, effect size.
3. The re-estimated sample size is taken as $\max(n, n_1)$.

The estimate of the variance could be made through a third-party unblinded analysis or an estimate of the variance could made in a blinded manner using the between-group difference used in the sample size calculation and taking this away from the total variance (obtained from a blind analysis) to get an estimate of the within-group variance.

Note the sample size is not reduced to protect the Type I error as without the restriction the Type I error could increase. To explain why this is true imagine that our trial is to have one interim analysis such that the data are collected in two parts (1 and 2) with no restriction on the sample size.

If the estimated variance from the first part is low compared to what we planned for trial, then we would reduce the amount of data collected in part 2. Conversely, if the estimated variance in part 1 is large compared to what we planned, then we would increase the sample size.

Now for the final analysis with standard statistical methods, ignoring the sample size re-estimation, the estimate of the variability in the data is biased downwards.

- If by chance part 1 has a small observed variance, then we have increased its importance by reducing the amount of data in part 2.
- If by chance part 1 has a larger observed variance, then we down-weight this by increasing the size of part 2.

This means that the estimate of overall variance is biased downwards, and the Type I error is inflated. Hence, if we use the "restricted" approach and look at the characteristic of the procedure when actual variance is the same as the prior variance we still have the same problem of downweighting the part I data when the observed variance is high. However, when the observed variance in the part 1 data is low we give it equal weight with the part 2 data. Hence, the effect on the overall variance estimate is less extreme than that in the other direction as we are using equal weight (using original size n) if observed variance is low, so we have removed "half" the problem.

Hence, having a restriction in the sample size re-estimation reduces but does not totally remove issues with the Type I error. Suppose we estimate the within-group variance using the between-group difference used in the sample size calculation. In a blinded sample size re-estimation, therefore, if the separation between observed location parameters (sample means) is larger than planned the variance will be overestimated, and the sample size will be increased. If it is smaller the estimated variance will be lower, and a smaller overall sample size will be used. Under the null hypothesis therefore the sample size will remain the same with a restricted approach. Also under the null hypothesis, if by chance the difference between means is large we downplay part 1; if it is by chance small, we overplay part 1; this has the effect of reducing the Type I error.

3.10 Cluster Randomised Trials

In this book there is a focus on trials in a regulatory setting. In such trials subjects are randomised at the individual level to receive treatment. For health technology assessments it may not always be possible to randomise at the individual level due to pragmatic considerations. Instead, subjects are randomised at the level of hospital, primary care practice or practitioner level or time window; hence subjects are cluster randomised.

Cluster-randomised trials are therefore experiments in which intact social units rather than independent individuals are randomly allocated to intervention groups. Examples include communities selected as the experimental unit in trials evaluating mass education programs, schools selected as the experimental unit in trials evaluating smoking prevention programs and families selected as the experimental unit in trials evaluating the efficacy of dietary interventions.

The reasons for adopting a cluster randomisation include administrative convenience, to enhance subject compliance and to avoid treatment group contamination. The last is of particular importance for instance for education initiative given in a primary care setting, for which it may not be feasible to give the intervention to one subject without other subjects in the same practice also being exposed.

There are disadvantages of cluster-randomised trials particularly if there is a between-cluster variation, the presence of which has the effect of reducing the effective sample size. The extent of the problem depends on the degree of within-cluster correlation and on average cluster size. There are a number of possible reasons for between-cluster variation. For example, subjects frequently select the clusters to which they belong (e.g. patient characteristics could be related to the primary care practice); important covariates at the cluster level affect all individuals within the cluster in the same manner; individuals within clusters frequently interact and as a result may respond similarly; finally there is a tendency for infectious diseases to spread more rapidly within rather than among families or communities.

A consequence of the issues associated with cluster-randomised trials is that standard approaches for sample size estimation and statistical analysis do not apply as standard sample size approaches would lead to an under-powered study, and applying standard statistical methods would generally tend to biased estimates.

An important consideration in designing cluster-randomised clinical trials is the estimation of the intracluster correlation coefficient (ICC) ς, such that the more similar the individuals in the same cluster are, the bigger the ICC will be. In terms of variance components the overall response variance σ^2 may be expressed as the sum of two components, that is,

$$\sigma^2 = \sigma_B^2 + \sigma_w^2, \tag{3.35}$$

where here σ_B^2 is defined as the between-cluster component of variance and σ_w^2 as the within-cluster component of variance. Now

$$\varsigma = \frac{\sigma^2}{\sigma_B^2 + \sigma_w^2}. \tag{3.36}$$

Note that $\sigma_w^2 = \sigma^2(1-\varsigma)$.

3.10.1   Quantifying the Effect of Clustering

Consider a trial in which k clusters of size m are randomly assigned to each of experimental and control groups. Also, assume the response variable Y is Normally distributed with common variance σ^2. The study is being designed as a superiority trial with the objective to test H_0: $\mu_A = \mu_B$.

Appropriate estimates of μ_A and μ_B are $\bar{x}_A^2$ and $\bar{x}_B^2$ the sample means, which have the common variance

$$\frac{[1+(m-1)\varsigma]\sigma^2}{km}, \tag{3.37}$$

where ς is the ICC, k is the number of clusters and m here is the average sample size per cluster.

3.10.2 Sample Size Requirements for Cluster-Randomised Designs

Suppose k clusters of size m are to be assigned to each of two intervention groups. Recall from (3.3) under the Normal approximation assumption the sample size for an individually randomised trial can be estimated from

$$n_A = \frac{2\sigma^2(Z_{1-\alpha/2} + Z_{1-\beta})^2}{d^2}. \tag{3.38}$$

To account for the effect of clustering the sample size for the number of subjects per intervention from (3.37) and (3.38) can be estimated from (Donner and Klar, 2000)

$$n_A = \frac{2\sigma^2(Z_{1-\alpha/2} + Z_{1-\beta})^2[1 + (m-1)\varsigma]}{d^2}. \tag{3.39}$$

From taking the ratio of (3.38) over (3.39) an IF can be estimated,

$$IF = 1 + (m-1)\,\varsigma, \tag{3.40}$$

to account for the cluster randomisation. Alternatively, in terms of clusters the sample size is estimated to be

$$k = \frac{2\sigma^2(Z_{1-\alpha/2} + Z_{1-\beta})^2[1 + (m-1)\varsigma]}{md^2}. \tag{3.41}$$

Actually, the results from (3.38) and (3.39) are not too dissimilar. Remember the chapter discussion regarding the effect of covariates on the sample size such that if a single baseline was collected that was correlated with outcome by ρ the sample size could be estimated from

$$n_A = \frac{2\sigma^2(Z_{1-\alpha/2} + Z_{1-\beta})^2(1 - \rho^2)}{d^2}. \tag{3.42}$$

In practice the result (3.42) is seldom used because for individually randomised trials a variance is used for sample size calculations appropriate for the study planned. Chapter 2 discussed how to assess the variance such that if the design, population and analysis from the study from which it is taken are similar to the one being planned then (3.38) could be applied. Similar principles should be considered for cluster-randomised trials; if variance estimates are from trials ostensibly similar to the trial planned, then (3.38) could be used.

Key Messages

- The variance used in the sample size calculation should reflect the planned analysis.
- Using an inappropriate variance could lead to a substantial over- (or under-) estimate in the sample size.
- Spending time to obtain an optimal variance estimate could have a substantial benefit for the design of the trial in terms of the sample size.
- Consideration should be given to investigating the sensitivity of the sample size calculations to the assumptions in the calculations, particularly around the variance.
- When undertaking a sample size re-estimation for a blinded trial it may actually be possible to estimate the within-group variance and possibly unblind the trial.

4

Sample Size Calculations for Superiority Cross-over Trials with Normal Data

4.1 Introduction

This chapter describes the calculations for cross-over clinical trials in which the expectation is that the data will take a plausibly Normal form. The emphasis in this chapter is on sample size calculations for trials in which the objective is to determine superiority.

4.2 Sample Sizes Estimated Assuming the Population Variance to Be Known

For the analysis of cross-over trial data this chapter concentrates on the case when an analysis of variance (ANOVA) is the primary analysis, fitting terms for subject, period and treatment. The assumption is that we are undertaking an AB/BA cross-over trial, although the methodology described can be extended to a pairwise comparison in a multiperiod cross-over trial (with appropriate adjustment to the degrees of freedom). With the analysis it is the within-subject residual errors that are assumed to be sampled from a Normal distribution.

There are alternative approaches for analysing cross-over trial data: the paired t test and the period adjusted t test. We now briefly describe these methods and the ANOVA approach.

4.2.1 Analysis of Variance

Suppose we have two groups of paired observations: $x_{11}, x_{12}, \ldots, x_{1n}$ in group 1 and $x_{21}, x_{22}, \ldots, x_{2n}$ in group 2 such that each group is measured on n subjects in two periods so that each subject receives both treatments, and it is the mean difference that is of interest $\bar{x}_1 - \bar{x}_2$. To undertake this analysis we would need to fit a general linear model and then use contrasts to estimate the difference in means.

The test statistic will be constructed using the within-subject standard deviation (SD) s_w from the residual line of the ANOVA

$$t = \frac{\bar{x}_1 - \bar{x}_2}{(\sqrt{2}s_w)/\sqrt{n}}. \tag{4.1}$$

Under the null hypothesis, t is distributed as Student's t, with $n - 2$ degrees of freedom.

4.2.2   Paired t-tests

For a paired t-test we simply place the observed individual effects on the two treatments in two columns, ignoring any ordering. For each subject a treatment difference is calculated d_i and consequently a mean of these differences $\bar{d}$, equivalent to $\mu_A - \mu_B$, and a SD of the differences σ_d. The test statistic is thus

$$\frac{\bar{d}\sqrt{n}}{s_d}, \tag{4.2}$$

which is compared to the t-distribution on $n - 1$ degrees of freedom.

   Note if the period is not fitted into the model with the ANOVA approach then this would be equivalent to the paired t-test; that is, (4.2) would be equivalent to (4.1).

4.2.3   Period-Adjusted t-tests

In a period-adjusted t-test for each treatment sequence (AB or BA) a mean difference is calculated $\bar{d}_{AB}$, equivalent to $\mu_A - \mu_B$, and $\bar{d}_{BA}$, equivalent to $\mu_B - \mu_A$. Assuming that the allocation to each sequence $n_{AB} = n_{BA} = n/2$ and the within-sequence variances $s_{d_{AB}}^2 = s_{d_{BA}}^2 = s_d^2$ are equal, then the mean difference of interest $(\bar{d}_{AB} - \bar{d}_{BA})/2$ has the variance $s_d^2(1/n_{AB} + 1/n_{AB})/4 /= s_d^2/\sqrt{n}$. Thus, the test statistic is

$$\frac{1/2(\bar{d}_{AB} - \bar{d}_{BA})}{s_d/\sqrt{n}}, \tag{4.3}$$

which is compared to the t-distribution on $n - 2$ degrees of freedom.

   Note if period is fitted into the model with the ANOVA approach then this would be equivalent to the period-adjusted t-test; that is, (4.3) would be equivalent to (4.1).

   If there is truly no period effect,

$$\frac{1/2(\bar{d}_{AB} - \bar{d}_{BA})}{s_d/\sqrt{n}} \approx \frac{1/2((\mu_A - \mu_B) - (\mu_B - \mu_A))}{s_d/\sqrt{n}} \approx \frac{\bar{d}\sqrt{n}}{s_d}, \tag{4.4}$$

and thus we would have an equivalent test to a paired t-test but with one less degree of freedom.

The reason why the approaches are the same is because $s_d^2 = 2\, s_w^2$; hence from inspection of (4.1), (4.2) and (4.3) we can see how the inference is the same.

4.2.4   Summary of Statistical Analysis Approaches

As highlighted, the three different statistical analysis approaches are approximately equivalent especially if there is period effect. So why highlight them? As with other chapters it is important to use a variance appropriate to the analysis that will be undertaken in the study being designed.

All the results in this chapter assume that an ANOVA will be the final analysis, and thus a within-subject variance is used in sample size estimation σ_w^2. If a variance is being estimated from a previous study in which a paired t-test was applied, then the variance of the difference σ_d^2 would be estimated. Thus, for this example it would be important to convert the estimate of σ_d^2 to σ_w^2 or the sample size would be overestimated by a factor of two.

4.2.5   Sample Size Calculations

To estimate a sample size for a cross-over trial as well as quantify the within-subject estimate of the difference in treatment means that is of interest, the effect size, we also need an estimate of the within- (intra-) subject SD σ_w. The within-subject SD is taken from the residual line of an ANOVA model and quantifies the expected variation among repeated measurements on the same individual (Julious, Campbell and Altman, 1999). With an estimate of both the within-subject SD and the effect size a sample size can be calculated similar to parallel group studies discussed in Chapter 3

$$n = \frac{2(Z_{1-\beta} + Z_{1-\alpha/2})^2 \sigma_w^2}{d^2},$$
(4.5)

where n here is the total sample size.

Note that with cross-over trials, unlike parallel group trials, there is no allocation ratio because in a cross-over trial the meaning of r would be the allocation ratio per treatment sequence AB and BA. The assumption in (4.5) is that subjects will be equally assigned to each sequence. If a sample variance is to be used in the analysis, then we can rewrite (4.5) as

$$n \geq \frac{2\,(Z_{1-\beta} + t_{1-\alpha/2,\,n-2})^2 \sigma_w^2}{d^2},$$
(4.6)

which in turn can be rewritten in terms of power to solve iteratively for n

$$1 - \beta = \Phi\left(\sqrt{\frac{nd^2}{2\sigma_w^2}} - t_{1-\alpha/2,n-2}\right).$$
(4.7)

Similar to parallel group trials, when the population variance is considered unknown for the statistical analysis, under H_1: $d \neq 0$ the Type II error (and hence the power) should be calculated under the assumption of a non-central t-distribution with degrees of freedom $n - 2$ and non-centrality parameter $\sqrt{nd^2/2\sigma_w^2}$ (Senn, 1993; Kupper and Hafner, 1989; Julious, 2004d). Thus, (4.7) can be rewritten as

$$1 - \beta = \text{Prob}t\left(t_{1-\alpha/2,n-2}, \quad n-2, \quad \sqrt{\frac{nd^2}{2\sigma_w^2}} \right). \tag{4.8}$$

In the same manner as a parallel group study we can add a correction factor of $Z_{1-\alpha/2}^2/2$ to (4.5) to allow for the Normal approximation and use this for initial calculations in (4.8) (Guenther, 1981):

$$n = \frac{2(Z_{1-\beta} + Z_{1-\alpha/2})^2 \sigma_w^2}{d^2} + \frac{Z_{1-\alpha/2}^2}{2}. \tag{4.9}$$

For quick calculations we can adapt (4.5) for the calculation of sample sizes with 90% power and a two-sided 5% Type I error rate.

$$n = \frac{21\sigma_w^2}{d^2}. \tag{4.10}$$

The sample size results (4.9) and (4.10) are slightly smaller than from (4.8); also compared to (4.8), (4.7) will mostly give the same sample size—occasionally underestimating by 1. Table 4.1 gives sample sizes using (4.8) for various standardised differences ($\delta = d/\sigma$).

The total sample sizes for a cross-over trial is nearly equivalent to that for one arm of parallel group studies, for each standardised difference δ in Chapter 3. The slight differences are accounted for by the different degrees of freedom used in (4.8) and the equivalent result from Chapter 3 for parallel group trials. Practically, though, they are the same. It should be noted, however, that the standardised differences in Table 4.1 represent different quantities from those for parallel group trials. The within-subject variance in a cross-over trial can be derived from

$$\sigma_w^2 = \sigma^2(1-\rho), \tag{4.11}$$

where σ^2 is the population variance from a conventional parallel group design, and ρ is the Pearson correlation coefficient estimated between two measures on the same subject. For a relatively modest correlation of 0.5, the within-subject variance would be half the population variance, and as a consequence the equivalent standardised difference would be 40% larger in a cross-over compared to a parallel group study. Parallel group and cross-over trials will only have an equivalent standardised difference for a zero correlation.

TABLE 4.1

Total Sample Sizes for a Cross-over
Study for Different Standardised
Differences for 90% Power and
Two-Sided Type I Error Rate of 5%

δ	n
0.05	8,408
0.10	2,104
0.15	936
0.20	528
0.25	339
0.30	236
0.35	174
0.40	134
0.45	106
0.50	87
0.55	72
0.60	61
0.65	52
0.70	45
0.75	40
0.80	35
0.85	32
0.90	29
0.95	26
1.00	24
1.05	22
1.10	20
1.15	19
1.20	17
1.25	16
1.30	15
1.35	14
1.40	13
1.45	13
1.50	12

4.2.6   Worked Example 4.1

Pollock et al. (2005) described a cross-over trial in patients with symptoms of hypothyroidism. The intervention arm was compared to placebo in a double-blind manner.

Suppose we wished to repeat the same trial but with a single primary endpoint of thyroid-stimulating hormone, taking the effect size to be 1 (mU/l) and assuming 85% of patients will complete the trial. The study is to be analysed through an ANOVA. Assume a two-tailed Type I error of 5% and 90% power using the data for the variability from Table 4.2.

TABLE 4.2

Summary of Results from a Cross-over Trial

Outcome	Thyroxitine	Placebo	Adjusted Difference (95% CI)	P-value
Thyroid-stimulating hormone (mU/l)	0.66 (0.77)	1.77 (1.21)	−1.17 (−1.76 to −0.59)	<0.001
Free thyroxine (ρmol/l)	17.95 (3.03)	13.68 (3.37)	4.75 (2.67 to 6.83)	<0.001
Free tri-iodothyronine (ρmol/l)	3.72 (0.66)	3.50 (0.54)	−0.23 (−0.11 to 0.56)	0.177
Cholesterol (mmol/l)	6.33 (1.17)	6.27 (1.25)	0.05 (−0.27 to 0.37)	0.739
Prolactin (mU/l)	250 (156)	307 (331)	−37 (−189 to 116)	0.622

Note: CI = confidence interval.

First we need to estimate the within-subject SD s_w. We have from the confidence interval around thyroid-stimulating hormone that

$$s_w = \frac{\text{Upper CI bound} - \text{Lower CI bound}}{2Z_{1-\alpha/2}\sqrt{2/n}} = \frac{1.76 - 0.59}{2 \times 1.96\sqrt{2/22}} = 0.99$$

while using *t*-values we would have

$$s_w = \frac{\text{Upper CI bound} - \text{Lower CI bound}}{2t_{n-2,1-\alpha/2}\sqrt{2/n}} = \frac{1.76 - 0.59}{2 \times 2.09\sqrt{2/22}} = 0.93.$$

Using the larger s_w estimate of 0.99 the total evaluable sample size from (4.8) is 24 subjects. Alternatively we could use Table 4.1. The standardised difference is $1/0.99 \approx 1$. From Table 4.1 the evaluable sample size is the same as the calculation.

If we had used 0.93 for the SD the evaluable sample size estimate from (4.8) would be a little lower at 22 subjects.

Note that for both these calculations (4.8) would give a sample size 1 less than (i.e. 23 and 21 subjects per arm).

The sample size calculation has given us the total evaluable sample size calculation. Suppose we only expected 85% of subjects to complete the trial; we thus require

- With an SD of 99 the total sample would become 24/0.85 = 28.3 or 29 subjects.
- With an SD of 0.93 the total sample size would be 22/0.85 = 25.9 or 26 subjects.

4.2.7   Worked Example 4.2

Suppose free tri-iodothyronine is the primary endpoint and all that we had for the calculation were mean difference and the *P*-value. The wish is to estimate the sample size to be able to detect a difference of 0.20 pmol/l with 90% power for a two-sided significance level of 5%.

The P-value is 0.177; hence from Normal tables the Z-value for this is 1.38 (note again with t-values this SD would be a little smaller):

$$s_p = \frac{(\bar{x}_A - \bar{x}_B)}{Z_{P-value}\sqrt{2/n}} = \frac{0.23}{1.38\sqrt{2/22}} = 0.55$$

The sample size estimate is 162 patients total from (4.8).

If we had used a standardised difference we would have 0.20/0.55 = 0.36. Approximating this as 0.35 Table 4.1 gives a sample size estimate of 174 patients in total.

4.2.8 Worked Example 4.3

As with Worked Example 4.2 often we have suboptimal data on which to base our sample sizes. Suppose it was possible to undertake a similar study to that of Yardley et al. (2004) described in Chapter 3 as a cross-over trial. The wish is to have the same primary endpoint of Dizziness Handicap Inventory assuming the same effect size of 5 to be of importance as for the parallel group trial and hence an estimate of the sample size to detect this difference (assuming a two-tailed Type I error of 5% and 90%).

Here of course we are designing a cross-over trial but only have data from a parallel group trial to assist us, a not uncommon problem.

We know from Chapter 3 that the variance formula for analysis of covariance for various numbers of baseline measures is

$$\text{Variance} = \sigma^2 \left(1 - \frac{p\rho^2}{1+(p-1)\rho} \right) \tag{4.12}$$

where ρ is the Pearson correlation coefficient between observations—assuming compound symmetry—and p is the number of baseline measures taken per individual. We also know that the within-subject variance is defined from (4.11).

In Chapter 3 we estimated the pooled variance σ^2 to be 447.01 and the variance estimate when accounting for baseline [i.e. (4.12)] to be 13.95 × 13.95 = 194.60. From (4.12) we therefore have

$$194.6 = 447.01(1 - \rho^2).$$

Hence we have that the correlation between consecutive measures can be estimated as 0.75. The within-subject variance can be estimated as

$$\sigma_w^2 = 447.01(1 - 0.75) = 111.75.$$

Using this as an estimate of the within-subject variance (within-subject SD of 10.57) the sample size can be estimated as 96 patients in total from (4.8). The result from (4.9) also gives a sample size of 96 patients.

4.3 Sensitivity Analysis about the Variance Used in the Sample Size Calculations

As with parallel group trials the sensitivity of the sample size estimate in a cross-over trial is relatively straightforward to investigate. The following result

$$s_w^2(95) < \frac{df}{\chi_{0.05,df}^2} s_w^2 \qquad (4.13)$$

can be used to assess the sensitivity of the sample size calculations to the assumptions about the variance.

4.3.1 Worked Example 4.4

The original trial from Pollock had 22 subjects total. Hence the variance was estimated with 20 degrees of freedom. For thyroid-stimulating hormone 0.99 was used as an estimate of the within-subject standard for the sample size calculations. A highly plausible value for the variance could be taken as

$$s_w^2(95) < \frac{20}{\chi_{0.05,20}^2} 0.99^2 = \frac{20}{10.85} 0.98 = 1.81.$$

Hence, a highly plausible value for the within-subject SD is 1.34. If the true variance was nearer to 1.34 then with 24 subjects total the study has 70% power. This is a decrease from 90% power. It would be recommended to have this calculation in the protocol and to communicate the sensitivity to the wider team, but the calculations could be considered to be reasonably robust to the assumption about the variance.

4.4 Calculations Taking Account of the Imprecision of the Variance Used in the Sample Size Calculations

To account for the imprecision of the variance used in the sample size calculations the results for parallel group trials can be generalised to give the following formula

$$n \geq \frac{2s_w^2[tinv(1-\beta, m, t_{1-\alpha/2,n-2})]^2}{d^2}, \qquad (4.14)$$

where n is the least integer value for (4.14) to hold, and m is the degrees of freedom about the estimate variance s_w^2. We can rewrite (4.14) in terms of power to obtain the following result:

$$1 - \beta = \text{Probt}\left(\sqrt{\frac{nd^2}{2s_w^2}}, m, t_{1-\alpha/2, n-2}\right). \tag{4.15}$$

Replacing the *t*-statistic with a *Z*-statistic gives the following result:

$$n = \frac{2s_w^2[tinv(1-\beta, m, Z_{1-\alpha/2})]^2}{d^2}, \tag{4.16}$$

which allows us to have a direct estimate of the sample size and gives an initial value for iterations for (4.14).

By taking the ratio of (4.16) to (4.5) inflation factors can be calculated independent of s_w and d and dependent only on α, β and m. These inflation factors are the same as Table 3.10 in Chapter 3 and are not repeated here.

 Key Message

- The sample size calculations in the chapter use the within-subject variance σ_w^2 and care should be given regarding whether a variance estimate obtained from a previous study for calculations is a within-subject variance or a variance of the difference σ_d^2.

5

Sample Size Calculations for Equivalence Clinical Trials with Normal Data

5.1 Introduction

The sample size calculations described so far in this book have concentrated on when we wish to determine whether one treatment is superior to another treatment. As discussed in Chapter 1, however, we do not always wish to show that two treatments are different. An objective of a trial can be to show that they are clinically the same.

In this chapter we discuss calculations for when a trial is being designed for which we wish to show two treatments are equivalent and the primary outcome is assumed to take a Normal form. Subsequent chapters discuss the related topics of non-inferiority and bioequivalence.

5.2 Parallel Group Trials

5.2.1 Sample Sizes Estimated Assuming the Population Variance to Be Known

5.2.1.1 General Case

Recall from Chapter 1 that the total Type II error (defined as $\beta = \beta_1 + \beta_2$) is derived from the following result:

$$Z_{1-\beta_1} = \frac{-d - \Delta}{\sqrt{Var(S)}} - Z_{1-\alpha} \quad \text{and} \quad Z_{1-\beta_2} = \frac{d - \Delta}{\sqrt{Var(S)}} - Z_{1-\alpha}. \tag{5.1}$$

For equivalence trials for the general case when the expected true mean difference is not fixed to be zero the sample size cannot be derived directly. This is because the total Type II error is the sum of the Type II errors associated with each one-tailed test. As is the case with superiority trials $Var(S)$ can be defined as

$$Var(S) = \frac{\sigma^2}{n_A} + \frac{\sigma^2}{n_B} = \frac{r+1}{r} \cdot \frac{\sigma^2}{n_A}, \tag{5.2}$$

where σ^2 is the population variance estimate and $n_B = rn_A$. From this and the fact that $\beta = \beta_1 + \beta_2$, the following can be used to derive the Type II error (and power)

$$1 - \beta = \Phi\left(\sqrt{\frac{((\mu_A - \mu_B) - d)^2 \, rn_A}{(r+1)\sigma^2}} - Z_{1-\alpha}\right) + \Phi\left(\sqrt{\frac{((\mu_A - \mu_B) + d)^2 \, rn_A}{(r+1)\sigma^2}} - Z_{1-\alpha}\right) - 1.$$

(5.3)

The sample size cannot be derived directly; instead we have to iterate until a sample size is reached that gives the required Type II error (and power). If the variance is to be considered unknown for the statistical analysis (5.4) can be used:

$$1 - \beta = \Phi\left(\sqrt{\frac{((\mu_A - \mu_B) - d)^2 \, rn_A}{(r+1)\sigma^2}} - t_{1-\alpha, n_A(r+1)-2}\right)$$

$$+ \Phi\left(\sqrt{\frac{((\mu_A - \mu_B) + d)^2 \, rn_A}{(r+1)\sigma^2}} - t_{1-\alpha, n_A(r+1)-2}\right) - 1.$$

(5.4)

As with superiority trials discussed in Chapters 3 and 4 it is best to assume a non-central t-distribution to calculate the Type II error and power. Under the assumption of a non-central t-distribution the power can be calculated using the following (Owen, 1965; Diletti, Hauschke and Steinijans, 1991; Julious, 2004d):

$$1 - \beta = \Pr\mathrm{ob}t(-t_{1-\alpha, n_A(r+1)-2}, n_A(r+1) - 2, \tau_2) - \Pr\mathrm{ob}t(t_{1-\alpha, n_A(r+1)-2}, n_A(r+1) - 2, \tau_1),$$

(5.5)

where τ_1 and τ_2 are non-centrality parameters defined respectively as

$$\tau_1 = \frac{((\mu_A - \mu_B) + d)\sqrt{rn_A}}{\sqrt{(r+1)\sigma^2}} \quad \text{and} \quad \tau_2 = \frac{((\mu_A - \mu_B) - d)\sqrt{rn_A}}{\sqrt{(r+1)\sigma^2}}.$$

(5.6)

For quick calculations, and to provide an initial value for the sample size in the iterations, an estimate of the sample size can be obtained from the following:

$$n_A = \frac{(r+1)\sigma^2(Z_{1-\beta} + Z_{1-\alpha})^2}{r\left((\mu_A - \mu_B) - d\right)^2}.$$

(5.7)

This provides reasonable approximations for the case of $\mu_A - \mu_B > 0$, especially when the mean difference approaches d. For very quick calculations, for 90% power and Type I error of 2.5%, the following formula can be used

$$n_A = \frac{10.5\sigma^2(r+1)}{((\mu_A - \mu_B) - d)^2 r},$$ (5.8)

or for $r = 1$

$$n_A = \frac{21\sigma^2}{((\mu_A - \mu_B) - d)^2}.$$ (5.9)

5.2.1.2 Special Case of No Treatment Difference

For the special case of no treatment difference, $\mu_A - \mu_B = 0$, (5.3) can be rewritten to obtain a direct estimate of the sample size:

$$n_A = \frac{(r+1)\sigma^2(Z_{1-\beta/2} + Z_{1-\alpha})^2}{rd^2}.$$ (5.10)

Here we have $\beta_1 = \beta_2$, and as we have $\beta = \beta_1 + \beta_2$ we hence have $\beta = 2\beta_1$ and $\beta/2 = \beta_1 = \beta_2$. Thus for the special case of no treatment difference an equal proportion of the Type II error is assigned to each one-tailed test from which the power is derived in (5.3). It is because of this that (5.10) is derived, giving a direct estimate of the sample size.

When the variance is considered unknown for the statistical analysis, (5.10) can be written in terms of

$$n_A \geq \frac{(r+1)\sigma^2(Z_{1-\beta/2} + t_{1-\alpha,n_A(r+1)-2})^2}{rd^2}.$$ (5.11)

Equation (5.11) can be rewritten to give power in terms of the sample size:

$$1 - \beta = 2\Phi\left(\sqrt{\frac{rd^2 n_A}{(r+1)\sigma^2}} - t_{1-\alpha,n_A(r+1)-2}\right) - 1,$$ (5.12)

and, similar to (5.12), under the assumption of a non-central t-distribution, the power can be derived from

$$1 - \beta = 2 \, \text{Probt}(-t_{1-\alpha,n_A(r+1)-2}, n_A(r+1) - 2, \tau) - 1,$$ (5.13)

where τ is defined as

$$\tau = \frac{-\sqrt{rn_A}\,d}{\sqrt{(r+1)\sigma^2}}.$$ (5.14)

For quick calculations, for 90% power and Type I error of 2.5%, the following formula, similar to (5.8), can be used

$$n_A = \frac{13\sigma^2(r+1)}{d^2 r},$$ (5.15)

or, for $r = 1$,

$$n_A = \frac{26\sigma^2}{d^2}.$$ (5.16)

The quick equations give reasonable estimates of the sample size, underestimating by one or two, and thus provide reasonable initial values for (5.5) and (5.13). It is worth noticing the difference between (5.15) and (5.16) compared to (5.8) and (5.9). The difference in the coefficients 10.5 and 21 compared to 13 and 26 has to do with the non-symmetric allocation of the Type II error if the population mean difference is non-zero.

Table 5.1 gives sample sizes for equivalence trials using (5.5) for different standardised equivalent limits ($\delta = d/\sigma$).

TABLE 5.1

Sample Sizes (n_A) for One Arm of a Parallel Group Equivalence Study with Equal Allocation ($r = 1$) for Different Standardised Equivalence Limits ($\delta = d/\sigma$) and True Mean Differences (as a percentage of the equivalence limit) for 90% Power and Type I Error Rate of 2.5%

	Percentage Mean Difference				
δ	0%	10%	15%	20%	25%
0.05	10,397	11,042	11,915	13,218	14,960
0.10	2,600	2,762	2,980	3,306	3,741
0.15	1,157	1,228	1,325	1,470	1,664
0.20	651	691	746	827	936
0.25	417	443	478	530	600
0.30	290	308	332	369	417
0.35	214	227	245	271	307
0.40	164	174	188	208	235
0.45	130	138	149	165	186
0.50	105	112	121	134	151
0.55	87	93	100	111	125
0.60	74	78	84	93	105
0.65	63	67	72	80	90
0.70	55	58	62	69	78
0.75	48	51	54	60	68
0.80	42	45	48	53	60
0.85	37	40	43	47	53
0.90	34	36	38	42	48
0.95	30	32	34	38	43
1.00	27	29	31	35	39

5.2.1.3   *Worked Example 5.1*

Suppose we wish to design a pain trial to compare two different treatments for osteoarthritis pain relief; the objective is to demonstrate equivalence between two treatments. The largest clinically acceptable effect for which equivalence can be declared is a mean difference in visual analogue scale (VAS) assessed pain of 10 mm (d). There is to be equal allocation between groups. The true mean difference between the treatments is thought to be zero, and the expected standard deviation in the population in which the trial is to be undertaken is 100 mm (σ). The Types I and II errors are fixed at 2.5% and 10%, respectively.

From (5.10), using the Normal approximation, the sample size is estimated as 2,599.2 or 2,600 subjects per arm. If we compare this calculation with the sample size given in Table 5.1 calculated using the non-central t approach we can see the table also gives a sample size estimate of 2,600 subjects per arm.

Taking 2,600 as the evaluable sample size required, we need a sufficient number of subjects to ensure that we have 2,600 for the analysis. For an equivalence trial the co-primary data set is the per protocol data set. Suppose we only expect 80% of subjects to be both in this data set and evaluable. Therefore we would need to recruit 2,600/0.80 = 3,250 subjects on each arm.

5.2.1.4   *Worked Example 5.2*

For the same worked example suppose that the true mean difference is thought to be 2 mm. This equates to 20% of the equivalence limits of 10 mm, that is, 0.2 = 2/10. We can see now that the sample size from Table 5.1 is increased to 3,306 subjects per arm.

It should be noted therefore that with equivalence trials our calculations are relatively sensitive to assumptions about the mean as well as the variance, which we now discuss.

5.2.2   Sensitivity Analysis about the Variance Used in the Sample Size Calculations

As with superiority trials described in Chapter 3 the sensitivity of the sample size estimate to the variance used in the calculations is relatively straightforward to investigate. For example, using the degrees of freedom for the variance we can estimate a high plausible value for the variance as an investigation into the sensitivity of the study to the assumptions about the variance used in the sample size calculations.

However, with equivalence trials we further have to investigate the sensitivity of calculations about the true mean difference. If we have assumed no difference between the treatments when this difference is truly non-zero, then this will have an effect on the power of the study.

TABLE 5.2

Worked Example of a
Sensitivity Analysis for an
Individual Equivalence Study

True Difference (%)	Power
0	0.57
5	0.57
10	0.56
15	0.54
20	0.51
25	0.47

5.2.2.1   Worked Example 5.3

Revisiting Worked Example 5.1, where we estimated the sample size to be 2,600 patients per arm. Here we assumed there was no difference between the treatments. However, suppose the variance used in the calculations was estimated with 25 degrees of freedom, and we wished to investigate the sensitivity of the study to the assumptions about both the mean and the variance.

Table 5.2 shows the sensitivity of the study's original calculations for different mean differences. We can see for this study that if there truly is no mean difference but the true variance is higher than used in the calculations, then our power may be nearer to 57%. However, if our assumptions were out for both the mean and the variance, then the power may be more adversely affected.

5.2.3   Calculations Taking Account of the Imprecision of the Variances Used in the Sample Size Calculations

5.2.3.1   General Case

Extending the arguments from superiority trials discussed in Chapters 3 and 4, to account for the degrees of freedom of the sample variance used in the calculations the following equation could be used to calculate the power:

$$1 - \beta = \text{probt}(\tau_1, m, t_{1-\alpha, n_A(r+1)-2}) + \text{probt}(\tau_2, m, t_{1-\alpha, n_A(r+1)-2}) - 1, \quad (5.17)$$

where m is the degrees of freedom about the estimate variance s^2, and τ_1 and τ_1 are the absolute standardised equivalence limits, defined respectively as

$$\tau_1 = \frac{|(\mu_A - \mu_B) - d|\sqrt{rn_A}}{\sqrt{(r+1)s^2}} \quad \text{and} \quad \tau_2 = \frac{|(\mu_A - \mu_B) + d|\sqrt{rn_A}}{\sqrt{(r+1)s^2}}. \quad (5.18)$$

To calculate the sample size we would need to iterate to find the minimum value that would give the required power from (5.17).

For non-zero treatment differences (i.e. for $\mu_A - \mu_B > 0$) most of the Type II error would come from just one tail; hence the power could be estimated from

$$1 - \beta = \text{Prob} \, t \left(\frac{|(\mu_A - \mu_B) - d| \sqrt{rn_A}}{\sqrt{(r+1)s^2}}, m, t_{1-\alpha, n_A(r+1)-2} \right). \tag{5.19}$$

which when written in terms of n becomes

$$n_A \geq \frac{(r+1)s^2 [tinv(1-\beta, m, t_{1-\alpha, n_A(r+1)-2})]^2}{r((\mu_A - \mu_B) - d)^2}. \tag{5.20}$$

Replacing the t statistic with a Z-statistic, (5.20) can in turn be approximated from the following equation to give a direct estimate of the sample size:

$$n_A = \frac{(r+1)s^2 [tinv(1-\beta, m, Z_{1-\alpha})]^2}{r((\mu_A - \mu_B) - d)^2}. \tag{5.21}$$

This direct estimate could be used to provide initial estimates of the sample size for (5.17).

5.2.3.2   Special Case of No Treatment Difference

For the special case of no treatment difference the power can be estimated from

$$1 - \beta = 2 \, \text{Prob} \, t(\tau, m, t_{1-\alpha, n_A(r+1)-2}) - 1, \tag{5.22}$$

where τ is defined as

$$\tau = \frac{\sqrt{rn_A} \, d}{\sqrt{(r+1)s^2}}, \tag{5.23}$$

which when written in terms of n_A becomes

$$n_A \geq \frac{(r+1)s^2 [tinv(1-\beta/2, m, t_{1-\alpha, n_A(r+1)-2})]^2}{rd^2}. \tag{5.24}$$

Replacing the t-statistic with a Z-statistic, (5.24) can in turn be approximated from the following equation to give a direct estimate of the sample size:

$$n_A = \frac{(r+1)s^2 [tinv(1-\beta/2, m, Z_{1-\alpha})]^2}{rd^2}. \tag{5.25}$$

Table 5.3 is produced for the special case of no mean difference between treatments. It gives the multiplication factors, compared to calculations assuming the population variance, for various degrees of freedom and Types I and II errors. Similar to superiority trials (5.25) converges to (5.12); however,

TABLE 5.3

Multiplication Factors for Different Levels of One-Sided
Significance, Type II Error and Degrees of Freedom

		Significance Level (α)			
m	β	0.010	0.025	0.050	0.100
5	0.05	2.649	2.509	2.385	2.238
	0.10	2.167	2.068	1.980	1.875
	0.15	1.929	1.850	1.780	1.696
	0.20	1.776	1.711	1.652	1.581
	0.50	1.367	1.337	1.311	1.278
10	0.05	1.611	1.562	1.520	1.470
	0.10	1.463	1.425	1.392	1.353
	0.15	1.382	1.351	1.323	1.290
	0.20	1.328	1.301	1.276	1.248
	0.50	1.166	1.153	1.141	1.127
25	0.05	1.208	1.192	1.178	1.162
	0.10	1.163	1.150	1.139	1.125
	0.15	1.137	1.126	1.116	1.105
	0.20	1.119	1.109	1.101	1.091
	0.50	1.062	1.058	1.053	1.058
50	0.05	1.099	1.091	1.085	1.077
	0.10	1.078	1.072	1.067	1.060
	0.15	1.066	1.061	1.056	1.051
	0.20	1.058	1.053	1.049	1.044
	0.50	1.031	1.028	1.026	1.024
75	0.05	1.065	1.060	1.056	1.051
	0.10	1.052	1.047	1.044	1.040
	0.15	1.044	1.040	1.037	1.033
	0.20	1.038	1.035	1.032	1.029
	0.50	1.020	1.019	1.017	1.016
100	0.05	1.048	1.044	1.041	1.038
	0.10	1.038	1.035	1.033	1.030
	0.15	1.033	1.030	1.028	1.025
	0.20	1.029	1.026	1.024	1.022
	0.50	1.015	1.014	1.013	1.012

the multiplication factors can be used regardless of the original formula for
sample size calculations.

5.3   Cross-over Trials

The methodologies and assumptions for an equivalence trial with a cross-
over design are the same as those for parallel group equivalence trials (for
the methodologies) and superiority cross-over trials (for assumptions about

the parameters). This section therefore only briefly goes through the sample size calculations for an equivalence trial with a cross-over design.

5.3.1   Sample Size Estimated Assuming the Population Variance to Be Known

5.3.1.1   General Case

The Type II error (and power) can be estimated from

$$1-\beta = \Phi\left(\sqrt{\frac{((\mu_A - \mu_B) - d)^2 n}{2\sigma_w^2}} - Z_{1-\alpha}\right) + \Phi\left(\sqrt{\frac{((\mu_A - \mu_B) + d)^2 n}{2\sigma_w^2}} - Z_{1-\alpha}\right) - 1,$$

(5.26)

where n here is the total sample size. If the variance is to be considered unknown for the statistical analysis, then (5.26) can be rewritten as

$$1-\beta = \Phi\left(\sqrt{\frac{((\mu_A - \mu_B) - d)^2 n}{2\sigma_w^2}} - t_{1-\alpha,n-2}\right) + \Phi\left(\sqrt{\frac{((\mu_A - \mu_B) + d)^2 n}{2\sigma_w^2}} - t_{1-\alpha,n-2}\right) - 1,$$

(5.27)

and under the assumption of a non-central t-distribution the power (Owen, 1965; Diletti, Hauschke and Steinijans, 1991) for the sample size can be estimated from

$$1-\beta = \text{Prob}\, t(-t_{1-\alpha,n-2}, n-2, \tau_2) - \text{Prob}\, t(t_{1-\alpha,n-2}, n-2, \tau_1),$$

(5.28)

where τ_1 and τ_2 are defined respectively as

$$\tau_1 = \frac{((\mu_A - \mu_B) + d)\sqrt{n}}{\sqrt{2\sigma_w^2}} \quad \text{and} \quad \tau_2 = \frac{((\mu_A - \mu_B) - d)\sqrt{n}}{\sqrt{2\sigma_w^2}}.$$

(5.29)

For quick calculations we can estimate the sample size from

$$n = \frac{2\sigma_w^2(Z_{1-\beta} + Z_{1-\alpha})^2}{((\mu_A - \mu_B) - d)^2},$$

(5.30)

and for very quick calculations, for 90% power and Type I error of 2.5%, we can use the following:

$$n = \frac{21\sigma_w^2}{((\mu_A - \mu_B) - d)^2}.$$

(5.31)

5.3.1.2   *Special Case of No Treatment Difference*

For the special case of $\mu_A - \mu_B = 0$ a direct estimate of the sample size can be obtained from

$$n = \frac{2\sigma_w^2(Z_{1-\beta/2} + Z_{1-\alpha})^2}{d^2}, \tag{5.32}$$

which, if the variance is to be considered unknown for the statistical analysis, can be rewritten as

$$n \geq \frac{2\sigma_w^2(Z_{1-\beta/2} + t_{1-\alpha,n-2})^2}{d^2}. \tag{5.33}$$

Equation (5.33) can in turn be rewritten as

$$1 - \beta = 2\Phi\left(\sqrt{\frac{d^2 n}{2\sigma_w^2}} - t_{1-\alpha,n-2}\right) - 1, \tag{5.34}$$

which in turn, under the assumption of a non-central t-distribution, can also be rewritten as

$$1 - \beta = 2\,\text{probt}(-t_{1-\alpha,n-2}, n-2, \tau) - 1, \tag{5.35}$$

where τ is defined as

$$\tau = \frac{\sqrt{nd}}{\sqrt{2\sigma_w^2}}. \tag{5.36}$$

For quick calculations, for 90% power and Type I error of 2.5%, the following result can be used:

$$n = \frac{26\sigma_w^2}{d^2}. \tag{5.37}$$

As with parallel group trials the quick equations give reasonable estimates of the sample size, underestimating the sample size by just one or two subjects, and thus provide reasonable initial values for iterations. Table 5.4 gives sample sizes using (5.17) for various standardised equivalence limits ($\delta = d/\sigma$) and mean differences.

5.3.2   Calculations Taking Account of the Imprecision of the Variance Used in the Sample Size Calculations

5.3.2.1   *General Case*

To account for the degrees of freedom of the within-subject sample variance the following equation could be used to calculate the power:

$$1 - \beta = \text{Probt}(\tau_1, m, t_{1-\alpha,n-2}) + \text{Probt}(\tau_2, m, t_{1-\alpha,n-2}) - 1, \tag{5.38}$$

TABLE 5.4

Total Sample Sizes (n) for Cross-over Equivalence Study for Different Standardised Equivalence Limits ($\delta = d/\sigma$) and True Mean Differences (as a percentage of the equivalence limit) for 90% Power and Type I Error Rate of 2.5%

δ	Percentage Mean Difference				
	0%	10%	15%	20%	25%
0.05	10,398	11,043	11,916	13,219	14,961
0.10	2,601	2,763	2,981	3,307	3,742
0.15	1,158	1,229	1,326	1,471	1,665
0.20	652	692	747	828	937
0.25	418	444	479	531	601
0.30	291	309	333	370	418
0.35	215	228	246	272	308
0.40	165	175	189	209	236
0.45	131	139	150	166	187
0.50	106	113	122	135	152
0.55	88	94	101	112	126
0.60	75	79	85	94	106
0.65	64	68	73	81	91
0.70	56	59	63	70	79
0.75	49	52	55	61	69
0.80	43	46	49	54	61
0.85	39	41	44	48	54
0.90	35	37	39	43	49
0.95	31	33	36	39	44
1.00	29	30	32	36	40

where m is the degrees of freedom about the estimate of the variance s_w^2, and τ_1 and τ_2 are non-centrally parameters defined respectively as

$$\tau_1 = \frac{|(\mu_A - \mu_B) - d|\sqrt{n}}{\sqrt{2}s_w} \quad \text{and} \quad \tau_2 = \frac{|(\mu_A - \mu_B) + d|\sqrt{n}}{\sqrt{2}s_w}. \tag{5.39}$$

To calculate the sample size we need to iterate to find the minimum value that would give the required power from (5.38).

For non-zero treatment differences (i.e. for $\mu_A - \mu_B > 0$) the power could be estimated from

$$1 - \beta = \Pr\text{obt}\left(\frac{|(\mu_A - \mu_B) - d|\sqrt{n}}{\sqrt{2}s_w}, m, t_{1-\alpha,n-2}\right), \tag{5.40}$$

which when written in terms of n becomes

$$n \geq \frac{2s_w^2[tinv(1-\beta, m, t_{1-\alpha,n-2})]^2}{((\mu_A - \mu_B) - d)^2}. \tag{5.41}$$

Replacing the t-statistic with a Z-statistic, (5.41) can in turn be approximated from

$$n = \frac{2s_w^2[tinv(1-\beta, m, Z_{1-\alpha})]^2}{((\mu_A - \mu_B)-d)^2}. \tag{5.42}$$

This direct estimate could be used to provide initial estimates of the sample size for (5.38).

5.3.2.2   Special Case of No Treatment Difference

For the special case of no treatment difference the power can be estimated from

$$1-\beta = 2\operatorname{Prob}t(\tau, m, t_{1-\alpha, n-2}) - 1, \tag{5.43}$$

where τ is defined as

$$\tau = \frac{\sqrt{n}d}{\sqrt{2}s_w}, \tag{5.44}$$

which when written in terms of n becomes

$$n \geq \frac{2s_w^2[tinv(1-\beta/2, m, t_{1-\alpha, n-2})]^2}{d^2}. \tag{5.45}$$

Replacing the t-statistic with a Z-statistic, then (5.45) can in turn be approximated from

$$n = \frac{2s_w^2[tinv(1-\beta/2, m, Z_{1-\alpha})]^2}{d^2}. \tag{5.46}$$

Multiplication factors can be produced for the special case of no mean difference. For cross-over trials these would be the same as parallel group (given in Table 5.3) and are not repeated here.

Key Message

- When designing an equivalence trial the sample size is sensitive to assumptions about both the variance and the true mean difference.

6

Sample Size Calculations for Non-inferiority Clinical Trials with Normal Data

6.1 Introduction

In Chapter 5 calculations were discussed for trials in which the objective is to demonstrate that two treatments are clinically the same. In this chapter calculations are described when the objective is to show one treatment is no worse than another, with one treatment an investigative, or new, treatment and the other a standard treatment.

The main difference between non-inferiority and equivalence trials is that with equivalence trials we wish to show that two treatments are the same such that we wish to prove the difference between treatments is wholly contained within the interval $(-d, d)$. However, with non-inferiority trials we are only concerned with one of the margins, for example $-d$, and demonstrating that the difference between investigative and standard treatment is sufficiently far enough away from this to declare non-inferiority. Moreover, the further away the better, and if we are sufficiently far away also to be able to declare the investigative treatment is statistically superior (i.e. greater than zero), this is also a good result. Such trials, "as-good-as-or-better" trials, were introduced in Chapter 1 and are revisited towards the end of this chapter.

6.2 Parallel Group Trials

6.2.1 Sample Size Estimated Assuming the Population Variance to Be Known

Recall from Chapter 1 we require

$$Var(S) = \frac{(d - \Delta)^2}{(Z_{1-\alpha} + Z_{1-\beta})^2}, \tag{6.1}$$

and as with superiority and equivalence trials $Var(S)$ can be defined as

$$Var(S) = \frac{r+1}{r} \cdot \frac{\sigma^2}{n_A}, \tag{6.2}$$

where σ^2 is the population variance estimate, and $n_B = rn_A$. When (6.2) is substituted into (6.1) (also replacing Δ with $\mu_A - \mu_B$), it gives a direct estimate of the sample size:

$$n_A = \frac{(r+1)\sigma^2(Z_{1-\beta} + Z_{1-\alpha})^2}{r((\mu_A - \mu_B) - d)^2}. \tag{6.3}$$

Rewriting (6.2) to give the power for a given sample size we have the following result:

$$1 - \beta = \Phi\left(\sqrt{\frac{((\mu_A - \mu_B) - d)^2 \, rn_A}{(r+1)\sigma^2}} - Z_{1-\alpha} \right). \tag{6.4}$$

The equivalent for the case when the variance is considered unknown for the analysis is

$$1 - \beta = \Phi\left(\sqrt{\frac{((\mu_A - \mu_B) - d)^2 \, rn_A}{(r+1)\sigma^2}} - t_{1-\alpha, n_A(r+1)-2} \right). \tag{6.5}$$

As with the chapters on equivalence and superiority trials it is best to calculate the power under the assumption of a non-central t-distribution (Julious, 2004d):

$$1 - \beta = \text{Prob} t(t_{1-\alpha, n_A(r+1)-2}, n_A(r+1) - 2, \tau), \tag{6.6}$$

where τ is defined as

$$\tau = \left| \frac{((\mu_A - \mu_B) - d)\sqrt{rn_A}}{\sqrt{(r+1)\sigma^2}} \right|. \tag{6.7}$$

For quick calculations, for 90% power and Type I error of 2.5%, the following formula can be used:

$$n_A = \frac{10.5\sigma^2(r+1)}{((\mu_A - \mu_B) - d)^2 r}. \tag{6.8}$$

For the case of $r = 1$ (6.8) resolves to

$$n_A = \frac{21\sigma^2}{((\mu_A - \mu_B) - d)^2}. \tag{6.9}$$

TABLE 6.1

Sample Sizes (n_A) for One Arm of a Parallel Group Non-inferiority Study with Equal Allocation for Different Standardised Non-inferiority Limits ($\delta = d/\sigma$) and True Mean Differences (as a percentage of the non-inferiority limit) for 90% Power and Type I Error Rate of 2.5%

	Percentage Mean Difference										
δ	−25%	−20%	−15%	−10%	−5%	0%	5%	10%	15%	20%	25%
0.05	5,381	5,839	6,358	6,949	7,626	8,407	9,316	10,379	11,636	13,136	14,945
0.10	1,346	1,461	1,590	1,738	1,908	2,103	2,330	2,596	2,910	3,285	3,737
0.15	599	650	708	773	849	935	1,036	1,155	1,294	1,461	1,662
0.20	338	366	399	436	478	527	584	650	729	822	935
0.25	217	235	256	279	306	338	374	417	467	527	599
0.30	151	164	178	194	213	235	260	290	325	366	417
0.35	111	121	131	143	157	173	192	213	239	270	306
0.40	86	93	101	110	121	133	147	164	183	207	235
0.45	68	74	80	87	96	105	116	130	145	164	186
0.50	55	60	65	71	78	86	95	105	118	133	151
0.55	46	50	54	59	64	71	78	87	98	110	125
0.60	39	42	46	50	54	60	66	74	82	93	105
0.65	33	36	39	43	47	51	57	63	70	79	90
0.70	29	31	34	37	40	44	49	54	61	68	78
0.75	25	27	30	32	35	39	43	48	53	60	68
0.80	23	24	26	29	31	34	38	42	47	53	60
0.85	20	22	23	26	28	31	34	37	42	47	53
0.90	18	20	21	23	25	27	30	34	37	42	48
0.95	16	18	19	21	23	25	27	30	34	38	43
1.00	15	16	17	19	21	23	25	27	31	34	39

The quick equations give reasonable estimates of the sample size, although with slight underestimation. Table 6.1 gives sample sizes using (6.6) for various standardised non-inferiority limits ($\delta = d/\sigma$) and standardised mean differences assuming equal allocation between groups.

One feature to highlight in Table 6.1 and Table 6.4 (described in the next section on cross-over trials) is the asymmetric effect on the sample size for different values of the true mean difference. In equivalence trials because we have two, usually symmetric, margins, when we move away from a zero mean difference in any direction the sample size is inflated. However, in non-inferiority trials the sample size is inflated only if the true mean difference moves towards the non-inferiority margin. If it is expected that the true mean difference is in favour of the comparator regimen (compared to control), then the sample size is significantly reduced.

6.2.2 Non-inferiority versus Superiority Trials

The asymmetric effect of the mean difference on the sample size is not trivial. There is a perception that non-inferiority trials require greater sample sizes than superiority trials. This is due to the non-inferiority margin often being set at some fraction of an effect seen previously in a placebo-controlled superiority trial of the active control being used in the current trial. Hence, if d_s is the effect seen in a retrospective placebo-controlled superiority trial and the non-inferiority margin d is set at $d = 0.5\,d_s$, then the inference is that we would require four times the sample size compared to setting the trial as a superiority. The logic comes from the following result for a superiority sample size calculation:

$$n_A = \frac{(r+1)\sigma^2(Z_{1-\beta} + Z_{1-\alpha/2})^2}{rd_s^2}, \tag{6.10}$$

which for a one-tailed Type I error (where the Type I error is set at half that for a two-tailed test) becomes

$$n_A = \frac{(r+1)\sigma^2(Z_{1-\beta} + Z_{1-\alpha})^2}{rd_s^2}. \tag{6.11}$$

The equivalent result to (6.11) for non-inferiority studies, (6.3) with $d = 0 \cdot S\,ds$ can be rewritten as

$$n_A = \frac{(r+1)\sigma^2(Z_{1-\beta} + Z_{1-\alpha})^2}{r((\mu_A - \mu_B) - 0.5d_s)^2}, \tag{6.12}$$

which for the special case of $\mu_A - \mu_B = 0$ becomes

$$n_A = \frac{4(r+1)\sigma^2(Z_{1-\beta} + Z_{1-\alpha})^2}{rd_s^2}. \tag{6.13}$$

Therefore, on the face of it (6.13) estimates the sample size to be four times greater than for (6.10). However, the d_s in question in (6.10) is for a trial powered to show an effect of active over placebo, while (6.13) is for a trial powered to show an effect of an active over an active control. This point is often lost. It is not uncommon when designing an active controlled trial for it to be designed as a superiority trial due to the misbelief that non-inferiority trials are unfeasibly large.

In fact if a study is being set up as a superiority study in effect it is a non-inferiority study but with a margin equal to zero (i.e. $d = 0$), that is,

$$n_A = \frac{(r+1)\sigma^2(Z_{1-\beta} + Z_{1-\alpha})^2}{r(\mu_A - \mu_B)^2}. \tag{6.14}$$

It could be argued, therefore, that it is harder to show superiority (lower bound greater than 0) than non-inferiority (lower bound greater than $-d$). Furthermore, it could argued if we were confident that $\mu_A > \mu_B$, such that a superiority study could be designed, then the effect of having a margin $-d$ in (6.14) and a non-inferiority study is to greatly reduce the sample size.

This asymmetric effect of the mean difference on the sample size should be considered when designing non-inferiority trials as even only a small expected mean difference in favour of the comparator could have a marked effect on the sample size.

One thing to highlight with non-zero mean differences is that it is only the evaluable sample size that may be comparable between a non-inferiority and a superiority trial. A co-primary data set for analysis for a non-inferiority trial is the per protocol (PP) data set, so a greater number of subjects may need to be recruited to ensure a sufficient number of evaluable subjects for this data set.

The concepts of superiority and non-inferiority are of course interrelated. Indeed there may be instances when instead of designing a study to show an investigative treatment is no worse than an active control at the 2.5% level of significance we may wish to design a superiority study but at a level of statistical significance greater than the nominal two-sided 5% (one-sided 2.5%) level. Such a study would give more assurance regarding the investigative treatment being no worse than the active control. The Committee for Medicinal Products for Human Use (CHMP) (2005) commented on this:

> It might be an acceptable approach, in extreme situations, to run a superiority trial using a less stringent significance level than P = 0.05, weighing up the increased risk of a false positive result against the risk of rejecting a drug with a valuable efficacy advantage. It might be more acceptable, and easier from an ethical perspective, to specify a level of confidence we require in the superiority of a drug, than to specify an extra number of deaths that is of no clinical importance.

The CHMP further expanded that

> For example with a data-set where the lower bound of an 85% confidence interval (by definition narrower than a 95% interval) touches zero, it might be that the 95% interval touches –5. If delta had been defined to be –5 then achieving non-inferiority in this example would correspond to having demonstrated superiority at the 15% level of significance.

Table 6.2 gives sample sizes using (6.6) for various standardised mean differences ($\mu_A - \mu_B/\sigma$) and significance levels assuming equal allocation between groups assuming the non-inferiority margin is set at zero.

6.2.3 Worked Example 6.1

An investigator wishes to design a trial to compare two treatments for hypertension; the objective is to demonstrate that one treatment (an investigative therapy) is non-inferior to another (a standard therapy). The largest clinically acceptable effect to be able to declare non-inferiority is a change in blood pressure of 2.5 mmHg (*d*). The true mean difference between the treatments is thought to be zero with an expected standard deviation in the trial population of 10 mmHg (σ). There is to be equal allocation between groups ($r = 1$), and the

TABLE 6.2

Sample Sizes (n_A) for One Arm of a Parallel Group Non-inferiority Study with Equal Allocation for Different Standardised True Mean Differences for 90% Power and Various One-Sided Type I Error Rates Assuming the Non-inferiority Margin Is Set at Zero

$(\mu_A - \mu_B)/\sigma$	One-Sided Significance Levels					
	0.025	0.050	0.075	0.100	0.125	0.150
0.05	8,407	6,852	5,924	5,257	4,732	4,299
0.10	2,103	1,714	1,482	1,315	1,184	1,075
0.15	935	762	659	585	527	478
0.20	527	429	371	329	297	269
0.25	338	275	238	211	190	173
0.30	235	191	166	147	132	120
0.35	173	141	122	108	97	88
0.40	133	108	94	83	75	68
0.45	105	86	74	66	59	54
0.50	86	70	60	53	48	44
0.55	71	58	50	44	40	36
0.60	60	49	42	37	34	31
0.65	51	42	36	32	29	26
0.70	44	36	31	28	25	23
0.75	39	32	27	24	22	20
0.80	34	28	24	21	19	18
0.85	31	25	22	19	17	16
0.90	27	22	19	17	15	14
0.95	25	20	17	16	14	13
1.00	23	18	16	14	13	12

Type I and Type II errors are to be fixed at 2.5% and 10%, respectively. From Table 6.1 the sample size required is estimated to be 338 patients per arm.

Suppose, though, we believe that the investigative therapy is a little superior to the standard such that the true mean difference is thought to be 0.5 mmHg. This would equate to 20% (0.2 = 0.5/2.5) of the non-inferiority limit. From Table 6.1 the sample size is reduced to 235 patients per arm.

Taking 235 as the sample size we now need to calculate the total sample size to ensure that we have this number of evaluable patients. Remember the PP data set is co-primary and suppose we only expect 75% of subjects to be in this data set and evaluable. The total sample size is therefore 235/0.75 = 313.33 or 314 patients on each arm.

6.2.4 Sensitivity Analysis about the Mean Difference Used in the Sample Size Calculations

As with superiority and equivalence trials described in previous chapters we can estimate a plausibly large value for the population variance. As with equivalence trials, however, we also need to investigate the sensitivity of calculations to the assumption about the true mean difference. If we assume there is no mean difference $(\mu_A - \mu_B = 0)$ when the mean difference is truly non-zero, then this will have an effect on the power of the study. As discussed in this chapter the effect of the mean difference on the power is not symmetric, and if there is a difference in favour of the investigative treatment there will be a positive effect on the power.

6.2.5 Worked Example 6.2

In Worked Example 6.1 we assumed that there was a small difference between treatments of 0.5 mmHg in favour of the investigative treatment. However, suppose that this is a little optimistic, and the true difference is actually zero $(\mu_A - \mu_B = 0)$; then, we only have 77% power in the study.

6.2.6 Calculations Taking Account of the Imprecision of the Variance Used in the Sample Size Calculations

To account for the imprecision of the sample variance used in the sample size calculations the results given in the chapter on superiority trials can be extended to give

$$n_A \geq \frac{(r+1)s^2[tinv(1-\beta, m, t_{1-\alpha, n_A(r+1)-2})]^2}{r((\mu_A - \mu_B) - d)^2}, \tag{6.15}$$

where m is the degrees of freedom about the estimate variance s^2, and the sample size required is the least integer value for (6.15) to hold. We can rewrite (6.15) in terms of power to obtain the following result:

$$1 - \beta = \text{Prob}t(\tau, m, t_{1-\alpha, n_A(r+1)-2}), \tag{6.16}$$

where τ is defined as

$$\tau = \left| \frac{((\mu_A - \mu_B) - d)\sqrt{rn_A}}{\sqrt{(r+1)s^2}} \right|. \tag{6.17}$$

As (6.15) can only be solved by numerical iteration by replacing the t-statistic with a Z-statistic we have

$$n_A = \frac{(r+1)s^2[tinv(1-\beta, m, Z_{1-\alpha/2})]^2}{r((\mu_A - \mu_B) - d)^2}, \tag{6.18}$$

which allows us to have a direct estimate of the sample size and gives an initial value for iterations for (6.15).

Table 6.3 gives the multiplication factors, compared to assuming we have the population variance, for various degrees of freedom and Types I and II errors. It is produced for the special case of no mean difference between treatments, that is, $\mu_A - \mu_B = 0$. These multiplication factors can be used to inflate a sample size to account for the imprecision in the variance.

TABLE 6.3

Multiplication Factors for Different Levels of One-Sided
Significance, Type II Error and Degrees of Freedom

		Significance Level (α)			
m	β	0.010	0.025	0.050	0.100
5	0.05	2.167	2.068	1.980	1.875
	0.10	1.776	1.711	1.652	1.581
	0.15	1.582	1.533	1.489	1.436
	0.20	1.457	1.419	1.385	1.344
	0.50	1.120	1.117	1.114	1.111
10	0.05	1.463	1.425	1.392	1.353
	0.10	1.328	1.301	1.276	1.248
	0.15	1.254	1.233	1.214	1.192
	0.20	1.204	1.187	1.172	1.154
	0.50	1.055	1.054	1.053	1.053
25	0.05	1.163	1.150	1.139	1.125
	0.10	1.119	1.109	1.101	1.091
	0.15	1.094	1.086	1.079	1.071
	0.20	1.076	1.070	1.065	1.058
	0.50	1.021	1.021	1.021	1.020
50	0.05	1.078	1.072	1.067	1.060
	0.10	1.058	1.053	1.049	1.044
	0.15	1.046	1.042	1.039	1.035
	0.20	1.037	1.034	1.032	1.028
	0.50	1.010	1.010	1.010	1.010
75	0.05	1.052	1.047	1.044	1.040
	0.10	1.038	1.035	1.032	1.029
	0.15	1.030	1.028	1.026	1.023
	0.20	1.025	1.023	1.021	1.019
	0.50	1.007	1.007	1.007	1.007
100	0.05	1.038	1.035	1.033	1.030
	0.10	1.029	1.026	1.024	1.022
	0.15	1.023	1.021	1.019	1.017
	0.20	1.019	1.017	1.016	1.014
	0.50	1.005	1.005	1.005	1.005

6.3 Cross-over Trials

6.3.1 Sample Size Estimated Assuming the Population Variance to Be Known

The equivalent sample size formula to (6.3) for cross-over trials is

$$n = \frac{2\sigma_w^2 (Z_{1-\beta} + Z_{1-\alpha})^2}{((\mu_A - \mu_B) - d)^2},$$ (6.19)

where n here is the total sample size. When rewritten in terms of power, this becomes

$$1 - \beta = \Phi\left(\sqrt{\frac{((\mu_A - \mu_B) - d)^2 n}{2\sigma_w^2}} - Z_{1-\alpha}\right). \tag{6.20}$$

The equivalent formula replacing the Z-statistic with the t-statistic is

$$1 - \beta = \Phi\left(\sqrt{\frac{((\mu_A - \mu_B) - d)^2 n}{2\sigma_w^2}} - t_{1-\alpha,n-2}\right). \tag{6.21}$$

As with parallel group designs it is preferable to calculate the Type II error (and power) under the assumption of a non-central t-distribution; thus (6.21) is rewritten as (Julious, 2004d)

$$1 - \beta = \text{Prob}t(t_{1-\alpha,n-2}, n-2, \tau), \tag{6.22}$$

where τ is defined as

$$\tau = \left|\frac{((\mu_A - \mu_B) - d)\sqrt{n}}{\sqrt{2\sigma_w^2}}\right|. \tag{6.23}$$

For quick calculations, for 90% power and Type I error of 2.5%, the following formula can be utilised:

$$n = \frac{21\sigma_w^2}{((\mu_A - \mu_B) - d)^2}. \tag{6.24}$$

As with parallel group estimation the quick equation slightly underestimates the sample size compared to (6.22). Table 6.4 gives sample sizes using (6.22) for various standardised non-inferiority limits ($\delta = d/\sigma$) and standardised mean differences assuming equal allocation between groups.

Table 6.5 gives sample sizes using (6.22) for various standardised mean differences $[(\mu_A - \mu_B)/\sigma]$ and significance levels assuming the non-inferiority margin is set at zero.

6.3.2 Calculations Taking Account of the Imprecision of the Variance Used in the Sample Size Calculations

To account for the imprecision of the variance used in the sample size calculations the results for parallel group trials can be generalised to

$$n \geq \frac{s_w^2 [tinv(1-\beta, m, t_{1-\alpha,n-2})]^2}{[(\mu_A - \mu_B) - d]^2}, \tag{6.25}$$

TABLE 6.4

Total Sample Sizes (n) for a Cross-over Non-inferiority Study with Equal Allocation for Different Standardised Non-inferiority Limits ($\delta = d/\sigma$) and True Mean Differences (as a percentage of the equivalence limit) for 90% Power and Type I Error Rate of 2.5%

	Percentage Mean Difference										
δ	−25%	−20%	−15%	−10%	−5%	0%	5%	10%	15%	20%	25%
0.05	5,382	5,840	6,359	6,949	7,627	8,408	9,316	10,380	11,637	13,137	14,946
0.10	1,347	1,462	1,591	1,739	1,909	2,104	2,331	2,597	2,911	3,286	3,738
0.15	600	651	709	774	850	936	1,037	1,156	1,295	1,462	1,663
0.20	339	367	400	437	479	528	585	651	730	823	936
0.25	218	236	257	280	307	339	375	418	468	528	600
0.30	152	165	179	195	214	236	261	291	326	367	418
0.35	112	122	132	144	158	174	193	214	240	270	307
0.40	87	94	102	111	122	134	148	165	184	208	236
0.45	69	75	81	88	97	106	117	131	146	165	187
0.50	56	61	66	72	79	87	96	106	119	134	152
0.55	47	51	55	60	65	72	79	88	99	111	126
0.60	40	43	47	51	55	61	67	75	83	94	106
0.65	34	37	40	44	48	52	58	64	71	80	91
0.70	30	32	35	38	41	45	50	55	62	69	79
0.75	26	29	31	33	36	40	44	49	54	61	69
0.80	24	25	27	30	32	35	39	43	48	54	61
0.85	21	23	25	27	29	32	35	38	43	48	54
0.90	19	21	22	24	26	29	31	35	38	43	49
0.95	18	19	20	22	24	26	28	31	35	39	44
1.00	16	17	19	20	22	24	26	29	32	35	40

where n is the least integer value for (6.25) to hold, and m is the degrees of freedom about the estimate variance s_w^2. We can rewrite (6.25) in terms of power

$$1 - \beta = \text{Prob}t\left(\frac{\sqrt{n}\,|(\mu_A - \mu_B) - d|}{\sqrt{2}s_w^2}, m, t_{1-\alpha, n-2}\right). \tag{6.26}$$

Replacing the t-statistic with a Z-statistic gives the following result:

$$n = \frac{2s_w^2[tinv(1 - \beta, m, Z_{1-\alpha/2})]^2}{[(\mu_A - \mu_B) - d]^2} \tag{6.27}$$

which allows us to have a direct estimate of the sample size and gives an initial value for (6.25).

As with parallel group trials multiplication factors can be calculated to allow us to account for the imprecision in the mean. As these factors depend only on the Type I error, Type II error and degrees of freedom they are the same for both parallel and cross-over trials. Please see Table 6.3 for more details.

TABLE 6.5

Total Sample Sizes (n_A) for a Cross-over Non-inferiority Study for Different Standardised True Mean Differences for 90% Power and Various Type I Error Rates of 2.5% Assuming the Non-inferiority Limit Is Set to Zero

Standardised Difference	Significance Levels					
	0.025	0.050	0.075	0.100	0.125	0.150
0.05	8,408	6,853	5,925	5,257	4,732	4,299
0.10	2,104	1,715	1,482	1,315	1,184	1,076
0.15	936	763	660	585	527	479
0.20	528	430	372	330	297	270
0.25	339	276	238	212	190	173
0.30	236	192	166	147	133	120
0.35	174	142	122	109	98	89
0.40	134	109	94	83	75	68
0.45	106	86	75	66	60	54
0.50	87	70	61	54	48	44
0.55	72	59	51	45	40	37
0.60	61	49	43	38	34	31
0.65	52	42	37	32	29	26
0.70	45	37	32	28	25	23
0.75	40	32	28	25	22	20
0.80	35	29	25	22	20	18
0.85	32	26	22	20	18	16
0.90	28	23	20	18	16	14
0.95	26	21	18	16	14	13
1.00	24	19	16	15	13	12

6.4 As-Good-as-or-Better Trials

To calculate the sample size required for an as-good-as-or-better trial we should apply the methodologies described in Chapters 3 and 4 for superiority trials as well as those in the current chapter.

For as-good-as-or-better trials therefore given that we are also investigating superiority, it may be appropriate to power for non-inferiority assuming a small difference between the two groups in favour of the investigative therapy. As discussed in this chapter this assumption would have marked effect in the sample size calculation, but then the calculation would be very sensitive to the assumptions made about the mean difference. The non-inferiority calculation in this context could be the main consideration in determining the sample size with maybe a statement in the sample size section regarding the expected power for superiority.

A further consideration in as-good-as-or-better trials is the choice of data set to have as primary, which adds a further complication. For a superiority trial the primary data set would be that based on intention to treat (ITT); for a non-inferiority trial the primary data set would be both the PP data set and the ITT (Committee for Proprietary Medicinal Products [CPMP], 2000). Hence, an appropriate sample size would need to be estimated to give an evaluable number of patients in both the PP and ITT data sets.

6.4.1   Worked Example 6.3

Extending Worked Example 6.1, suppose an investigator wished to design a parallel group trial in hypertensive patients with the objective of demonstrating that one treatment (an investigative therapy) is non-inferior to another (a standard therapy). The largest clinically acceptable effect to be able to declare non-inferiority is a change in blood pressure of 2.5 mmHg (d) and the standard deviation is taken as 10 mmHg. There is to be equal allocation between groups, and the Type I and Type II errors are to be fixed at 2.5% and 10%, respectively.

Suppose it was truly believed that the investigative therapy was a little superior to the standard such that the true mean difference is thought to be 0.5 mmHg, so (from Table 6.1) the sample size is taken as 235 patients per arm.

With 235 as the evaluable sample size and only expecting 75% of subjects to be in the PP data set and evaluable, the total sample size is therefore 314 subjects total to ensure 235 evaluable patients per arm.

Suppose, however, we expect 90% of subjects to be evaluable in the ITT population. The total sample size in this data set would be $314 \times 0.90 = 282.6$ or 283 subjects. With this sample size for a difference of 0.5 mmHg the study would have 9.1% power for the test of superiority. Obviously if a greater difference between treatments was expected (or even is true) the greater the power will be for the study.

   Key Messages

- When designing a non-inferiority study a key assumption is one made about the true mean difference. Even a small difference in favour of the investigative treatment can substantially reduce the estimate of the sample size.
- Non-inferiority studies can require fewer subjects than a superiority study depending on the assumptions about the mean difference.

7

Sample Size Calculations
for Bioequivalence Trials

7.1 Introduction

In Chapter 1 bioequivalence trials were first described. For such trials pharmacokinetics are used as a surrogate for safety and efficacy such that equivalence in the pharmacokinetics would be assumed to equate to equivalence in terms of safety and efficacy.

This chapter describes the sample size calculations for bioequivalence; in a reversal from previous chapters this chapter starts with cross-over trials, which are the most common type of bioequivalence trial.

7.2 Cross-over Trials

7.2.1 Sample Sizes Estimated Assuming the Population Variance to Be Known

7.2.1.1 General Case

The derivation of the sample size equations is similar to that for equivalence trials described in Chapter 6. For the general case for which the expected true mean difference is not fixed to be unity the sample size cannot be directly derived. We instead have to iterate until a sample size is reached that gives the required Type II error and power.

To calculate the power for the two one-sided test procedure at the 5% significance level with bioequivalence acceptance limits of (0.80, 1.25) for any given value for the true ratio μ_T/μ_R, the following formula can be used:

$$
1 - \beta = \Phi\left(\sqrt{\frac{(\log(\mu_T/\mu_R) - \log(1.25))^2 n}{2\sigma_w^2}} - Z_{1-\alpha} \right)
$$

$$
+ \Phi\left(\sqrt{\frac{(\log(\mu_T/\mu_R) - \log(0.80))^2 n}{2\sigma_w^2}} - Z_{1-\alpha} \right) - 1.
$$

(7.1)

where σ_w is the within-subject variability on the log scale, and n is the total sample size. Replacing the Z-statistic with the t-statistic, (7.1) can be rewritten as

$$1-\beta = \Phi\left(\sqrt{\frac{(\log(\mu_T/\mu_R)-\log(1.25))^2 n}{2\sigma_w^2}}-t_{1-\alpha,n-2}\right)$$

$$+\Phi\left(\sqrt{\frac{(\log(\mu_T/\mu_R)-\log(0.80))^2 n}{2\sigma_w^2}}-t_{1-\alpha,n-2}\right)-1. \tag{7.2}$$

As with superiority, equivalence and non-inferiority trials discussed earlier in this book it is best to calculate the power using a non-central t-distribution of the power as outlined by Owen (1965), rewriting (7.2) to the following (Owen, 1965; Diletti, Hauschke and Steinijans, 1991; Julious, 2004d):

$$1-\beta = \text{prob}t(t_{1-\alpha,n-2},n-2,\tau_1)-\text{prob}t(t_{1-\alpha,n-2},n-2,\tau_2), \tag{7.3}$$

where τ_1 and τ_2 are non-centrality parameters defined respectively as

$$\tau_1 = \frac{\sqrt{n}(\log(\mu_T/\mu_R)-\log(0.80))}{\sqrt{2\sigma_w^2}} \quad \text{and} \quad \tau_2 = \frac{\sqrt{n}(\log(\mu_T/\mu_R)-\log(1.25))}{\sqrt{2\sigma_w^2}}. \tag{7.4}$$

An estimate of the sample size for μ_T/μ_R greater than unity can be obtained from

$$n = \frac{2\sigma_w^2(Z_{1-\beta}+Z_{1-\alpha})^2}{(\log(\mu_T/\mu_R)-\log(1.25))^2}, \tag{7.5}$$

which can be used to provide an initial value for the iterations. This equation provides reasonable approximations for $\mu_T/\mu_R \neq 1$, especially when the mean ratio becomes large relative to (0.80 to 1.25) as in such circumstances most of the Type II error comes from one of the two one-sided tests. For quick calculations, for 90% power and a Type I error of 5%, the following can be used:

$$n = \frac{17\sigma_w^2}{(\log(\mu_T/\mu_R)-\log(1.25))^2}. \tag{7.6}$$

Obviously, for true ratios less than unity $\log(1.25)$ should be replaced by $\log(0.80)$.

7.2.1.2 Special Case of the Mean Ratio Equalling Unity

For the special case when the true mean difference is expected to be unity the sample size can be directly derived from the following formula:

$$n = \frac{2\sigma_w^2(Z_{1-\beta/2}+Z_{1-\alpha})^2}{(\log(1.25))^2}. \tag{7.7}$$

By replacing the Z-statistic with the t-statistic (7.7) can be rewritten to give the sample size as

$$n \geq \frac{2\sigma_w^2 (Z_{1-\beta/2} + t_{1-\alpha,n-2})^2}{(\log(1.25))^2}. \tag{7.8}$$

In turn (7.8) can be rewritten as

$$1 - \beta = 2\Phi\left(\sqrt{\frac{(\log(1.25))^2 n}{2\sigma_w^2}} - t_{1-\alpha,n-2} \right) - 1. \tag{7.9}$$

Estimating the power from a non-central t-distribution, (7.9) can be rewritten as

$$1 - \beta = 2 \operatorname{Probt}(t_{1-\alpha,n-2}, n-2, \tau) - 1, \tag{7.10}$$

where τ is the non-centrality parameter defined as

$$\tau = \frac{\sqrt{n}(\log(1.25))}{\sqrt{2\sigma_w^2}}. \tag{7.11}$$

Equation (7.7) can be used to obtain initial estimates of the sample size to use in (7.10). For quick calculations for 90% power, 5% Type I error rate and 20% acceptance criteria we could use

$$n = 433\sigma_w^2. \tag{7.12}$$

Table 7.1 gives sample size estimates using (7.3) for different within subject coefficients of variability (CVs), mean ratios and acceptance criteria 10% (0.90 to 1.11), 15% (0.85 to 1.18), 20% (0.80 to 1.25), and so on for a Type I error rate of 5% and 90% power. The simpler equations provide good estimates of the total sample size, underestimating the sample size by one or two, and hence good initial values for iteration.

7.2.2 Replicate Designs

For compounds with high variability the standard *AB/BA* can require a relatively large sample size, especially if the mean ratio is not expected to be unity. Among the designs that can partially overcome this problem are replicate cross-over designs. By adding an extra arm to the study such that the sequences are *ABB/BAA* we can reduce the sample size by 25% compared to a standard *AB/BA* design; an *ABBA/BAAB* design can reduce the sample size by 50% (Liu, 1995). This option may not be practical for certain compounds, for example, those with a long half-life, but it is a possible solution for compounds with high pharmacokinetic variability.

Another type of replicate design is a two-period replicate design *AA/AB/BA/BB*, also known as Balaam's design (Jones and Kenward, 2003). This design allows for an intra-subject estimate of variability for a given compound without increasing the number of periods beyond two. To consider

TABLE 7.1

Total Sample Sizes (*n*) for Bioequivalence Cross-over Study
for Different within Subject CVs, Levels of Bioequivalence
and True Mean Ratios for 90% Power and Type I Error of 5%

CV (%)	Ratio	Levels of Bioequivalence				
		10%	15%	20%	25%	30%
10	0.80				43	12
	0.85			48	13	7
	0.90		54	14	8	5
	0.95	60	16	8	6	5
	1.00	21	10	7	5	5
	1.05	55	15	8	6	5
	1.10		40	13	7	5
	1.15			26	10	6
	1.20			104	17	8
15	0.80				93	23
	0.85			106	26	12
	0.90		119	29	14	8
	0.95	132	33	15	9	7
	1.00	45	20	12	8	6
	1.05	121	31	15	9	7
	1.10		86	25	12	8
	1.15			57	19	10
	1.20			231	36	15
20	0.80				163	40
	0.85			185	45	20
	0.90		207	50	22	13
	0.95	232	56	25	14	10
	1.00	78	34	19	12	9
	1.05	212	54	24	14	10
	1.10		151	43	20	12
	1.15			99	33	16
	1.20			405	62	24
25	0.80				251	60
	0.85			284	68	30
	0.90		320	77	33	18
	0.95	357	86	37	21	14
	1.00	120	52	28	18	12
	1.05	326	82	36	21	14
	1.10		232	65	30	17
	1.15			151	49	24
	1.20			625	95	36

TABLE 7.1 (CONTINUED)

Total Sample Sizes (*n*) for Bioequivalence Cross-over Study
for Different within Subject CVs, Levels of Bioequivalence
and True Mean Ratios for 90% Power and Type I Error of 5%

CV (%)	Ratio	Levels of Bioequivalence				
		10%	15%	20%	25%	30%
30	0.80				356	85
	0.85			403	96	41
	0.90		454	108	46	25
	0.95	507	121	52	29	18
	1.00	170	73	39	25	17
	1.05	463	116	51	28	18
	1.10		329	92	42	24
	1.15			214	69	33
	1.20			888	135	50
35	0.80				477	113
	0.85			540	128	54
	0.90		608	145	61	33
	0.95	679	162	69	38	24
	1.00	227	97	52	32	22
	1.05	620	155	67	37	24
	1.10		440	123	55	31
	1.15			287	92	44
	1.20			1,190	180	67
40	0.80				612	144
	0.85			694	164	69
	0.90		780	185	78	42
	0.95	871	207	88	48	30
	1.00	291	124	66	41	27
	1.05	796	198	86	47	30
	1.10		565	157	71	39
	1.15			367	118	56
	1.20			1,527	231	86
45	0.80				760	179
	0.85			861	203	86
	0.90		969	230	97	52
	0.95	1082	257	109	60	37
	1.00	361	153	82	50	33
	1.05	989	246	106	59	37
	1.10		701	195	87	48
	1.15			456	146	69
	1.20			1,897	286	106

the effect such a design has on the sample size we must consider the derivation of the total variance $\sigma^2 = \sigma_b^2 + \sigma_w^2$, where σ_w^2 is the within-subject component of variation and σ_b^2 is the between-subject component of variation. Both these variance components can be estimated from previous cross-over

TABLE 7.2

Multiplication Factors for
Different Values of k for a
Two-Period Replicate Cross-
over Design

k	$\dfrac{2k+1}{k+1}$
2	1.67
4	1.80
6	1.86
8	1.89
10	1.91

trials with the test and reference compounds. Now suppose $\sigma_b^2 = k\sigma_w^2$; it can be shown, assuming an equal allocation to each sequence, that the sample size required for a two-period replicate design can be derived by multiplying the sample size for standard AB/BA design as follows (Julious, 2004d):

$$n_{AA/AB/BA/BB} = \left(\frac{2k+1}{k+1} \right) n_{AB/BA}. \tag{7.13}$$

Table 7.2 gives inflation factors for different values of k. It is evident from both Table 7.2 and (7.1) that a two-period replicate design will always require more subjects than a standard AB/BA requiring the same sample size only for $k = 0$. However, no matter how much larger k becomes it will only require twice as many subjects at most. This is because as k becomes large virtually all the information, in the comparison of the mean ratio, comes from the AB/BA sequences, and with twice as many subjects there will be as many people in these sequences as in a standard AB/BA design.

7.2.3   Worked Example 7.1

A bioequivalence study is to be planned for a new formulation for a compound being developed. Standard Food and Drug Administration (FDA) bioequivalence criteria are to be used such that bioequivalence will be declared if the 90% confidence interval is wholly contained within (0.80, 1.25). Two previous studies have been conducted with the compound; the variability data are summarised in Table 7.3. For the planned study bioequivalence

TABLE 7.3

CVs (degrees of freedom) for
AUC and C_{max}

	AUC	C_{max}
Study 1	33% (13)	20% (13)
Study 2	24% (15)	23% (15)

will be declared if the area under the concentration curve (AUC) and C_{max} are equivalent for the two formulations.

The corresponding within-subjects standard deviation (SD) of the logs for the AUC are (from $\sigma_w = \sqrt{\log(CV_w^2 + 1)}$) 0.32 and 0.24. Hence, an overall estimate of the SD can be obtained from

$$s_w = \sqrt{\frac{\sum_{i=1}^k df_i s_i^2}{\sum_{i=1}^k df_i}} = \sqrt{\frac{13 \times 0.32^2 + 15 \times 0.24^2}{13 + 15}} = \sqrt{0.0784} = 0.28.$$

Likewise for the C_{max} an overall estimate of the SD is 0.22.

The AUC has the larger of the two variances, so the sample size will be estimated from this. In terms of CV_w we have

$$CV_w = \sqrt{e^{\sigma_w^2} - 1} = \sqrt{e^{0.28^2} - 1} = 0.29.$$

Using AUC, and taking the CV to be 30%, Table 7.1 gives the sample size to be 39 subjects. As the trial will be an AB/BA cross this would equate to 20 subjects per sequence (or 40 total).

With a cross-over trial only subjects who complete will contribute to the analysis, and it is anticipated that 15% of subjects will not complete the trial. Hence the total sample size required to ensure completion by 40 subjects is $40/0.85 = 47.1 = 48$ subjects total.

Suppose an *ABBA/BAAB* replicate design is proposed as a way to reduce the sample size. Now the evaluable sample size would become half of 40, that is, 20 subjects.

7.2.4 Sensitivity Analysis about the Variance Used in the Sample Size Calculations

Bioequivalence and other early phase trials, such as food effect, drug interaction studies, and the like, maybe be particularly sensitive to the assumptions in the design of the trial as often by definition these trials may be designed early in clinical development with very little information on the variance to power the current trial.

As with other types of trial described in this book a plausibly large value for the population variance can be used to assess the sensitivity of the study to the assumptions in the calculations. For bioequivalence-type studies these calculations are particularly recommended.

7.2.5 Worked Example 7.2

For AUC in the worked example a highly plausible value for the variance could be estimated from

$$s_w^2(95) < \frac{df}{\chi_{0.05,df}^2} s_w^2 = \frac{28}{16.93} \times 0.28^2 = 0.36.$$

TABLE 7.4

Sensitivity Analysis for the Planned Study (%)

	CV_w	95th	Power for 95th percentile
AUC	29	37	71
C_{max}	27	35	76

From this the CV_w is estimated to be 37% (from the 95th percentile for this variance). Likewise a highly plausible value for the C_{max} variance could be estimated to be 35%. With these highly plausible values the variance (7.3) could be used to assess the loss of power if the true variance was nearer to these plausibly high variances (Table 7.4). This study up front therefore seems quite robust to the assumptions made about the variance.

7.2.6 Calculations Taking Account of the Imprecision of the Variance Used in the Sample Size Calculations

7.2.6.1 General Case

Extending the arguments for equivalence trials given in previous chapters the sample size for a bioequivalence study, taking into account the degrees of freedom about the sample variance study, can be derived from

$$1-\beta = \text{Prob}t\left(\sqrt{\frac{(\log(\mu_T/\mu_R)-\log(1.25))^2 n}{2s_w^2}}, m, t_{1-\alpha,n-2}\right)$$
$$+ \text{Prob}t\left(\sqrt{\frac{(\log(\mu_T/\mu_R)-\log(0.80))^2 n}{2s_w^2}}, m, t_{1-\alpha,n-2}\right) - 1, \tag{7.14}$$

where s_w^2 is a sample estimate of the within-subject population variance, and m is the degrees of freedom for this variance. Replacing the t-statistic with the Z-statistic, (7.14) becomes

$$1-\beta = \text{Prob}t\left(\sqrt{\frac{(\log(\mu_T/\mu_R)-\log(1.25))^2 n}{2s_w^2}}, m, Z_{1-\alpha}\right)$$
$$+ \text{Prob}t\left(\sqrt{\frac{(\log(\mu_T/\mu_R)-\log(0.80))^2 n}{2s_w^2}}, m, Z_{1-\alpha}\right) - 1. \tag{7.15}$$

A direct estimate of the sample size can be obtained if the expected true mean ratio is expected to be large, $\mu_T/\mu_R \geq 1.05$. Hence, the following quick formula can be used to obtain direct initial estimates of the sample size for the general case of $\mu_T/\mu_R \neq 1$:

$$n = \frac{2s_w^2[tinv(1-\beta, m, Z_{1-\alpha})]^2}{[\log(1.25)-\log(\mu_T/\mu_R)]^2}. \tag{7.16}$$

7.2.6.2 Special Case of the Mean Ratio Equalling Unity

For the special case of μ_T/μ_R (7.14) can be rewritten as

$$1 - \beta = 2 \operatorname{Prob}t\left(\sqrt{\frac{(\log\log(1.25))^2 n}{2s_w^2}}, m, t_{1-\alpha, n-2}\right) - 1, \tag{7.17}$$

which when replacing the t-statistic with the Z-statistic becomes

$$1 - \beta = 2 \operatorname{Prob}t\left(\sqrt{\frac{(\log\log(1.25))^2 n}{2s_w^2}}, m, Z_{1-\alpha}\right) - 1. \tag{7.18}$$

TABLE 7.5

Multiplication Factors for Different Levels of One-Sided
Significance, Type II Error and Degrees of Freedom

		Significance Level (α)			
m	β	0.010	0.025	0.050	0.100
5	0.05	2.649	2.509	2.385	2.238
	0.10	2.167	2.068	1.980	1.875
	0.15	1.929	1.850	1.780	1.696
	0.20	1.776	1.711	1.652	1.581
	0.50	1.367	1.337	1.311	1.278
10	0.05	1.611	1.562	1.520	1.470
	0.10	1.463	1.425	1.392	1.353
	0.15	1.382	1.351	1.323	1.290
	0.20	1.328	1.301	1.276	1.248
	0.50	1.166	1.153	1.141	1.127
25	0.05	1.208	1.192	1.178	1.162
	0.10	1.163	1.150	1.139	1.125
	0.15	1.137	1.126	1.116	1.105
	0.20	1.119	1.109	1.101	1.091
	0.50	1.062	1.058	1.053	1.058
50	0.05	1.099	1.091	1.085	1.077
	0.10	1.078	1.072	1.067	1.060
	0.15	1.066	1.061	1.056	1.051
	0.20	1.058	1.053	1.049	1.044
	0.50	1.031	1.028	1.026	1.024
75	0.05	1.065	1.060	1.056	1.051
	0.10	1.052	1.047	1.044	1.040
	0.15	1.044	1.040	1.037	1.033
	0.20	1.038	1.035	1.032	1.029
	0.50	1.020	1.019	1.017	1.016
100	0.05	1.048	1.044	1.041	1.038
	0.10	1.038	1.035	1.033	1.030
	0.15	1.033	1.030	1.028	1.025
	0.20	1.029	1.026	1.024	1.022
	0.50	1.015	1.014	1.013	1.012

Hence, a direct estimate of the sample size can be obtained from

$$n = \frac{2s_w^2 [tinv(1 - \beta/2,\ m,\ Z_{1-\alpha})]^2}{(\log(1.25))^2}. \tag{7.19}$$

Table 7.5 gives the multiplication factors, compared to assuming we have the population variance, for various degrees of freedom and Type I and II errors assuming a mean ratio of unity using (7.19) and (7.7).

7.3 Parallel Group Studies

Although cross-over trials are the 'norm' for the assessment of bioequivalence sometimes, particularly with very long half-life compounds, these designs are not practical. This section briefly describes the methodology for sample size calculation for parallel group bioequivalence trials.

7.3.1 Sample Size Estimated Assuming the Population Variance to Be Known

7.3.1.1 General Case

The power for a bioequivalence trial with acceptance limits of (0.80, 1.25) for given values of the any true ratio is given by

$$1 - \beta = \Phi\left(\sqrt{\frac{(\log(\mu_T/\mu_R) - \log(1.25))^2\, rn_T}{(r+1)\sigma^2}} - Z_{1-\alpha}\right)$$

$$+ \Phi\left(\sqrt{\frac{(\log(\mu_T/\mu_R) - \log(0.80)^2\, rn_T}{(r+1)\sigma^2}} - Z_{1-\alpha}\right) - 1, \tag{7.20}$$

where σ is the between-subject variability on the log scale, r is the allocation ratio, and n_T is the sample size in the test group—assuming here $n_T = n_R$. Replacing the Z-statistic with a t-statistic, (7.20) can be rewritten as

$$1 - \beta = \Phi\left(\sqrt{\frac{(\log(\mu_T/\mu_R) - \log(1.25))^2\, rn_T}{(r+1)\sigma^2}} - t_{1-\alpha, n_T(r+1)-2}\right)$$

$$+ \Phi\left(\sqrt{\frac{(\log(\mu_T/\mu_R) - \log(0.80)^2\, rn_T}{(r+1)\sigma^2}} - t_{1-\alpha, n_T(r+1)-2}\right) - 1. \tag{7.21}$$

and under the assumption of a non-central t-distribution the power is estimated from

$$1 - \beta = \text{Prob}t(t_{1-\alpha,n_T(r+1)-2}, n_T(r+1)-2, \tau_1) - \text{Prob}t(t_{1-\alpha,n_T(r+1)-2}, n_T(r+1)-2, \tau_2),$$

(7.22)

where τ_1 and τ_2 are non-centrality parameters defined respectively as

$$\tau_1 = \frac{\sqrt{rn_T}(\log(\mu_T/\mu_R) - \log(0.80))}{\sqrt{(r+1)\sigma^2}} \quad \text{and} \quad \tau_2 = \frac{\sqrt{rn_T}(\log(\mu_T/\mu_R) - \log(1.25))}{\sqrt{(r+1)\sigma^2}}.$$

As with a cross-over trial a direct estimate of the sample size for a mean ratio greater than unity can be obtained from

$$n_T = \frac{(r+1)\sigma^2(Z_{1-\beta} + Z_{1-\alpha})^2}{r(\log(\mu_T/\mu_R) - \log(1.25))^2},$$

(7.23)

and for quick calculations we could use

$$n_T = \frac{17(r+1)\sigma^2}{r(\log(\mu_T/\mu_R) - \log(1.25))^2}.$$

(7.24)

If the mean ratio is expected to be less than unity, then replace $\log(1.25)$ with $\log(0.80)$ in (7.23) and (7.24).

7.3.1.2 Special Case of the Ratio Equalling Unity

When the mean ratio is expected to be unity the sample size can be derived directly from

$$n_T = \frac{(r+1)\sigma^2(Z_{1-\beta/2} + Z_{1-\alpha})^2}{r(\log(1.25))^2}.$$

(7.25)

Replacing the Z-statistic with the t-statistic, (7.25) can be rewritten as

$$n_T = \frac{(r+1)\sigma^2(Z_{1-\beta/2} + t_{1-\alpha,n_T(r+1)-2})^2}{r(\log(1.25))^2}.$$

(7.26)

Equation (7.26) can in turn be rewritten as

$$1 - \beta = 2\Phi\left(\sqrt{\frac{(\log(1.25))^2 rn_T}{(r+1)\sigma^2}} - t_{1-\alpha,n_T(r+1)-2}\right) - 1,$$

(7.27)

and under the assumption of a non-central t-distribution the power can be derived from

$$1 - \beta = 2 \; \mathrm{Prob}t(t_{1-\alpha,n_T(r+1)-2}, n_T(r+1) - 2, \tau) - 1, \tag{7.28}$$

where τ is the non-centrality parameter defined as

$$\tau = \frac{\sqrt{rn_T}\,(\log(1.25))}{\sqrt{(r+1)\sigma^2}}. \tag{7.29}$$

Equation (7.25) can be used for initial estimates of the sample size to use in (7.28). For quick calculations of the sample size for 90% power, 5% Type I error rate and 20% we could use

$$10.75(k+1)\sigma^2/r. \tag{7.30}$$

As with cross-over trials the simpler equations provide good estimates for initial calculations. Table 7.6 gives sample size estimates using (7.22) for different CVs, mean ratios and acceptance criteria 10% (0.90 to 1.11), 15% (0.85 to 1.18), 20% (0.80 to 1.25), and so on for a Type I error rate of 5%, 90% power and an allocation ratio of one.

7.3.2 Calculations Taking Account of the Imprecision of the Variance Used in the Sample Size Calculations

7.3.2.1 General Case

For a parallel group bioequivalence study the sample size can be derived from

$$1 - \beta = \mathrm{Prob}t\left(\sqrt{\frac{(\log(\mu_T/\mu_R) - \log(1.25))^2\,rn_T}{(r+1)s^2}}, mt_{1-\alpha,n_T(r+1)-2}\right)$$

$$+ \mathrm{Prob}t\left(\sqrt{\frac{(\log(\mu_T/\mu_R) - \log(0.80))^2\,rn_T}{(r+1)s^2}}, m, t_{1-\alpha,n_T(r+1)-2}\right) - 1, \tag{7.31}$$

where s^2 is a sample estimate of the population variance, and m is the degrees of freedom for this variance. Replacing the t-statistic with the Z-statistic, (7.31) becomes

$$1 - \beta = \mathrm{Prob}t\left(\sqrt{\frac{(\log(\mu_T/\mu_R) - \log(1.25))^2\,rn_T}{(r+1)s^2}}, m, Z_{1-\alpha}\right),$$

$$+ \mathrm{Prob}t\left(\sqrt{\frac{(\log(\mu_T/\mu_R) - \log(0.80))^2\,rn_T}{(r+1)s^2}}, m, Z_{1-\alpha}\right) - 1. \tag{7.32}$$

TABLE 7.6

Sample Sizes for One Arm of a Bioequivalence Parallel Group Study for Different CVs, Levels of Bioequivalence and True Mean Ratios for 90% Power and a Type I Error Rate of 5%

CV (%)	Ratio	Levels of Bioequivalence				
		10%	15%	20%	25%	30%
30	0.80				356	84
	0.85			403	95	40
	0.90		453	108	46	25
	0.95	506	121	51	28	18
	1.00	169	72	39	24	16
	1.05	462	115	50	28	17
	1.10		328	92	41	23
	1.15			213	69	33
	1.20			887	134	50
35	0.80				476	112
	0.85			540	128	54
	0.90		607	144	61	33
	0.95	678	161	69	37	23
	1.00	226	96	51	31	21
	1.05	620	154	67	37	23
	1.10		439	122	55	30
	1.15			286	92	43
	1.20			1,189	179	66
40	0.80				611	144
	0.85			693	163	69
	0.90		779	184	78	41
	0.95	871	207	88	48	30
	1.00	291	123	66	40	26
	1.05	796	198	85	47	29
	1.10		564	157	70	38
	1.15			367	117	55
	1.20			1,527	230	85
45	0.80				759	178
	0.85			861	203	85
	0.90		968	229	96	51
	0.95	1,082	257	109	59	36
	1.00	361	152	81	49	33
	1.05	988	245	106	58	36
	1.10		700	194	87	47
	1.15			455	146	68
	1.20			1,896	286	105

(Continued)

TABLE 7.6 (CONTINUED)

Sample Sizes for One Arm of a Bioequivalence Parallel Group
Study for Different CVs, Levels of Bioequivalence and True
Mean Ratios for 90% Power and a Type I Error Rate of 5%

CV (%)	Ratio	\multicolumn{5}{c}{Levels of Bioequivalence}
		10%	15%	20%	25%	30%
50	0.80				919	216
	0.85			1,041	245	103
	0.90		1,171	277	116	62
	0.95	1,309	310	131	71	44
	1.00	436	184	98	60	39
	1.05	1,195	297	128	70	43
	1.10		847	235	104	57
	1.15			551	176	82
	1.20			2,295	345	127
55	0.80				1,088	255
	0.85			1,233	290	121
	0.90		1,387	327	137	73
	0.95	1,550	367	155	84	52
	1.00	516	218	116	70	46
	1.05	1,416	351	151	82	51
	1.10		1,003	278	124	68
	1.15			652	208	97
	1.20			2,718	409	150
60	0.80				1,266	297
	0.85			1,434	337	141
	0.90		1,613	381	160	85
	0.95	1,803	427	180	97	60
	1.00	601	253	135	82	54
	1.05	1,647	408	176	96	59
	1.10		1,167	323	144	78
	1.15			759	242	113
	1.20			3,162	476	174
65	0.80				1,450	340
	0.85			1,643	386	161
	0.90		1,849	436	183	97
	0.95	2,066	489	207	111	68
	1.00	688	290	154	93	61
	1.05	1,887	468	201	109	68
	1.10		1,337	371	164	90
	1.15			869	277	129
	1.20			3,623	545	200

For $\mu_T/\mu_R \geq 1.05$ a direct estimate of the sample size to start iterations can be obtained from

$$n_T = \frac{(r+1)s^2[tinv(1-\beta,\ m,\ Z_{1-\alpha})]^2}{r[\log(1.25) - \log(\mu_T/\mu_R)]^2}. \tag{7.33}$$

7.3.2.2 Special Case of the Mean Ratio Equalling Unity

For the special case of $\mu_T = \mu_R$ (7.31) can be rewritten as

$$1 - \beta = 2\ \text{Prob}t\left(\sqrt{\frac{(\log\log(1.25))^2\, r n_T}{(r+1)s^2}},\, m, t_{1-\alpha,\, n_T(r+1)-2}\right) - 1, \tag{7.34}$$

which when replacing the t-statistic with the Z-statistic becomes

$$1 - \beta = 2\ \text{Prob}t\left(\sqrt{\frac{(\log\log(1.25))^2\, r n_T}{(r+1)s^2}},\, m, Z_{1-\alpha}\right) - 1. \tag{7.35}$$

Hence, a direct estimate of the sample size can be obtained from

$$n_T = \frac{2s_w^2[tinv(1-\beta/2,\ m,\ Z_{1-\alpha})]^2}{(\log(1.25))^2}. \tag{7.36}$$

Table 7.5 (for cross-over trials) can be used for multiplication factors as these depend only on degrees of freedom and Type I and II errors.

 Key Messages

- For studies in which the variance is anticipated to be high then a replicate design may be an option to reduce the sample size.
- Bioequivalence trials may be particularly sensitive to assumptions about the estimates used in sample size calculations.

8

Sample Size Calculations for Precision-Based Clinical Trials with Normal Data

8.1 Introduction

So far the book has concentrated on trials in which we are powering a study to investigate a null hypothesis. As discussed in Chapter 1, however, often we may be designing a trial in which the objective is not to formally investigate a hypothesis—and hence whether a treatment difference truly exists—but to estimate plausible differences with a view to design a definitive study afterwards (Julious and Patterson, 2004).

All trials however have to have some form of sample size justification provided. For an exploratory trial what is proposed is to estimate a sample size that provides a given level of precision for any estimates. Hence, we are not powering in the traditional fashion for a (in truth unknown) desirable and prespecified difference of interest.

Simply when analysing a trial you have a point estimate of effect and a confidence interval. If you take a half-width (w) of the confidence interval, then this could be taken as a measure of precision for the trial. This measure of precision could in turn be used to design a clinical trial.

For precision-based studies, rather than testing a formal hypothesis, an estimation approach through the provision of confidence intervals around a possible effect may be more appropriate. Here, therefore, the concentration will not be on assessing statistical significance but on estimation. It is important however that if the sample size is based on estimation calculations, then the protocol should clearly state this as the study's objective and as the basis for the sample size of the study.

The precision-based approach may also be useful for secondary or tertiary objectives. An example is when a trial is designed to test an overall effect but there is also an interest to investigate effects in possible subgroups. Here, instead, the study would have little power in the subgroups, so we can calculate what precision we may have when estimating possible effects.

8.2   Parallel Group Trials

8.2.1   Sample Size Estimated Assuming the Population Variance to Be Known

As discussed in Chapter 1 a $(1 - \alpha)$ 100% confidence interval for $f(\mu)$ has half-width

$$w = Z_{\alpha/2}\sqrt{Var(S)}, \tag{8.1}$$

so defining $Var(S)$ as per the equation

$$Var(S) = \frac{\sigma^2}{n_A} + \frac{\sigma^2}{n_B} = \frac{r+1}{r} \cdot \frac{\sigma^2}{n_A},$$

where σ^2 is the population variance estimate, and $n_B = rn_A$. We can solve (8.1) to give (Julious and Patterson, 2004)

$$n_A = \frac{(r+1)Z^2_{1-\alpha/2}\sigma^2}{rw^2}. \tag{8.2}$$

If the population variance is assumed unknown in the statistical analysis, (8.2) can be rewritten as (Julious and Patterson, 2004)

$$n_A \geq \frac{(r+1)t^2_{1-\alpha/2,\,n_A(r+1)-2}\sigma^2}{rw^2}. \tag{8.3}$$

Result (8.3) can be solved iteratively to find a value of n_A for which the left-hand side of the equation is greater than the right. An alternative equation to solve for n_A would be

$$0.5 \geq \Phi\left(\sqrt{\frac{rn_A w^2}{(r+1)\sigma^2}} - t_{1-\alpha/2,\,n_A(r+1)-2}\right). \tag{8.4}$$

Actually, (8.4) holds; if we were to rewrite it in terms of n_A, we would initially have

$$Z_{0.5} = 0 \geq \sqrt{\frac{rn_A w^2}{(r+1)\sigma^2}} - t_{1-\alpha/2,\,n_A(r+1)-2}, \tag{8.5}$$

and hence

$$n_A \geq \frac{(r+1)\sigma^2(t_{1-\alpha/2,\,n_A(r+1)-2} + Z_{0.5})^2}{rw^2}. \tag{8.6}$$

The result (8.6) holds as $Z_{0.5} = 0$, and hence it becomes (8.3). The result (8.6) is in fact the same as the results for superiority trials but with the Type II error set at 0.5—although obviously as precision trials are not powered they cannot have any Type II error. The practical application of this result is given later in the section on sample sizes for which the population variance is assumed unknown for sample size calculations.

To allow for the Normal approximation (8.2) can have a correction factor added to assist in initial calculations (Guenther, 1981; Julious and Patterson, 2004)

$$n_A = \frac{(r+1)\sigma^2 Z_{1-\alpha/2}^2}{rw^2} + \frac{Z_{1-\alpha/2}^2}{4}, \tag{8.7}$$

while the following quick formula can be used assuming we wish to have a 95% confidence interval for the precision estimates:

$$n_A = \frac{4\sigma^2}{w^2} \frac{(r+1)}{r}, \tag{8.8}$$

or for $r = 1$:

$$n_A = \frac{8\sigma^2}{w^2}. \tag{8.9}$$

Table 8.1 gives sample sizes using (8.3) for various standardised widths ($\delta = w/\sigma$). The simpler equations slightly underestimate the sample size.

If we compare Table 8.1 to the sample sizes using (8.1) for these calculations, then the sample size estimates are about two smaller when using (8.1) over Table 8.1. The correction factor of $Z_{1-\alpha/2}^2/4$ given in (8.7) could be added to account for part of this underestimation.

8.2.1.1 Worked Example 8.1: Standard Results

A parallel two-arm precision-based study is being designed. The primary endpoint is systolic blood pressure, and the standard deviation (SD) is assumed to be 10 mmHg. Suppose the precision we required for a half-width of a 95% confidence interval is 2.5 mmHg; then the sample size would be estimated as 122.9 or 123 patients per arm if the sample size had been estimated using the Normal approximation approach from (8.2).

8.2.1.2 Worked Example 8.2: Using Results from Superiority Trials

Remember the Normal approximation sample size result from Chapter 3

$$n_A = \frac{(r+1)(Z_{1-\beta} + Z_{1-\alpha/2})^2 \sigma^2}{rd^2}. \tag{8.10}$$

TABLE 8.1

Sample Sizes for One Group, n_A ($n_B = rn_A$), in a Parallel
Group Study for Different Standardised Widths
($\delta = w/\sigma$) and Allocation Ratios with 95% Confidence
Intervals for the Precision Estimates

	Allocation Ratios (r)			
δ	1	2	3	4
0.05	3,075	2,306	2,050	1,922
0.10	770	578	513	481
0.15	343	257	229	214
0.20	194	145	129	121
0.25	125	94	83	78
0.30	87	65	58	54
0.35	64	48	43	40
0.40	50	37	33	31
0.45	40	30	26	25
0.50	32	24	22	20
0.55	27	20	18	17
0.60	23	17	15	14
0.65	20	15	13	12
0.70	17	13	12	11
0.75	15	12	10	10
0.80	14	10	9	9
0.85	12	9	8	8
0.90	11	8	7	7
0.95	10	8	7	6
1.00	9	7	6	6

Imagine we did calculations using the superiority sample size formula from
Chapter 3 but using 50% power. Now we have $Z_{1-\beta} = 0$, and hence we would
have (8.2). Thus the sample size would remain the same.

8.2.1.3 Worked Example 8.3: Sample Size Is Based on Feasibility

A trial is being designed in which the sample size of 12 per group is based
on feasibility and is fixed *a priori*. However, you have a previous estimate
10 for the SD. Now, with n fixed we could calculate the precision that could
be anticipated if a 95% confidence interval is to be used. Hence, the width
would be

$$w = t_{1-\alpha/2,2(n-1)}\sqrt{2s^2/n} = 2.07387\sqrt{2 \times 10^2/12} = 8.47 \text{ mmHg}.$$

An alternative calculation is to say what difference could be detected for a
requisite power and significance level. For the same trial with 90% power and

a two-sided significance level of 5% the difference, rewriting (8.10), would be estimated from

$$d = \sqrt{\frac{2(Z_{1-\alpha/2} + Z_{1-\beta})^2 \sigma^2}{n_A}}. \tag{8.11}$$

Hence, a difference that could be detected with 90% power is 13.2 mmHg.

8.2.2 Sensitivity Analysis about the Variance Used in the Sample Size Calculations

Precision-based studies are usually undertaken early in the development of a compound when, by definition, there is little variability information available. Hence, a sensitivity analysis of the study may be quite important.

When undertaking a sensitivity analysis in a precision-based study designed to estimate effects to a given precision, however, it is not the power we investigate against a highly plausible value for the variance but the precision itself. Hence, from (8.2) or (8.3) we estimate the required sample size and then use the same results to quantify the precision the study will have supposing the variance is nearer to a larger plausible variance for the same sample size.

8.2.3 Worked Example 8.4

Revisiting Worked Example 8.3, the sample size was estimated to be 123 patients using the Normal approximation method based on a width of 2.5 and an SD of 10. Now suppose the variance used in the calculations was estimated with 10 degrees of freedom from Chapter 3, a highly plausible value for the variance $\chi^2_{0.05,10} = 3.94$:

$$s_p(95) < \sqrt{\frac{10}{3.94} \times 10^2} = 15.93.$$

Hence, for this highly plausible value for the variance the precision for the trial would be 3.98—about 60% worse than the width on which the sample size calculations were based.

8.2.4 Accounting for the Imprecision of the Variance in the Future Trial

When undertaking conventional powered trials we are in effect accounting for the imprecision in the future trials' variance (and mean). This is because we are supposing we have the population responses for the sample size calculation and that we will be undertaking a trial that will give estimates of the population response. However, in these future trials there will be random variability in our estimates from trial to trial such that even if there truly is a difference between treatment groups we still have a chance of not observing a statistically significant effect. This is when we have the concepts of Type II error and power.

In the context of precision-based trials with (8.2) or (8.3) we have a good chance of not achieving the desired precision because in a large proportion of trials the observed study variance will be greater than the population variance simply due to random sampling. To overcome this problem we can estimate the sample size from the following result (Grieve, 1989, 1990, 1991):

$$\text{Probability} = \text{Probchi}\left(\frac{w^2 r n_A(n_A(r+1)-2)}{(r+1)t^2_{1-\alpha/2,\,n_A(r+1)-2}\sigma^2}, n_A(r+1)-2\right), \quad (8.12)$$

where probchi$(\bullet, n_A(r+1)-2)$ is a cumulative density distribution (using the same notation as SAS) of a χ^2 distribution on $n_A(r+1)-2$ degrees of freedom. To estimate a sample size we have to iterate until a required level of probability is reached.

The probability here is the probability of the confidence interval having the required precision for the variance estimated in the planned trial for a given sample size. This result accounts for the fact that, at random, the sample variance in the study may be bigger (or smaller) than the population variance. An important point to emphasise is that this probability is not a power.

Table 8.2 gives sample sizes from (8.12) for given probabilities and various standardised widths ($\delta = w/\sigma$). From visual inspection of this table and Table 8.1 [estimated from (8.2)] it is clear that for a probability of 0.5 (8.12) gives the same results as (8.2), allowing for a little rounding error. Also from inspection, it seems that to ensure a greater probability of having the required precision it does not require a great increase in the required sample size.

8.2.4.1 Worked Example 8.5: Accounting for the Imprecision in the Variance in the Future Trial

In Worked Example 8.1 for a standardised precision of 0.25 the sample size required was estimated as 125 using Table 8.1 and (8.3). From Table 8.2 we can see that if we wish just to be 50% certain of having the requisite precision we would also need 125 patients per arm. However, if we wish to have a bit more certainty, say 90%, the sample size would increase by about 11% to 139 patients per arm.

8.2.5 Calculations Taking Account of the Imprecision of the Variance Used in the Sample Size Calculations

To account for the imprecision of the variance used in the sample size calculations for parallel group precision-based trials, the results from superiority

TABLE 8.2

Sample Sizes for One Group, n_A ($n_B = n_A$), in a Parallel Group Study for Different Standardised Widths and Probabilities for 95% Confidence Intervals for the Precision Estimates

	Probabilities			
δ	0.50	0.80	0.90	0.95
0.05	3,075	3,121	3,145	3,165
0.10	770	793	805	815
0.15	343	358	366	373
0.20	193	205	211	216
0.25	124	134	138	142
0.30	87	94	98	102
0.35	64	71	74	77
0.40	49	55	58	60
0.45	39	44	47	49
0.50	32	37	39	41
0.55	27	31	33	35
0.60	23	27	28	30
0.65	20	23	25	26
0.70	17	20	22	23
0.75	15	18	20	21
0.80	13	16	18	19
0.85	12	15	16	17
0.90	11	13	15	16
0.95	10	12	14	15
1.00	9	11	13	13

trials given in Chapter 3 can be generalised to give

$$n_A \geq \frac{(r+1)s^2[tinv(0.5, m, t_{1-\alpha/2, n_A(r+1)-2})]^2}{rd^2}, \tag{8.13}$$

where n_A is the least integer value for (8.13) to hold, and m is the degrees of freedom about the estimate variance s^2. This equation can in turn be rewritten as

$$0.5 \geq probt\left(\sqrt{\frac{rn_A d^2}{(r+1)s^2}}, m, t_{1-\alpha/2, n_A(r+1)-2}\right). \tag{8.14}$$

Replacing the t-statistic with a Z-statistic gives

$$n_A = \frac{(r+1)s^2[tinv(0.5, m, Z_{1-\alpha/2})]^2}{rd^2}, \tag{8.15}$$

TABLE 8.3

Sample Sizes for One Group, n_A ($n_B = rn_A$), in a Parallel Group Precision Study for Different Standardised Widths and Degrees of Freedom Using (8.13) for a 5% Level of Significance

Degrees of Freedom	Standardised Widths					
	0.05	0.10	0.25	0.50	0.75	1.00
5	3,434	860	139	36	17	10
10	3,242	812	131	34	16	10
25	3,138	786	127	33	16	10
50	3,106	778	126	33	16	10
100	3,090	774	125	33	15	10
∞	3,075	770	125	32	15	9

Note: Sample sizes with "infinite" degrees of freedom were estimated from (8.3).

which allows a direct estimate for the sample size and gives an initial value for iterations for (8.13).

Table 8.3 gives the sample sizes required for 95% confidence interval precision estimates and for a range of degrees of freedom m and standardised widths w/s.

Table 8.4 gives the multiplication factors for different levels of statistical significance. What is interesting to note is that for precision-based studies the impact on the sample size is not as great as that for formally powered studies. From Table 8.4 the largest impact only increases the sample size by 12%.

8.2.5.1 Worked Example 8.6: Accounting for the Imprecision in the Variance of the Variance Used in Calculations

In Worked Example 8.1 for a standardised precision of 0.25 the sample size per arm required was estimated as 125 using Table 8.1 and (8.3). Suppose

TABLE 8.4

Multiplication Factors for Different Levels of Two-Sided Statistical Significance

m	Significance Level (α)			
	0.010	0.025	0.050	0.100
5	1.122	1.120	1.117	1.114
10	1.056	1.055	1.054	1.053
25	1.021	1.021	1.021	1.021
50	1.010	1.010	1.010	1.010
75	1.007	1.007	1.007	1.007
100	1.005	1.005	1.005	1.005

the variance used in the sample size calculation was estimated with just 10 degrees of freedom. Thus, from Table 8.3 we would need to increase the sample size to 131 patients per arm to account for this imprecision, around a 5% increase in the sample size.

8.2.6 Allowing for the Imprecision in the Variance Used in the Sample Size Calculations and in Future Trials

In an elegant solution Grieve (1991) demonstrated that if there was prior uncertainty around the variance used in the precision sample size calculations, then the probability of seeing the required precision for a given sample size can be calculated from

$$\text{Probability} = \text{Prob}f\left(\frac{w^2 r n_A}{(r+1)t^2_{1-\alpha/2, \, n_A(r+1)-2}s^2}, n_A(r+1)-2, m \right), \tag{8.16}$$

where $\text{prob}f(\bullet, n_A(r+1)-2, m)$ is a cumulative density distribution (using the same notation as SAS) of an F-distribution on $n_A(r+1)-2$ and m degrees of freedom. This result was originally given without proof by Mood and Snedecor (1946).

Here s^2 is the estimate of the variance from a previous trial being used to plan the current trial, n_A is the sample size in the trial being planned, $n_A(r+1)-2$ is the degrees of freedom of the variance in this trial and m is the degrees of freedom for s^2. To solve for n_A you iterate (8.16) until the appropriate probability is reached.

The sample sizes from (8.16) are given in Table 8.5. For probabilities of 0.50 the table should be comparable to Table 8.3; however, the results from this table are a little conservative in comparison.

From observation of Table 8.5 there seems to be a marked effect on the sample size of having an imprecisely estimated variance for these calculations for various standardised widths ($\delta = w/\sigma$). There therefore needs to be a call regarding the value of these calculations. If we have a well-estimated variance (in terms of the number of degrees of freedom), then these calculations may be considered to add value. However, if the variance is poorly estimated, then a call could be made as to the value of the calculations as the objective of precision-based trials is to provide good estimates of the variance and possible treatment effects due to their exploratory nature.

8.2.6.1 *Worked Example 8.7: Allowing for the Imprecision in the Variance Used in the Sample Size Calculations and in Future Trials*

In Worked Example 8.5 a sample size was estimated that accounted for the imprecision in the future trials' variance while in Worked Example 8.6 we

TABLE 8.5

Sample Sizes for One Group, n_A ($n_B = n_A$) in a Parallel Group Precision Study for Different Standardised Widths, Probabilities (P) and Degrees of Freedom Using (8.16) for a 5% Level of Significance

Probability	Degrees of Freedom	Standardised Widths					
		0.05	0.10	0.25	0.50	0.75	1.00
0.5	5	3,533	884	143	37	17	10
	10	3,291	824	133	34	16	10
	25	3,158	791	128	33	15	9
	50	3,116	780	126	33	15	9
	100	3,095	775	125	32	15	9
	∞	3,075	770	124	32	15	9
0.8	5	6,561	1,642	264	67	31	18
	10	4,976	1,246	201	52	24	15
	25	4,059	1,017	165	43	21	13
	50	3,710	930	152	40	19	12
	100	3,499	878	144	39	19	12
	∞	3,121	793	134	37	18	11
0.9	5	9,544	2,388	384	97	44	26
	10	6,319	1,582	255	66	31	18
	25	4,667	1,169	190	50	24	15
	50	4,081	1,024	167	45	22	14
	100	3,737	938	155	42	21	13
	∞	3,145	805	138	39	20	13
0.95	5	13,417	3,356	539	136	62	36
	10	7,802	1,953	315	81	37	22
	25	5,262	1,318	214	56	27	17
	50	4,425	1,110	182	49	24	15
	100	3,950	993	164	45	22	14
	∞	3,165	815	142	41	21	13

Note: Sample sizes with "infinite" degrees of freedom were estimated from (8.12).

estimated the sample size that allowed for the imprecision of the variance used in the sample size calculations. Suppose we now wish to account for imprecision of the variance used both with respect to the sample size calculation and the future trial.

For a standardised precision of 0.25 the sample size per arm required was estimated as 255 using Table 8.5 and (8.16) assuming the variance is estimated with 10 degrees of freedom and we wish to be 90% sure that we will see the desired precision. This is nearly a twofold increase in the sample size. If we had 50 degrees of freedom for the variance estimate used in the sample size calculation the sample size would need to be increased to 167 patients per arm.

8.3 Cross-over Trials

8.3.1 Sample Size Estimated Assuming the Population Variance to Be Known

Similar to the parallel group case you can solve the following (Julious, 2004d)

$$n = \frac{2Z_{1-\alpha/2}^2 \sigma_w^2}{w^2},$$ (8.17)

to give an estimate of the sample size where n is the total sample size. If the population variance is considered unknown in the statistical analysis, then (8.17) can be rewritten as (Julious, 2004d)

$$n \geq \frac{2t_{1-\alpha/2,\,n-2}^2 \sigma_w^2}{w^2},$$ (8.18)

which can be solved iteratively. Alternatively as with parallel group trials the following formula could be used

$$0.5 \geq \Phi\left(\sqrt{\frac{nw^2}{2\sigma_w^2}} - t_{1-\alpha/2,n-2}\right).$$ (8.19)

To allow for the Normal approximation, (8.17) can be amended to have a correction factor (Guenther, 1981; Julious, 2004d)

$$n = \frac{2\sigma_w^2 Z_{1-\alpha/2}^2}{w^2} + \frac{Z_{1-\alpha/2}^2}{2}.$$ (8.20)

The following formula can be used assuming we wish to have 95% confidence interval precision estimates

$$n = \frac{8\sigma_w^2}{w^2}.$$ (8.21)

Table 8.6 gives sample sizes using (8.18) for various standardised widths ($\delta = w/\sigma$). As with parallel group trials the quick formula slightly underestimates the sample size.

8.3.2 Sensitivity Analysis about the Variance Used in the Sample Size Calculations

The methodology for assessing sensitivity is the same as for parallel group studies, described in Section 8.2.2, in which you assess the loss in the precision estimates for a highly plausible value for the variance.

TABLE 8.6

Total Sample Sizes for a Cross-over Study for
Different Standardised Widths with 95%
Confidence Intervals for the Precision Estimates

δ	n
0.05	3,076
0.10	771
0.15	344
0.20	195
0.25	126
0.30	88
0.35	66
0.40	51
0.45	41
0.50	34
0.55	28
0.60	24
0.65	21
0.70	19
0.75	17
0.80	15
0.85	14
0.90	13
0.95	12
1.00	11

8.3.3 Accounting for the Imprecision of the Variance in the Future Trial

The work of Grieve (1989, 1990, 1991) can be extended to cross-over trials such that the total sample size can be estimated from

$$\text{Probability} = \text{Probchi}\left(\frac{w^2 n(n-2)}{2t^2_{1-\alpha/2,\,n-2}\sigma^2_w}, n-2 \right) \quad (8.22)$$

As with parallel group trials to estimate a sample size you have to iterate until a required level of probability is reached. Table 8.7 gives sample sizes from (8.22) for given probabilities and various standardised widths ($\delta = w/\sigma$).

8.3.4 Calculations Taking Account of the Imprecision of the Variance Used in the Sample Size Calculations

To account for the imprecision in the estimate of the sample variance, the results from parallel group trials can be generalised to give

$$n \geq \frac{2s^2_w [tinv(0.5,\, m,\, t_{1-\alpha/2,n-2})]^2}{d^2}, \quad (8.23)$$

TABLE 8.7

Total Sample Sizes for a Cross-over Study for Different Standardised Widths and Probabilities for 95% Confidence Intervals for the Precision Estimates

	Probabilities			
δ	0.50	0.80	0.90	0.95
0.05	3,075	3,141	3,175	3,204
0.10	771	803	820	834
0.15	344	366	377	386
0.20	194	211	219	226
0.25	125	138	145	150
0.30	88	98	104	108
0.35	65	74	79	83
0.40	50	58	63	66
0.45	40	47	51	54
0.50	33	40	43	45
0.55	28	34	37	39
0.60	24	29	32	34
0.65	21	26	28	30
0.70	18	23	25	27
0.75	16	20	22	24
0.80	15	18	20	22
0.85	13	17	19	20
0.90	12	16	17	19
0.95	11	14	16	17
1.00	10	13	15	16

where m is the degrees of freedom about the estimate variance s_w^2. This equation can in turn be rewritten as

$$0.5 \geq \text{prob}t\left(\sqrt{\frac{nd^2}{2s_w^2}}, m, t_{1-\alpha/2, n-2}\right). \tag{8.24}$$

Replacing the *t*-statistic with a *Z*-statistic gives the following result:

$$n = \frac{2s_w^2[\text{tinv}(0.5, m, Z_{1-\alpha/2})]^2}{d^2}, \tag{8.25}$$

which allows a direct estimate for the sample size and gives an initial value for iterations for (8.23).

Table 8.8 gives the sample sizes required for 95% confidence interval precision estimates and for a range of degrees of freedom m and standardised widths w/s. The multiplication factors for a cross-over trial are the same as those for a parallel group study given in Table 8.4 for various standardised widths ($\delta = w/\sigma$).

TABLE 8.8

Total Sample Sizes for a Cross-over Precision Study for Different Standardised Widths and Degrees of Freedom Using (8.23) for a 5% Level of Significance

Degrees of Freedom	Standardised Widths					
	0.05	0.10	0.25	0.50	0.75	1.00
5	3,435	861	140	37	18	12
10	3,243	813	133	35	18	11
25	3,140	787	128	34	17	11
50	3,107	779	127	34	17	11
100	3,092	775	126	34	17	11
∞	3,076	771	126	34	17	11

Note: Sample sizes with "infinite" degrees of freedom were estimated from (8.18).

8.3.5 Allowing for the Imprecision in the Variance Used in the Sample Size Calculations and in Future Trials

By extending the parallel group result to allow for prior uncertainty around the variance used in the precision sample size calculations the probability of seeing the required precision for a given sample size can be

TABLE 8.9

Total Sample Sizes for a Cross-over Study for Different Standardised Widths, Probabilities (P) and Degrees of Freedom Using (8.26) for a 5% Level of Significance

Probability	Degrees of Freedom	Standardised Width					
		0.05	0.10	0.25	0.50	0.75	1.00
0.5	5	3,533	885	144	38	18	11
	10	3,292	825	134	35	17	11
	25	3,159	791	129	34	17	11
	50	3,117	781	127	34	16	10
	100	3,096	776	126	33	16	10
	250	3,084	773	126	33	16	10
	500	3,080	772	125	33	16	10
	1,000	3,077	771	125	33	16	10
	∞	3,075	771	125	33	16	10
0.8	5	6,563	1,643	266	69	32	20
	10	4,977	1,247	203	54	26	16
	25	4,061	1,019	167	45	23	14
	50	3,713	933	154	42	21	14
	100	3,502	881	147	41	21	14
	250	3,337	842	142	40	21	14
	500	3,262	825	140	40	20	13
	1,000	3,213	815	139	40	20	13
	∞	3,141	803	138	40	20	13

TABLE 8.9 (CONTINUED)

Total Sample Sizes for a Cross-over Study for Different Standardised Widths, Probabilities (*P*) and Degrees of Freedom Using (8.26) for a 5% Level of Significance

Probability	Degrees of Freedom	Standardised Width					
		0.05	0.10	0.25	0.50	0.75	1.00
0.9	5	9,546	2,389	385	99	46	28
	10	6,321	1,584	257	68	32	20
	25	4,670	1,172	193	52	26	17
	50	4,085	1,027	171	48	24	16
	100	3,742	943	159	45	23	15
	250	3,480	881	151	44	23	15
	500	3,362	855	148	43	23	15
	1,000	3,287	839	146	43	23	15
	∞	3,175	820	145	43	22	15
0.95	5	13,418	3,357	540	138	63	37
	10	7,804	1,955	317	83	39	24
	25	5,265	1,322	217	59	30	19
	50	4,430	1,114	186	52	27	18
	100	3,956	999	169	49	25	17
	250	3,603	914	158	47	25	16
	500	3,448	879	154	46	24	16
	1,000	3,349	859	152	46	24	16
	∞	3,204	834	150	45	24	16

Note: Sample sizes with "infinite" degrees of freedom were estimated from (8.22).

calculated from

$$\text{Probability} = \text{Prob}f\left(\frac{w^2 n}{t^2_{1-\alpha/2,\,n-2}s^2_w},\, n-2, m\right). \tag{8.26}$$

To solve for *n* you iterate (8.26) until the appropriate probability is reached. Table 8.9 gives sample size tables using (8.26) for various standardised widths ($\delta = w/\sigma$).

 Key Messages

- Precision-based trials are designed to assess if a treatment effect may exist.
- Type I and Type II errors are not formally considered when undertaking precision-based trials; however, sample sizes can be calculated to ensure we will have a given precision with a required probability.

9

Sample Size Calculations for Parallel Group Superiority Clinical Trials with Binary Data

9.1 Introduction

This chapter describes the sample size calculations for trials in which the primary outcome is binary. As discussed in Chapter 1 binary outcomes are common endpoints in clinical trials and appear when the outcome of interest is a two-point response variable such as presence/absence, alive/dead or yes/no.

The sample size calculations are described in this chapter for situations in which the trial design is a parallel group. The conventional calculations are first introduced for each trial design and objective, followed by calculations, which account for the imprecision of the estimates.

9.2 Inference and Analysis of Clinical Trials with Binary Data

There is a saying in statistics that "as ye shall design is as ye shall analyse". The meaning of this is that if for example you allow, say, for stratification by treatment centre in your design then you should also allow for centre in the analysis. The reverse is also true: "As ye shall analyse is as ye shall design".

We have previously, although not specifically, touched on this when discussing appropriate estimates of the variance. The maxim is particularly true for a trial in which the primary outcome is a binary response.

For a clinical trial in which the primary outcome is a binary response the data may take the form summarised in Table 9.1 where p_A and p_B are the responses anticipated on treatments A and B, respectively; $\bar{p}$ is the average response across treatments; n_A and n_B are the sample sizes in each treatment group, respectively; and n is the total sample size.

So far, so straightforward, and indeed in the face of it a binary response is a relatively easy outcome to summarise as all the data from a trial can be put simply into a table of the form of Table 9.1 for analyses.

TABLE 9.1

Summary for a Clinical Trial with a Binary Outcome

Treatment	Outcome		Sample Size
	0	**1**	**Sample Size**
A	$1 - p_A$	p_A	n_A
B	$1 - p_B$	p_B	n_B
Overall response	$1 - \bar{p}$	$\bar{p} = (p_A + p_B)/2$	$n = (n_A + n_B)$

TABLE 9.2

Summary Measures for a Binary Outcome

Measure	Abbreviation	Definition
Absolute risk difference		$p_A - p_B$
Odds ratio	OR	$\dfrac{p_A(1 - p_B)}{p_B(1 - p_A)}$
Relative risk	RR	$\dfrac{p_A}{p_B}$
Number needed to treat	NNT	$\dfrac{1}{p_A - p_B}$

Once you have an observed response (p_A and p_B) for the two treatments you may then wish to summarise the effect appropriately. Table 9.2 gives definitions of the most common summary measures. For this chapter we concentrate on the absolute risk difference and the odds ratio.

9.3 π's or p's

Being someone from the north of England I like my π's and p's, but in the context of designing clinical trials with a binary response a thing to be conscious of when reading this chapter is the flip-flopping between π's or p's. To a degree this is unavoidable although admittedly a little confusing. For inference π's are taken as the known population estimates for the absolute risks, while p's are taken as sample estimates (from a trial) of π. Hence, in the discussion of confidence intervals we give p's in the results as we are talking about sample estimates.

For sample size calculations we mainly assume absolute response is known for the sample size calculation, so we give π's. This is contradicted of course by our need to do a trial to try to quantify them. It is further contradicted by the fact we often take for π's estimates (p's) from a retrospective study.

It is a Gordian knot. Making assumptions about the population parameter is something that we need to do in all sample size calculations and one to which sample size calculations are very sensitive, as discussed throughout the book.

9.3.1   Absolute Risk Difference

The absolute risk reduction is probably the simplest way of summarising binary data. We simply take the risk of the event for each treatment, p_A and p_B, and take the absolute difference of these, $p_A - p_B$.

One drawback of working on the absolute risk scale is that the difference is bounded by (−1, 1). This bounding can adversely affect inference, especially when a response is near one of the bounds. The effect of bounding of the absolute risk scale is discussed throughout the chapter.

9.3.1.1   *Calculation of Confidence Intervals*

To calculate an estimate of the sample size you generally need an effect size and some estimate of the variation about the response.

9.3.1.2   *Normal Approximation*

Under Normal approximation the confidence interval for the difference in absolute risks is defined as

$$p_A - p_B \pm Z_{1-\alpha/2} se(p_A - p_B), \tag{9.1}$$

where

$$se(p_A - p_B) = \sqrt{\frac{p_A(1-p_A)}{n_A} + \frac{p_B(1-p_B)}{n_B}}. \tag{9.2}$$

This is referred to as the Wald method (Newcombe, 1998b). This confidence interval would be used in conjunction with a chi-squared test. Thus, if a chi-squared test is the planned analysis and the absolute risk difference will be the quantification of effect, then a sample size calculation consistent with (9.1) would be appropriate.

9.3.1.3   *Normal Approximation with Continuity Correction*

We can add a continuity correction to the confidence interval through addition to the right-hand side of (9.1) of $(1/n_A + 1/n_B)/2$ (Newcombe, 1998b; Fleiss, 1981) such that it takes the form

$$p_A - p_B \pm Z_{1-\alpha/2} se(p_A - p_B) + (1/n_A + 1/n_B)/2. \tag{9.3}$$

This confidence interval would be used in conjunction with a continuity corrected chi-squared test. Thus if a continuity corrected chi-squared test is the planned analysis, then the sample size calculation consistent with (9.3) would be appropriate.

Also, if a Fisher's exact test is the planned analysis, then a sample size calculation using a continuity correction maybe appropriate. This is discussed later in the chapter.

9.3.1.4   *Exact Confidence Intervals*

For two independent risks p_A (r_A events in n_A subjects) and p_B (r_B events in n_B subjects) the probability function for their difference $\theta = p_A - p_B$ can be expressed in terms of θ and a nuisance parameter p_B (Agresti, 2003; Agresti and Min, 2001; Newcombe, 1998b):

$$f(r_A, r_B; n_A, n_B, \theta, p_B) = \binom{n_A}{r_A}(\theta + p_B)^{r_A}(1 - \theta - p_B)^{(n_A - r_A)}\binom{n_B}{r_B}p_B^{r_B}(1 - p_B)^{(n_B - r_B)}.$$

(9.4)

To obtain the lower and upper bounds for the 95% confidence interval (9.4) could be used through iteration to obtain the 2.5th and 97.5th percentile. This confidence interval would be used if a Fisher's exact test is the planned analysis; again the sample size calculation should reflect this.

9.3.2   Odds Ratio

The difference between two absolute risks can also be expressed through the odds ratio (*OR*), which is defined as

$$OR = \frac{p_B(1 - p_A)}{p_A(1 - p_B)}.$$

(9.5)

Odds of 2:1 would mean that for every three subjects on a control regimen, for example, we would expect one event (i.e. non-events are twice as numerous as events). Odds of 4:1 on the investigative regimen would mean non-events are four times as numerous. An odds ratio is simply therefore a ratio of two odds and is an assessment of the likelihood of success on one treatment compared to another. Hence, this example odds ratio would be 2, indicating non-events relative to events are twice as numerous on the investigative regimen compared to control.

One of the main advantages of the odds ratio is that it is invariant to the definition of success (Olkin, 1998; Walker, 1998). An analysis based on the odds ratio also easily allows us to adjust for covariates such that estimates can be provided that are independent of, but adjusted for, any predictive factors of interest. As an analysis with covariate adjustment is often the standard analysis it is often used to summarise a trial.

The log odds ratio is also an attractive scale for analysis as it is both unbounded and likely to be additive across a wide range.

9.3.2.1 Calculation of Confidence Intervals

9.3.2.1.1 Normal Approximation

Under the Normal approximation the confidence interval for the log(*OR*) is defined as

$$\log(OR) \pm Z_{1-\alpha/2} se(\log(OR)), \tag{9.6}$$

where the confidence interval on the original odds ratio scale is obtained by back-transforming the confidence interval on the log scale. There are a number of ways of estimating the standard error for the odds ratio (McCullagh, 1980), although in this chapter we concentrate on just one, defined by Whitehead (1993) as

$$Var\ (\text{Log}(OR)) = \frac{12}{n\left(1 - \Sigma_{i=1}^2 \bar{p}_i^3\right)}, \tag{9.7}$$

where $\bar{p}_1 = (p_A + p_B)/2$ and $\bar{p}_2 = 1 - \bar{p}_1$. For just two categories (9.7) becomes

$$\frac{12}{n\left(1 - \Sigma_{i=1}^2 \bar{p}_i^3\right)} = \frac{12}{n\left((\bar{p}_1 + \bar{p}_2)^3 - \bar{p}_1^3 - \bar{p}_2^3\right)} = \frac{4}{n\bar{p}_1(1 - \bar{p}_1)}, \tag{9.8}$$

where

$$2\bar{p}_1(1 - \bar{p}_1) \approx p_A(1 - p_A) + p_B(1 - p_B). \tag{9.9}$$

Thus, the variance for the log(*OR*) is proportional to the reciprocal of the variance for the difference in absolute risks, that is,

$$Var\ \text{Log}(OR) \propto 1/Var(p_A - p_B). \tag{9.10}$$

This Normal approximation confidence interval would be used in conjunction with a chi-squared test. Thus, if a chi-squared test is the planned analysis and an odds ratio will be used to quantify effect, then a sample size calculation consistent with (9.6) would be appropriate.

9.3.2.1.2 Exact Confidence Intervals

Following the notation in Table 9.3, by conditioning on x a sufficient statistic for the odds ratio can be obtained (Fisher, 1935; Chan, 2003; Dunnett and

TABLE 9.3

Notation for Calculation Confidence Intervals about an Odds Ratio

	Number of Successes	Number of Failures	Total
Treatment A	X	$n_A - x$	n_A
Treatment B	Y	$n_B - y$	n_B
Total	n_1	n_2	n

Gent, 1977). Hence, the probability of observing an outcome in the top left cell equal to x can be calculated from a hypergeometric distribution (Troendle and Frank, 2001; Agresti and Min, 2001; Agresti, 2003):

$$P(x;OR) = \frac{\binom{n_A}{x}\binom{n_B}{n_1-x}OR^x}{\sum_{i=0}^{n_1}\binom{n_A}{i}\binom{n_B}{n_1-i}OR^i}. \tag{9.11}$$

In this calculation the assumption is that cell counts follow a multinomial distribution or are independent Poisson or independent binomial, conditioning on the row and column marginal totals (Agresti and Min, 2003).

Using this result therefore two one-sided confidence intervals, each of $\alpha/2$, can be calculated through iteration to find

$$\sum_{(x):OR(x)\leq OR_{obs}} P(x;OR_U) = \alpha/2 \quad \text{and} \quad \sum_{(x):OR(x)\geq OR_{obs}} P(x;OR_L) = \alpha/2, \tag{9.12}$$

to construct a $(1 - \alpha)\%$ confidence interval (Troendle and Frank, 2001). Note that unlike the difference in absolute risks we can compute exact confidence intervals for odds-ratios (Miettinen and Nurminen, 1985). Now the sum extends across all x that satisfy the condition and are possible for the totals n_1 and n_A.

Exact confidence intervals around the odds ratio should be used in conjunction with a Fisher's exact test, and any sample size calculation should reflect this.

9.4 Sample Sizes with the Population Effects Assumed Known

9.4.1 Odds Ratio

For a given binary response, π_A and π_B are defined as the proportion of responders expected on each of the two treatment groups A and B, respectively. Each of these expected responses can in turn be written in terms of odds, $\pi_A/(1 - \pi_A)$ and $\pi_B/(1 - \pi_B)$ (each odds is a ratio of responders over non-responders). As a consequence an odds-ratio can be used as assessment of the treatment difference (and effect size for sample size calculations) where the odds ratio is defined as in (9.5).

In a trial in which the objective is to determine whether there is evidence of a statistical difference between the regimens the null (H_0) and alternative (H_1) hypotheses may take the form

H_0: The two treatments have equal effect with respect to the odds ratio ($OR = 1$).

H_1: The two treatments are different with respect to the odds ratio ($OR \neq 1$).

From these null and alternative hypotheses a formula can be constructed to calculate a sample size per group (Julious et al., 1997, 2000; Campbell, Julious and Altman, 1995; Whitehead, 1993). As discussed in Chapter 1, in general terms for a two-tailed, α-level test the variance of the measure of effect must satisfy

$$Var(S) = \frac{d^2}{(Z_{1-\beta} + Z_{1-\alpha/2})^2},$$ (9.13)

and the variance of the log odds ratio ($S = \log OR$ in this instance) can be approximated by (Whitehead, 1993)

$$Var(S) = \frac{6}{n_A\left(1 - \Sigma_{i=1}^2 \bar{\pi}_i^3\right)},$$ (9.14)

where $\bar{\pi}_i$ is the average response across treatments for each outcome category (i.e. $\bar{\pi}_1 = (\pi_{1_A} + \pi_{2_B})/2$ and $\bar{\pi}_2 = 1 - \bar{\pi}_1$), and α and β are the overall Type I and Type II errors, respectively, with $Z_{1-\alpha/2}$ and $Z_{1-\beta}$, respectively, denoting the percentage points of a standard Normal distribution for these two errors. Here n_A is the sample size for treatment A, assuming equal allocation to treatment and $n_A = n/2$. Note that in this chapter the assumption will be that there is equal allocation to treatment.

Now by equating (9.13) with (9.14) we get

$$n_A = \frac{6[Z_{1-\beta} + Z_{1-\alpha/2}]^2/(\log OR)^2}{\left[1 - \Sigma_{i=1}^2 \bar{\pi}_i^3\right]}.$$ (9.15)

Table 9.4 provides sample sizes for various odds ratios and responses on a given treatment using (9.15). This table was calculated also using the result (9.31) and Table 9.10. A description of these will be given later in this chapter.

9.4.2 Absolute Risk Difference

Keeping the data on the absolute risk difference scale would have the effect expressed in terms of an absolute difference defined as $p_A - p_B$. On this scale the null and alternative hypothesis would be written as

TABLE 9.4

Sample Size Estimates for One Arm of a Parallel Group Trial for Various Expected Outcome Responses for a Given Treatment π_A and Odds Ratios for a Two-Sided Type I Error Rate of 5% and 90% Power

π_A	Odds Ratio					
	1.25	1.50	1.75	2.00	3.00	4.00
0.05	8,002	2,212	1,072	650	208	110
0.10	4,278	1,200	588	362	122	68
0.15	3,058	868	432	268	94	56
0.20	2,468	710	356	224	82	50
0.25	2,132	620	316	200	76	46
0.30	1,926	566	290	186	72	44
0.35	1,800	534	276	180	70	44
0.40	1,726	518	270	176	70	46
0.45	1,692	512	270	176	72	46
0.50	1,694	518	274	180	76	50
0.55	1,730	532	284	188	80	52
0.60	1,804	560	300	200	86	56
0.65	1,924	602	326	218	94	62
0.70	2,106	664	360	242	106	70
0.75	2,382	756	412	278	122	80
0.80	2,820	900	494	334	146	98
0.85	3,574	1,150	632	430	190	126
0.90	5,112	1,654	914	622	276	184
0.95	9,780	3,182	1,766	1,202	536	360

H_0: The two treatments have equal effect with respect to the absolute risk difference ($\pi_A = \pi_B$).

H_1: The two treatments are different with respect to the absolute risk difference ($\pi_A \neq \pi_B$).

There are a number of approaches to calculating a sample size which will now be described.

9.4.2.1 Method 1: Using the Anticipated Responses

A sample size formula using the anticipated responses under the alternative hypothesis—and following the same arguments as (9.13) and (9.14)—where an absolute difference is the response of interest can be derived (Julious et al., 1997; Campbell, Julious and Altman, 1995). For the difference in the response we have (as $n_A = n_B$)

$$Var(S) = \frac{\pi_A(1-\pi_A)+\pi_B(1-\pi_B)}{n_A}, \tag{9.16}$$

TABLE 9.5

Sample Size Estimates Using Method 1 for One Arm of a Parallel Group Trial for Various Expected Outcome Responses for a Given Treatment π_A and Comparator π_B for a Two-Sided Type I Error Rate of 5% and 90% Power

π_A	π_B								
	0.05	0.10	0.15	0.20	0.25	0.30	0.35	0.40	0.45
0.10	578								
0.15	184	915							
0.20	97	263	1,209						
0.25	63	120	331	1,461					
0.30	44	79	158	389	1,671				
0.35	33	54	94	182	437	1,839			
0.40	25	39	62	106	200	473	1,965		
0.45	20	29	44	69	115	214	500	2,048	
0.50	16	23	33	48	74	121	223	515	2,091

and hence equating (9.13) and (9.17) we have

$$n_A = \frac{[Z_{1-\beta} + Z_{1-\alpha/2}]^2 (\pi_A(1-\pi_A) + \pi_B(1-\pi_B))}{(\pi_A - \pi_B)^2}. \tag{9.17}$$

Table 9.5 gives the sample sizes using (9.17).

From (9.9) and (9.16) we can estimate the variance for the difference in absolute risk in terms of the average response. From this we can produce Figure 9.1, which gives the variance for the absolute risk difference for different mean absolute responses. As we can see from this figure, the variances take a "bell" shape in relation to the mean absolute response with a maximum when $\bar{p} = 0.5$.

Another feature to highlight is how the variance is relatively stable for a large range of the mean response (0.3 to 0.7), only varying greatly as the mean response approaches a boundary. From this fact and within this range for the average response a quick estimate of the sample size, for 90% power and a two-sided significance level of 5%, can be obtained from the following result:

$$n_A = \frac{5.25}{(\pi_A - \pi_B)^2}. \tag{9.18}$$

For 80% power and a two-sided significance level of 5% the sample size can be estimated from

$$n_A = \frac{4}{(\pi_A - \pi_B)^2}. \tag{9.19}$$

Both of these results will provide conservative "maximum" estimates of the sample size.

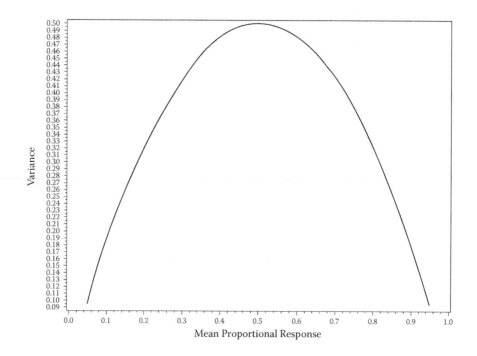

Variance

Mean Proportional Response

FIGURE 9.1 Plot of the variance of an absolute response for different responses.

9.4.2.2   Method 2: Using the Responses under the Null and Alternative Hypotheses

It could be argued that (9.17) is too simplistic as it assumes that we have the same variance under the null and alternative hypotheses. This is not the case, however, as under the null we have $\pi_A = \pi_B$ while under the alternative we have $\pi_A \neq \pi_B$, which give different variances. Hence, in the sample size calculation $Z_{1-\alpha/2}$ should be multiplied by the variance under the null hypothesis, while $Z_{1-\beta}$ should be multiplied by the variance under the alternative hypothesis, that is, something of the form

$$n_A = \frac{(Z_{1-\alpha/2}\sqrt{\text{Variance under Null}} + Z_{1-\beta}\sqrt{\text{Variance under the Alternative}})^2}{(\pi_A - \pi_B)^2}.$$

$$(9.20)$$

Therefore, the sample size can be estimated from

$$n_A = \frac{(Z_{1-\alpha/2}\sqrt{2\bar{\pi}_1(1-\bar{\pi}_1)} + Z_{1-\beta}\sqrt{\pi_A(1-\pi_A)+\pi_B(1-\pi_B)})^2}{(\pi_A - \pi_B)^2}, \qquad (9.21)$$

TABLE 9.6

Sample Size Estimates Using Method 2 for One Arm of a Parallel Group Trial for Various Expected Outcome Responses for a Given Treatment π_A and Comparator π_B for a Two-Sided Type I Error Rate of 5% and 90% Power

π_A	π_B								
	0.05	0.10	0.15	0.20	0.25	0.30	0.35	0.40	0.45
0.10	582								
0.15	188	918							
0.20	102	266	1,212						
0.25	66	134	336	1,464					
0.30	48	82	162	392	1,674				
0.35	36	58	98	186	440	1,842			
0.40	28	42	66	110	204	478	1,970		
0.45	24	34	48	72	118	218	504	2,054	
0.50	20	26	36	52	78	124	228	520	2,096

where $\bar{\pi}_1 = (\pi_A + \pi_B)/2$. Note that with a superiority under the null hypothesis the treatment responses are the same; hence $\pi_A = \pi_B$. An estimate of the response under the null hypothesis is therefore the average response across the two treatments $\bar{\pi}$. This is an estimate of the common response and is used to give an estimate of the variance under the null hypothesis. Sample sizes using (9.21) are given in Table 9.6.

The sample sizes in Table 9.6 are a little conservative compared to Table 9.5. Practically, however, use is often made of (9.9) to demonstrate that (9.17) approximately equates to (9.21) as evidenced empirically from Table 9.7. From this table we can see that for most practical effect sizes (within 0.30) (9.9) holds and hence (9.17) should be a reasonable estimate for (9.21). This is further evidenced through inspection of the sample sizes estimated in Table 9.6 and Table 9.5.

9.4.2.3 Accounting for Continuity Correction

If the final analysis was to be a continuity-corrected chi-squared analysis, then (9.17) and (9.21) should be increased to account for the conservative nature of this test by inflating the estimated sample size n_A to n_{cc}, to account for the continuity correction, from

$$n_{cc} = \frac{n_A}{4} \left[1 + \sqrt{1 + \frac{4}{n_A \delta}} \right]^2. \tag{9.22}$$

The result (9.22) could also be used to estimate the sample size for a Fisher's exact test. Table 9.8 gives estimates of the sample size using (9.22) with (9.21).

TABLE 9.7

Variances Estimated from Two Different Results for Different Expected
Treatment Responses π_A and π_B

a. $\pi_A (1 - \pi_A) + \pi_B (1 - \pi_B)$

					π_B				
π_A	0.10	0.20	0.30	0.40	0.50	0.60	0.70	0.80	0.90
0.1	0.18	0.25	0.30	0.33	0.34	0.33	0.30	0.25	0.18
0.2	0.25	0.32	0.37	0.40	0.41	0.40	0.37	0.32	0.25
0.3	0.30	0.37	0.42	0.45	0.46	0.45	0.42	0.37	0.30
0.4	0.33	0.40	0.45	0.48	0.49	0.48	0.45	0.40	0.33
0.5	0.34	0.41	0.46	0.49	0.50	0.49	0.46	0.41	0.34
0.6	0.33	0.40	0.45	0.48	0.49	0.48	0.45	0.40	0.33
0.7	0.30	0.37	0.42	0.45	0.46	0.45	0.42	0.37	0.30
0.8	0.25	0.32	0.37	0.40	0.41	0.40	0.37	0.32	0.25
0.9	0.18	0.25	0.30	0.33	0.34	0.33	0.30	0.25	0.18

b. $2\bar{\pi}_1 (1 - \bar{\pi})$

					π_B				
π_A	0.10	0.20	0.30	0.40	0.50	0.60	0.70	0.80	0.90
0.1	0.18	0.26	0.32	0.38	0.42	0.46	0.48	0.50	0.50
0.2	0.26	0.32	0.38	0.42	0.46	0.48	0.50	0.50	0.50
0.3	0.32	0.38	0.42	0.46	0.48	0.50	0.50	0.50	0.48
0.4	0.38	0.42	0.46	0.48	0.50	0.50	0.50	0.48	0.46
0.5	0.42	0.46	0.48	0.50	0.50	0.50	0.48	0.46	0.42
0.6	0.46	0.48	0.50	0.50	0.50	0.48	0.46	0.42	0.38
0.7	0.48	0.50	0.50	0.50	0.48	0.46	0.42	0.38	0.32
0.8	0.50	0.50	0.50	0.48	0.46	0.42	0.38	0.32	0.26
0.9	0.50	0.50	0.48	0.46	0.42	0.38	0.32	0.26	0.18

TABLE 9.8

Sample Size Estimates Using Method 2 for One Arm of a Parallel Group Trial for
Various Expected Outcome Responses for a Given Treatment π_A and Comparator
π_B for a Two-Sided Type I Error Rate of 5% and 90% Power

					π_B				
π_A	0.05	0.10	0.15	0.20	0.25	0.30	0.35	0.40	0.45
0.10	622								
0.15	208	958							
0.20	116	286	1,252						
0.25	76	148	356	1,504					
0.30	56	92	176	412	1,714				
0.35	44	66	108	200	460	1,882			
0.40	34	50	74	120	218	498	2,010		
0.45	30	40	56	80	128	232	524	2,094	
0.50	26	32	42	60	86	134	242	540	2,136

TABLE 9.9

Sample Size Estimates for One Arm of a Parallel Group Trial for Various Expected Outcome Responses for a Given Treatment π_A and Comparator π_B for a Two-Sided Type I Error Rate of 5% and 90% Power Assuming Fisher's Exact Test Is the Final Analysis

π_A	π_B								
	0.05	0.10	0.15	0.20	0.25	0.30	0.35	0.40	0.45
0.10	621								
0.15	207	957							
0.20	114	286	1,252						
0.25	69	146	354	1,504					
0.30	51	89	174	412	1,714				
0.35	38	62	107	198	460	1,882			
0.40	31	47	72	119	216	496	2,008		
0.45	24	36	53	79	128	230	523	2,092	
0.50	21	29	41	58	85	134	240	538	2,134

For completeness Table 9.9 is included; it gives sample sizes for Fisher's exact test (Hintze, 2007). We can see from inspection of this table and Table 9.8 that the result using the continuity correction is reasonably close to the Fisher's exact sample sizes provided that the absolute risk difference is less than 0.15 and outside of this is a little conservative.

The advantage of course of (9.22) is that we can calculate sample sizes by hand without recourse to use of a computer.

9.4.3   Equating Odds Ratios with Absolute Risks

Although (9.15) and (9.17) seem on the face of it to be quite different it can be shown that they are approximately algebraically the same (Julious and Campbell, 1996). This comes from the following two results:

$$\frac{6}{\left(1 - \Sigma_{i=1}^{2}\bar{\pi}_i^3\right)} = \frac{2}{\bar{\pi}_1(1-\bar{\pi}_1)}, \qquad (9.23)$$

and

$$\log(OR) \approx \frac{2(OR-1)}{OR+1}, \qquad (9.24)$$

which holds for $0.33 \leq OR \leq 3.00$ (i.e. for most practical differences). Thus,

$$\frac{2(OR-1)}{OR+1} = \frac{2\,(\pi_A - \pi_B)}{\pi_A(1-\pi_B)+\pi_A(1-\pi_B)} \approx \frac{\pi_A - \pi_B}{\bar{\pi}_1(1-\bar{\pi}_1)}, \qquad (9.25)$$

which if substituted back into (9.23) gives the result

$$n_A = (Z_{1-\alpha/2} + Z_{1-\beta})^2 \left(\frac{2}{\bar{\pi}_1(1-\bar{\pi}_1)} \right) \left(\frac{\bar{\pi}_1(1-\bar{\pi}_1)}{\pi_A - \pi_B} \right)^2 \tag{9.26}$$

$$= \frac{2\bar{\pi}_1(1-\bar{\pi}_1)(Z_{1-\alpha/2} + Z_{1-\beta})}{(\pi_A - \pi_B)^2} \tag{9.27}$$

$$\approx \frac{[Z_{1-\beta} + Z_{1-\alpha/2}]^2 (\pi_A(1-\pi_A) + \pi_B(1-\pi_B))}{(\pi_A - \pi_B)^2}. \tag{9.28}$$

Thus, (9.15) and (9.17) can be used interchangeably depending on preference. Due to this property we therefore require

$$\frac{2\bar{\pi}_1(1-\bar{\pi}_1)(Z_{1-\alpha/2} + Z_{1-\beta})}{(\pi_A - \pi_B)^2} \approx \frac{2(Z_{1-\alpha/2} + Z_{1-\beta})^2}{(\log(OR))^2 \bar{\pi}_1(1-\bar{\pi}_1)}. \tag{9.29}$$

Hence, from (9.29) the following approximate result can be derived:

$$\left| \bar{\pi}_A - \bar{\pi}_B \right| \approx \left| \log(OR) \right| (\bar{\pi}_1(1-\bar{\pi}_1)), \tag{9.30}$$

and therefore the absolute risk difference can be written in terms of the odds ratio and the mean overall response.

As a brief note a by-product of the results highlighted in this section is that as a result of (9.30) the null and alternative hypotheses on the absolute risk difference scale can be written as

H_0: The two treatments have equal effect with respect to the absolute risk responses $|\pi_A - \pi_B| = 0$.

H_1: The two treatments are different with respect to the absolute risk responses $|\pi_A - \pi_B| = |\log(OR)| (\bar{\pi}_1(1-\bar{\pi}_1))$.

The practical consequence of these results is that the formulae for the odds ratio and the absolute difference can be used, for all intents and purposes, interchangeably for the same effects sizes.

9.4.4   Equating Odds Ratios with Absolute Risks: Revisited

The result in Section 9.4.3 is quite reassuring in that it demonstrates that you can take two different routes to obtain (approximately) the same answer. A pragmatic approach is assuming we have an estimate of effect in terms of an odds ratio—from a logistic regression say—and an estimate of the control

TABLE 9.10

Expected Outcome Responses for an Investigative Treatment π_B for Various Comparator Response Rates π_A and Odds Ratios

	Odds Ratio					
π_A	1.25	1.50	1.75	2.00	3.00	4.00
0.05	0.06	0.07	0.08	0.10	0.14	0.17
0.10	0.12	0.14	0.16	0.18	0.25	0.31
0.15	0.18	0.21	0.24	0.26	0.35	0.41
0.20	0.24	0.27	0.30	0.33	0.43	0.50
0.25	0.29	0.33	0.37	0.40	0.50	0.57
0.30	0.35	0.39	0.43	0.46	0.56	0.63
0.35	0.40	0.45	0.49	0.52	0.62	0.68
0.40	0.45	0.50	0.54	0.57	0.67	0.73
0.45	0.51	0.55	0.59	0.62	0.71	0.77
0.50	0.56	0.60	0.64	0.67	0.75	0.80
0.55	0.60	0.65	0.68	0.71	0.79	0.83
0.60	0.65	0.69	0.72	0.75	0.82	0.86
0.65	0.70	0.74	0.76	0.79	0.85	0.88
0.70	0.74	0.78	0.80	0.82	0.88	0.90
0.75	0.79	0.82	0.84	0.86	0.90	0.92
0.80	0.83	0.86	0.88	0.89	0.92	0.94
0.85	0.88	0.89	0.91	0.92	0.94	0.96
0.90	0.92	0.93	0.94	0.95	0.96	0.97
0.95	0.96	0.97	0.97	0.97	0.98	0.99

response rate p_A then for $OR > 1$ we have

$$\pi_B = \frac{OR \times \pi_A}{1 - \pi_A + OR \times \pi_A}. \tag{9.31}$$

Hence, with an estimate of π_A and π_B we can use (9.17) [and (9.22)] to estimate the sample size required.

From (9.31) Table 9.10 can be estimated; it gives values for π_B for various π_A and odds ratios,

9.4.5   Worked Example 9.1

McIntyre et al. (2005) undertook a trial to compare the efficacy of buccal midazolam versus rectal diazepam for emergency treatment of epileptic seizures in children. For buccal midazolam the authors observed a therapeutic success rate of 56%. Suppose now we wish to design a new study to investigate a new treatment with buccal midazolam as the control. We expect this new treatment to increase the chances of success to 66%. We wish to have 90% power and a two-sided significance level of 5%.

The quick result to give a "top-end" estimate of the sample size from (9.18) gives an estimate of the sample size as 525 patients per arm. From method 1 and (9.17) the sample size is estimated to be 494.83 or 495 patients per arm. The quick result overestimates the sample size by 30 patients.

If we had used response rates of 35% and 45% (equivalent to 65% and 55%, respectively), then from Table 9.5 the sample size estimate would be 500 patients per arm. From Table 9.6 the sample size is 504 using method 2.

9.4.6   Worked Example 9.2

Taking the response rates to be 35% and 45% and using the estimate of the sample size of 504 we wish to quantify the increase in the sample size assuming a continuity correction is to be used in the final analysis.

If a continuity-corrected chi-squared analysis was planned, then the estimated sample size would be

$$n_{cc} = \frac{n_A}{4}\left[1+\sqrt{1+\frac{4}{n_A\delta}}\right]^2 = \frac{504}{4}\left[1+\sqrt{1+\frac{4}{504\times0.1}}\right]^2$$

$$= 523.8 \text{ or } 524 \text{ patients per arm}$$

or 20 patients more per arm to account for the more conservative nature of the test.

If a Fisher's exact test was to be the final analysis, then Table 9.9 estimates the sample size to be 523 patients per arm.

9.4.7   Worked Example 9.3

Suppose for the same response of 56% for buccal midazolam the effect size of interest is an odds ratio of 2 in favour of the new treatment with a sample size required to achieve a Type II error of 10% and a Type I error of 5%.

Now, from (9.31) an odds ratio of 2 and an expected control response of 0.56 would equate to the following response on the investigative treatment:

$$\pi_B = \frac{OR\pi_A}{(1-\pi_A+OR\pi_A)} = \frac{2\times0.56}{1-0.56+2\times0.56} = 0.72$$

and the sample size would be estimated as 183.9 or 184 patients per arm.

Taking the response on control as 0.55 [$\bar{\pi} = (0.56 + 0.72)/2 = 0.64 \approx 0.65$] then from Table 9.4 the sample size is 188.

Now if 194 subjects is taken as the evaluable sample size with 10% dropouts expected in the study the total sample size to ensure this evaluable sample size would be 188/0.9 = 209 patients per arm.

TABLE 9.11

Hypothetical Data from a Parallel Group Trial

a. Broken Down by Gender

Males

		Outcome			**Females**		Outcome		
		1	0	Total			1	0	Total
Treatment	A	225	75	300	Treatment	A	150	150	300
	B	150	150	300		B	75	225	300
	Total	375	225	600		Total	225	375	600

b. Overall

		Outcome		
		1	0	Total
Treatment	A	375	225	600
	B	225	375	600
	Total	600	600	1,200

9.5   Inclusion of Baselines or Covariates

To illustrate the issues of designing clinical trials when covariates are to be considered with binary data the hypothetical example in Table 9.11 is given.

This example illustrates the issue of covariate adjustment through a logistic regression with a binary response with these hypothetical data taken to be from a parallel group trial designed to compare the outcome of two treatments for which the outcome takes a binary form. There is a known prognostic factor, gender, that exists, and there is perfect balance with respect to this factor and no interaction between the factor and treatment (see Table 9.11a) with an odds ratio equal to 3 in each subgroup. If we collapsed the data and ignored the covariate the estimated odds ratio is biased down to 2.78 (see Table 9.11b). Hence the unadjusted collapsed response gives a biased (towards the null) estimate of treatment effect.

This hypothetical example nicely illustrates the issues as the unadjusted log odds ratio has a smaller standard error of 0.119 compared to 0.125 for a logistic regression. Hence, the standard error has increased by 5% through covariate adjustment. However, this effect is more than offset by the bias in the log odds ratio, with the unadjusted log odds ratio being 1.022 ($OR = 2.78$) compared to an adjusted 1.099 ($OR = 3.00$). A 7.5% increase occurs in the log odds ratio by adjusting. Thus, bias introduced by not adjusting it seems will pull the estimate nearer to the null despite any reduction in the standard error.

As discussed in Chapter 3 in the analysis of the results of a clinical trial, the effects of treatment on the response of interest are often adjusted for predictive factors, such as demographic or clinical covariates, by fitting them concurrently with the treatment variable. It was highlighted in this chapter how when adjusting for a highly predictive covariate, such as baseline, the sample size can be dramatically reduced due to a reduction in the variance estimate for data anticipated to take a Normal form.

With binary data we do not have such a marked effect. Not adjusting for covariates biases the estimate of effect towards the null response (in terms of odds ratios), although this is countered also by a reduction in the variance.

In the context of sample size calculations the saying "as ye shall analyse is as ye shall design" would need to be considered such that if a logistic regression is planned as the final analysis than an estimate of response from an equivalent analysis would be optimal to get estimates of treatment effect. However, such considerations are not as critical as with Normal data.

9.6   Sample Size Re-estimation

For binary data sample size re-estimation is relatively straightforward for we could use the average anticipated response rate $\bar{\pi}_1$, which we can estimate blind to the actual treatment allocation. From (9.9), (9.17) can be rewritten as

$$n_A = \frac{2[Z_{1-\beta} + Z_{1-\alpha/2}]^2 \bar{\pi}_s(1-\bar{\pi}_s)}{(\pi_A - \pi_B)^2}.$$ (9.32)

In the context of the problem here $\bar{\pi}_s$ is the average response used in the sample size calculation. Suppose now $\bar{\pi}_I$ is the average response estimate from the interim analysis; then all things being equal, assuming that the treatment effect is as per the sample size calculation, the sample size can be re-estimated as

$$n_A = \frac{2[Z_{1-\beta} + Z_{1-\alpha/2}]^2 \bar{\pi}_I(1-\bar{\pi}_I)}{(\pi_A - \pi_B)^2}.$$ (9.33)

The convention for the sample size re-assessment would be to have some form of restricted sample size re-estimation with the following procedure applied as for Normal data discussed in Chapter 3:

1. Take an initial estimate of the same size: n (say).
2. After a proportion of subjects has been enrolled (say $n/2$) recalculate the sample size n_1, using the same sample size criteria Type I error, power, effect size.
3. The re-estimated sample size is taken as max (n, n_1).

9.7 Sensitivity Analysis about the Estimates of the Population Effects Used in the Sample Size Calculations

In Chapter 3 the concept of a sensitivity analysis of a trial design was first introduced for data anticipated to take a Normal form in which the trial's sensitivity was assessed with respect to the variance estimate used in the calculations.

For binary data, however, it is the response rate on the control arm p_A, usually estimated from a previous clinical study as an estimate of population response, to which the study design is sensitive. This control response rate in turn feeds into the estimate of variance used in the calculations. Hence, any imprecision in the estimation of the control response rate will have an impact on the study design.

To investigate the effect the imprecision of the estimate of the control response rate will have on the study design a range of plausible values could be obtained through construction of a 95% confidence interval. From the two tails of this confidence interval a re-estimation of the variance could be made. The power could then be assessed using these new variance estimates through use of the following equation for absolute risk differences—(9.17) rewritten in terms of power

$$1 - \beta = \Phi\left(\sqrt{\frac{n(p_A - p_B)^2}{(p_A(1 - p_A) + p_B(1 - p_B))}} - Z_{1-\alpha/2} \right) \tag{9.34}$$

and the following for odds ratios[(9.15) rewritten in terms of power]

$$1 - \beta = \Phi\left(\sqrt{n(\log OR)^2 \left[1 - \sum_{i=1}^{2} \overline{p}_i^3 \right]/6} - Z_{1-\alpha/2} \right). \tag{9.35}$$

These calculations would assess the sensitivity of the study design to plausible values for the control response rate.

In truth due to the stability of the variance of the absolute risk within the range (0.3, 0.7) there would be less need to assess a study's sensitivity if the anticipated response is to be around 50%. Due to (9.10) the same is also true for the odds ratios. For anticipated responses outside of (0.3, 07), however, there may be a need to assess sensitivity.

9.7.1 Worked Example 9.4

Suppose previously we had conducted a trial in 50 patients in which the control event rate was estimated to be 50%. We wished with 90% power and two-sided significance to reduce this to 40%. The sample size from Table 9.6 was estimated to be 519 patients per arm.

TABLE 9.12

Sensitivity Analysis for Superiority Worked Example

a. Absolute Risk Scale

	Observed	95% Confidence Interval	
		Lower	Upper
Control response	0.50	0.36	0.64
Investigative response	0.40	0.26	0.53
Power	90%	94%	91%

b. Odds Ratio Scale

	Observed	95% Confidence Interval	
		Lower	Upper
Control response	0.50	0.36	0.64
Investigative response	0.40	0.28	0.54
Power	90%	86%	89%

A 95% confidence interval for this point estimate would give the true value as between 36% and 64%. Table 9.12a gives the equivalent calculations assuming the effect was fixed at an absolute difference of 10%. We can see from these results that if a lower or higher response rate than expected was observed the power would actually increase. The reason for this, recalling from discussion in this chapter, is that the maximum value the variance could possibly be on the absolute risk difference scale is when the response rate is expected to be in the middle of the range. This is a situation we approximately anticipate to observe here (although the pooled two-group variance is a little different as it accounts for the anticipated investigative response rate).

Table 9.4b gives the sensitivity of the study design using the odds ratio, which for this example is 1.5, to calculate the sample size, which from Table 9.4 is estimated as 517 patients per arm. Assuming the effect stays the same at 1.5 we can see from Table 9.4b that there is only a small loss in power of 4% if the control response rate is 36% and a nominal loss if the response of 64% was observed.

9.7.2   Worked Example 9.5

Worked Example 9.4 was a special case in that the response was anticipated to be towards the middle of the range. Suppose though that the control response was expected to be 20%, and this was estimated from a study with 50 patients on the control arm. The sample size from Table 9.4 required for an odds ratio of 1.5 is 900 patients per arm.

The equivalent calculation on the absolute risk scale gives a sample size of 917 (a control response rate of 20% and an odds ratio of 1.5 equates to an absolute difference of 5.7%).

TABLE 9.13

Sensitivity Analysis for Superiority Worked Example

A. Absolute Risk Scale

	Observed	95% Confidence Interval	
		Lower	Upper
Control response	0.200	0.089	0.311
Investigative response	0.143	0.034	0.254
Power	90%	>90%	77%

b. Odds ratio scale

	Observed	95% Confidence Iinterval	
		Lower	Upper
Control response	0.200	0.089	0.311
Investigative response	0.143	0.061	0.231
Power	90%	62%	>90%

Table 9.13 gives the same sensitivity analysis as conducted with Table 9.12. We can see here we get quite markedly different answers compared to Table 9.12 with the absolute risk difference scale quite sensitive to the assumptions around active response rate.

What these examples highlight is the complexity of investigating the sensitivity of a study with an uncertain control response rate. The sensitivity of the design varies according to the anticipated control response rate.

9.8 Calculations Taking Account of the Imprecision of the Estimates of the Population Effects Used in the Sample Size Calculations

As highlighted in Section 9.7 if a study has a primary endpoint that is binary then a study's design would not be relatively sensitive with respect to the variance of the anticipated response as long as the anticipated response is within the range (0.3, 0.7). Given this, the calculations that are now described may seem to be a little laborious as there are no general solutions, and numerical methods have to be applied.

However, although a study may be robust within the range (0.3, 0.7) outside this range they can be quite sensitive, and although the calculations may be a little time consuming they should be considered when designing clinical trials. Clinical trials are expensive and can take a long time to run, so spending a little time up front on optimising the sample size calculation could prove to be beneficial.

9.8.1 Odds Ratio

Assume in this instance that it is the control response rate p_A, estimated from a previous study, that is random, and that the effect size of interest is the odds ratio and is fixed. Using an appropriate confidence interval methodology an estimate of the first, second and third percentiles, say, of p_A can be made based on the previously observed p_A. In this instance these percentiles are estimated using a Normal approximation.

For each percentile the corresponding anticipated response on the investigative arm can be estimated from

$$p_B = \frac{1}{\exp\left(\log(OR) - \log\left(\frac{p_A}{1-p_A}\right)\right) + 1}. \tag{9.36}$$

Now for the case of the $\log(OR)$ remember the approximate result

$$Var\left(\log(OR)\right) = \frac{6}{n_A\left(1 - \Sigma_{i=1}^2 \bar{p}_i^3\right)} \tag{9.37}$$

and an estimate of the variance can be made for each percentile. If we took the average across all the percentiles, then for a given sample size n and imprecision around the estimate of p_A the power can be estimated from

$$1 - \beta = \frac{1}{0.998} \sum_{perc=0.001}^{0.998} 0.5 \left[\begin{array}{c} \Phi\left(\sqrt{n_A(\log OR)^2\left[1 - \Sigma_{i=1}^2 \bar{p}_{perc_i}^3\right]/6} - Z_{1-\alpha/2}\right) \\ + \Phi\left(\sqrt{n_A(\log OR)^2\left[1 - \Sigma_{i=1}^2 \bar{p}_{(perc+0.001)_i}^3\right]/6} - Z_{1-\alpha/2}\right) \end{array} \right]. \tag{9.38}$$

Then (9.38) can be iterated on n until the appropriate power has been reached.

9.8.2 Absolute Risk Difference

Remember that, for the difference in absolute risks $p_A - p_B$, the variance is defined as

$$Var(p_A - p_B) = \frac{p_A(1-p_A)}{n_A} + \frac{p_B(1-p_B)}{n_B}. \tag{9.39}$$

As described for an odds ratio using the Normal approximation percentiles for p_A can be estimated from previously observed p_A. Now assuming the effect size $p_A - p_B$ is fixed then for each percentile the corresponding anticipated response on the investigative arm can be estimated from

$$p_B = p_A + Effect \tag{9.40}$$

and an estimate of the variance made from (9.39). Correspondingly an estimate of the power for a given n and imprecision about p_A can be made from

$$1-\beta = \frac{1}{0.998} \sum_{perc=0.001}^{0.998} 0.5 \left[\Phi\left(\sqrt{\frac{n_A(p_A-p_B)^2}{(p_{perc_A}(1-p_{perc_A})+p_{perc_B}(1-p_{perc_B}))}} - Z_{1-\alpha/2}\right) + \Phi\left(\sqrt{\frac{n_A(p_A-p_B)^2}{(p_{(perc+0.001)_A}(1-p_{(perc+0.001)_A})+p_{(perc+0.001)_B}(1-p_{(perc+0.001)_B}))}} - Z_{1-\alpha/2}\right) \right].$$

(9.41)

The sample size can be estimated through iteration.

9.8.3   Worked Example 9.6

An investigator wishes to design a study in which the response anticipated on the control therapy is 20%. The effect of interest is an odds ratio of 2.0 "in favour" of the control therapy (i.e. the aim is to reduce the number of events), and the investigator wishes to design the study with Type I and II errors fixed at 5% and 10%, respectively. From (9.15) the sample size required would be 333 patients per arm of the trial.

Now suppose this estimate of the control response rate came from a trial with 50 patients receiving the control. To allow for the imprecision in the estimate of the control response rate the sample size [from (9.38)] would need to increase to 354 patients.

9.9   Calculations Taking Account of the Imprecision of the Estimates Used in the Sample Size Calculations: Bayesian Methods

If the primary endpoint is a binary response, then it is the uncertainty in the estimation of this response that adversely affects sample size calculations. The context now is to interrogate sample sizes for which a superiority study is being planned and a control response p_A had previously been observed. In the prospective trial being designed inference is to be made about the 'true' difference $\pi_A = \pi_B$.

The utility of Bayesian methods now is that they allow us to draw not only on retrospective data about the anticipated control response but also on our subjective belief regarding the response while accounting for the imprecision in the initial estimates.

In context with the problem here the effect size (whether an odds ratio or an absolute risk difference) is assumed known so that the variance for the odds ratio and absolute risk difference can be estimated from (9.36) and (9.39), respectively, as before.

For the given sample size what needs to be determined is the probability of observing a given control response p_{Ai} or greater for θ given that p_{A1} has already been observed, that is, $Prob(\theta > p_{Ai} \mid p_{A1})$.

For inference about an unknown binary parameter θ, what we are interested in is how our belief about θ would change. If the prior is expressed in the density $p(\theta)$ and if subsequently data x is observed then the posterior distribution is expressed in the density $p(\theta \mid x)$, where the Bayes rule for densities is

$$p(\theta \mid x) \propto \lambda(x \mid \theta) \, p(\theta), \tag{9.42}$$

where $\lambda(x \mid \theta)$ is the likelihood function.

For binary data the Beta distribution can be used for the prior responses such that

$$PROBBETA(p_A, a, b) \propto p_A{}^{a-1}(1 - p_A)^{b-1}, \tag{9.43}$$

where $PROBBETA(\bullet)$ is defined as a cumulative density distribution for a beta distribution. The Bayesian updating rules are now described. Although not directly comparable this chapter draws on the work of Johnson et al. (2004).

9.9.1   Prior Response

Prior values for $PROBBETA(p_{perc_A}, a_0, b_0)$ (and the corresponding $P_{perc_A} = BETAINV(perc, a_0, b_0)$) could be derived as follows. For an informative prior we could use the mode (or most likely value) and a percentile to build a prior. For a Beta distribution the mode is defined by

$$m = \frac{a_0 - 1}{a_0 + b_0 - 2}.$$

Hence, the a_0 (and consequently b_0) could be derived from

$$p_{percentile} = BETAINV(percentile, a_0, [a_0 - 1] / m - a_0 + 2) \tag{9.44}$$

if a percentile for the control response can be postulated. If we wished to use a non-informative prior, then a Jeffrey's prior could be used such that

$$P_{perc_A} = BETAINV(perc, 0.5, 0.5). \tag{9.45}$$

This Jeffrey's prior has the advantage of being invariant with respect to transformations.

9.9.2   Anticipated Response

The anticipated control response (and consequent variance) is defined as p_{A_1}. This value is taken from an objective value observed in a previous clinical trial. The control response equates to an observed number of successes a_1 and failures b_1.

9.9.3   Posterior Response

With the anticipated prior responses the posterior distribution can be calculated from the following result:

$$P_{perc_A} = BETAINV(perc, a_1 + a_0, b_1 + b_0) \tag{9.46}$$

These values for $P_{perc_A} = BETAINV(perc, a_1 + a_0, b_1 + b_0)$ can be used in (9.38) and (9.41) to obtain estimates of the sample size for an odds ratio and an absolute risk difference, respectively, accounting for the imprecision in the control response estimate.

9.9.4   Worked Example 9.7

Repeating Worked Example 9.6 in which an investigator wished to design a study in which the response anticipated on the control therapy was 20%. The effect size of interest is an odds ratio of 2.0 "in favour" of the control therapy with the investigator wishing to design the study with Type I and II errors fixed at 5% and 10%, respectively.

Now, again, suppose this estimate of the control response rate came from a trial with 50 patients receiving the control and the investigator wished to allow for this imprecision in the estimate of the control response rate in the estimation of the sample size.

9.9.4.1   Non-informative

If initially a non-informative prior was used, then the percentiles for our prior response would be estimated from (9.45). A plot of the prior is given in Figure 9.2a. The distribution of observed response would be estimated from $P_{perc_A} = BETAINV(perc, 10, 40)$ and is given in Figure 9.2b. Finally the posterior would be estimated from (9.46) as $P_{perc_A} = BETAINV(perc, 10.5, 40.5)$ and is given in Figure 9.2c. As we have a non-informative prior the posterior and the observed response would virtually be the same, as illustrated in Figure 9.2d.

To calculate the sample size we would use (9.46) in (9.38), which gives an estimate of 354 patients. The sample size is as calculated previously when allowing for the imprecision in the sample variance in Worked Example 9.6, which is not surprising given that the posterior and the observed response are virtually the same.

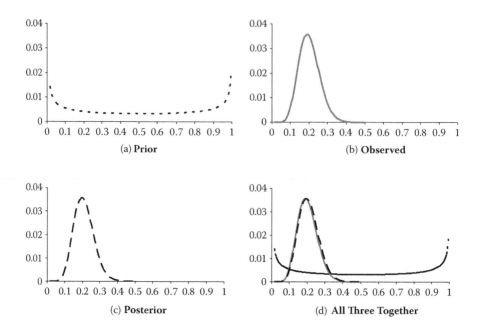

FIGURE 9.2 Plot of the prior, observed and anticipated responses for the control with a non-informative prior.

9.9.4.2 Sceptical Prior

Imagine now the investigator was sceptical regarding the control response being as high as 20% such that the belief was that the most likely response was 15% with at least 90% certainty that it was greater than 10%.

From (9.44) estimates of a_0 and b_0 of 7.899 and 40.094, respectively, are obtained. The prior for the percentiles for the control response would hence be $P_{perc_A} = BETAINV(perc, 7.899, 40.094)$. Figure 9.3a gives an illustration of the prior distribution.

The observed response would still be $P_{perc_A} = BETAINV(perc, 10, 40)$ and is given in Figure 9.3b although with a slightly rescaled y axis compared to Figure 9.2b. Finally the posterior would be taken from (9.46) as $P_{perc_A} = BETAINV(perc, 17.899, 80.094)$ and is given in Figure 9.2c. Figure 9.2d gives all three distributions together.

Hence, using (9.46) in (9.38) the estimate of the sample size is now 379, which is a little higher than before.

9.9.4.3 Optimistic

Now suppose the investigator is more optimistic about the control response, believing the most likely response to be 25%, and is at least 90% certain that

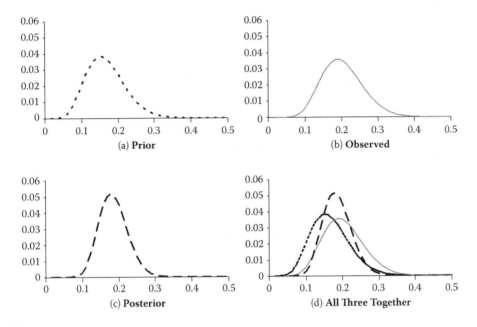

FIGURE 9.3 Plot of the prior, observed and anticipated responses for the control with a sceptical prior.

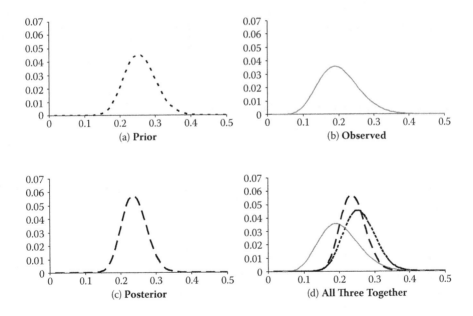

FIGURE 9.4 Plot of the prior, observed and anticipated responses for the control with an optimistic prior.

it was greater than 20%. From (9.44) estimates of a_0 and b_0 of 25.048 and 73.144, respectively, are obtained. Figure 9.4 gives an illustration of the different responses.

Hence, now using (9.46) in (9.38) a sample size estimate of 297 is calculated. This is less than the sample size calculated not allowing for impression in the variance.

Note here we have undertaken calculations using the odds ratio. Similar calculations could be done if calculations were based around an absolute difference in the responses. Here, though (in terms of the variance), an optimistic prior would be one for which the response is lower than 20%, and a pessimistic prior would be one for which the response is higher than 20%.

 Key Messages

- There are a number of approaches for calculating sample size when the primary endpoint is binary with the main deciding factor regarding which approach to use being the planned analysis.
- The study design is relatively robust with respect to assumptions about the variance of the anticipated response as long as the anticipated response is within the range (0.3, 0.7).
- Covariate adjustment has little effect on sample size calculations if the primary endpoint is binary.
- Sample size re-estimation is relatively straightforward with a binary primary endpoint.

10

Sample Size Calculations for Superiority Cross-over Clinical Trials with Binary Data

10.1 Introduction

When the data are paired, such as in a cross-over trial, there are two main summary measures that can be used: the difference in proportions and the odds ratio. This chapter concentrates on these two summary measures in considering sample size calculations. The methodologies are now discussed in detail.

10.2 Analysis of a Trial

For a cross-over trial with a binary primary endpoint the data could be summarised as per Table 10.1 and analysed by the McNemar test

$$\frac{(n_{10} - n_{01})^2}{n_{10} + n_{01}} \sim \chi_1^2,$$

where n_{10} and n_{01} are the number of responses expected in cells '10' and '01', respectively. The data in the final column and final row of the table give the overall responses for each treatment. These overall responses are the outcomes we may expect in a parallel group study.

In a cross-over trial only discordant responses are of interest for statistical comparisons (i.e. those subjects who respond '10' or '01'). A large proportion of subjects are thus discarded in constructing a statistical test as the test is conditional on subjects being discordant. This is quite intuitive, though, as in a superiority trial concordant responses agree with the null hypothesis of no treatment differences. Thus, what we are determining is whether for those subjects who only respond to one treatment if this response is more likely to be in favour of one treatment over the other.

TABLE 10.1

Summary of Hypothetical Cross-over Trial

		Treatment B		
		1	0	
Treatment A	1	n_{11}	n_{10}	n_{A1}
	0	n_{01}	n_{00}	n_{A0}
		n_{B1}	n_{B0}	n

10.2.1 Sample Size Estimation with the Population Effects Assumed Known

Table 10.1 can be rewritten in terms of proportions as per Table 10.2, where $\lambda_{10} = n_{10}/n$, $\lambda_{01} = n_{01}/n$, $\lambda_{11} = n_{11}/n$ and $\lambda_{00} = n_{00}/n$ and $p_A = n_{A1}/n$ and $p_B = n_{B1}/n$; the trial can be summarised with an odds ratio defined as

$$\psi = \frac{\lambda_{10}}{\lambda_{01}}. \tag{10.1}$$

This odds ratio is a conditional summary statistic, using just the discordant responses. A conditional odds ratio can be difficult to interpret. To assist in the interpretation the odds ratio can be approximated from the marginal totals (Royston, 1993),

$$\text{Odds ratio} = \psi \approx \frac{p_A(1-p_B)}{p_B(1-p_A)}, \tag{10.2}$$

where $\lambda_{10} \approx p_A(1-p_B)$, and $\lambda_{01} \approx p_B(1-p_A)$. Thus, the conditional odds ratio for a cross-over trial can be interpreted in terms of the odds ratio from a parallel group study (approximated from the marginal proportions). This is of particular use in the calculation of sample sizes as marginal totals could be used to estimate the conditional odds ratio, which in turn can be used to estimate the discordant sample size.

The discordant sample size n_d for a cross-over trial can be derived from (Royston, 1993; Julious, Campbell and Altman, 1999; Connett, Smith and

TABLE 10.2

Summary of Hypothetical Cross-over Trial

		Treatment B		
		1	0	
Treatment A	1	λ_{11}	λ_{10}	p_A
	0	λ_{01}	λ_{00}	$1 - p_A$
		p_B	$1 - p_B$	1

McHugh, 1987; Fleiss and Levin, 1988; Schesselman, 1982)

$$n_d = \frac{(Z_{1-\alpha/2}(\psi+1)+2Z_{1-\beta}\sqrt{\psi})^2}{(\psi-1)^2},$$ (10.3)

which has performed well in simulations (Julious and Campbell, 1998). The result (10.3) could be considered useful as the sample size is defined only in terms of the effect size ψ. There are no "unknowns" such as the anticipated proportion of responders on a given treatment.

Practically, therefore, a discordant sample size calculation could be estimated based around a clinically meaningful difference, and sufficient numbers of subjects could be recruited until this target discordant sample size is reached.

For budgetary and planning purposes there would need to be an estimate of the total sample size also, here the number of subjects needed to be enrolled to ensure a sufficient discordant sample size. To calculate the total sample size, the discordant sample size is divided by the proportion expected to be discordant (Julious, Campbell and Altman, 1999; Connett, Smith and McHugh, 1987), that is,

$$N_c = \frac{n_d}{\lambda_{01}+\lambda_{10}}.$$ (10.4)

Table 10.3 gives sample sizes for various odds ratios for (10.3).

TABLE 10.3

Discordant Sample Size for a
Cross-over Trial with 90% Power and
Two-Sided Significance Level of 5%

Odds Ratios	Sample Size
0.05	8
0.10	12
0.15	16
0.20	20
0.25	25
0.30	32
0.35	42
0.40	53
0.45	69
0.50	91
0.55	121
0.60	164
0.65	230
0.70	334
0.75	511
0.80	848
0.85	1,595
0.90	3,791
0.95	15,983

TABLE 10.4

Summary of Anticipated Responses for Worked Example

		Buccal Midazolam		
		1	0	
New treatment	1	0.40	0.32	0.72
	0	0.16	0.12	0.28
		0.56	0.44	

10.2.1.1 Worked Example 10.1

In Chapter 9 we introduced a trial to assess the effects of buccal midazo-lam that was designed as a parallel group trial. Suppose the trial could be run as a cross-over trial. Table 10.4 gives a summary of the antici-pated treatment responses for the two treatments. An odds ratio of 2 is of interest and we wish to have 90% power at the two-sided 5% level of significance.

The marginal totals in Chapter 9 and here are used to complete the table. Using (10.3) an estimate of the discordant sample size for the trial would be

$$n_d = \frac{(Z_{1-\alpha/2}(\varphi+1)+2Z_{1-\beta}\sqrt{\psi})^2}{(\psi-1)^2} = \frac{(1.96(2+1)+2\times1.282\sqrt{2})^2}{(2-1)^2} = 90.36.$$

The discordant sample size required is thus 91 subjects, which could be used for recruitment purposes (i.e. we would enrol sufficient numbers of patients until we observed 91 that were discordant).

We could have instead used Table 10.3. An odds ratio of 2 is equivalent (ignoring the sign of the effect) to an odds ratio of 0.5. From Table 10.3 we also get a sample size of 91 subjects.

For planning purposes we need to have an estimate of the total sample size, which we will estimate from (10.4). The total sample size is thus 91/0.48 = 189.6 or 190 subjects.

10.2.1.2 Worked Example 10.2

An investigator wishes to design a study in which the marginal response anticipated on the control therapy is 40%. The effect of interest is 2.0 in favour of the control therapy, and the investigator wishes to design the study with Type I and II errors fixed at 5% and 10%, respectively.

An anticipated control response of 40% and an odds ratio of 2.0 would equate to a response of 25% on the investigative therapy. Hence, the mar-ginal responses, as per Table 10.5, can be completed, as can the remain-ing entries in the table, through multiplying the marginal totals. From this

TABLE 10.5

Summary of Anticipated Responses for Worked Example

		Investigative		
		1	0	
Control	1	0.10	0.30	0.40
	0	0.15	0.45	0.60
		0.25	0.75	1

table it is evident that the odds ratio defined through (10.1) and (10.2) are the same.

The discordant sample size required would be 91 subjects, with the total sample size estimated as 203 subjects.

10.2.2 Comparison of Cross-over and Parallel Group Results

The sample size for one arm in a parallel group trial n_{pg} can be estimated from (10.5) (Campbell, Julious and Altman, 1995; Whitehead, 1993)

$$n_{pg} = \frac{6\,(Z_{1-\alpha/2}+Z_{1-\beta})^2/(\log OR)^2}{\left[1-\sum\limits_{i=0}^{1}\bar{\pi}_i^3\right]}, \tag{10.5}$$

where $\bar{\pi}_0$ and $\bar{\pi}_1$ are the responses across treatments for outcomes 0 and 1, respectively, such that $\bar{\pi}_1 = (\pi_A + \pi_B)/2$ and $\bar{\pi}_1 = 1 - \bar{\pi}_0$. On the face of it (10.3) and (10.4) are quite dissimilar to (10.5). However, (10.4) can be rewritten as

$$n_c = \frac{(Z_{1-\alpha/2}(\pi_{10}+\pi_{01})+2Z_{1-\beta}\sqrt{\pi_{10}\pi_{01}})^2}{(\pi_{10}+\pi_{01})(\pi_{10}-\pi_{01})^2}, \tag{10.6}$$

and in turn rewriting π_{10} and π_{01} in terms of the marginal totals $(\pi_{10} \approx \pi_A(1-\pi_B)$ and $\pi_{01} \approx \pi_B(1-\pi_A))$ (10.6) can be approximated by

$$n_c \approx \frac{(Z_{1-\alpha/2}(\pi_A(1-\pi_B)+\pi_B(1-\pi_A))+2Z_{1-\beta}\sqrt{\pi_A(1-\pi_B)\pi_B(1-\pi_A)})^2}{(\pi_A(1-\pi_B)+\pi_B(1-\pi_A))(\pi_A(1-\pi_B)-\pi_B(1-\pi_A))^2}. \tag{10.7}$$

Also, through the following results $\pi_A(1-\pi_B)\pi_B(1-\pi_A) \approx \bar{\pi}_0^2(1-\bar{\pi}_0)^2$ and $\pi_A(1-\pi_B)+\pi_B(1-\pi_A) \approx 2\bar{\pi}(1-\bar{\pi})$ (10.7) can be rewritten as

$$n_c \approx \frac{(Z_{1-\alpha/2}+Z_{1-\beta})^2\,2\bar{\pi}_0^2(1-\bar{\pi}_0)^2}{\bar{\pi}_0(1-\bar{\pi}_0)(\pi_A-\pi_B)^2}. \tag{10.8}$$

Returning to the case of a parallel group trial in which the odds ratio (*OR*) is defined as

$$OR = (\pi_A(1-\pi_B))/(\pi_B(1-\pi_A))$$

and remember

$$\log(OR) \approx \frac{\pi_A - \pi_B}{\bar{\pi}_0(1-\bar{\pi}_0)},$$

(10.9)

$$\frac{6}{\left(1-\sum\limits_{i=0}^{1}\bar{\pi}_i^3\right)} = \frac{2}{\bar{\pi}_0(1-\bar{\pi}_0)}.$$

(10.10)

Substituting (10.9) and (10.10) back into (10.8) we get

$$n_c \approx \frac{6(Z_{1-\alpha/2}+Z_{1-\beta})^2/(\log OR)^2}{\left[1-\sum\limits_{i=0}^{1}\bar{\pi}_i^3\right]} = n_{pg},$$

(10.11)

and the sample size formula for one arm in a parallel group study. Thus, the sample size required for a cross-over trial is approximately equivalent to that for one arm of a parallel group trial. An alternative way of phrasing this would be to say that the sample size required is half that required in total for a parallel group trial.

The practical application of this result is that when designing a clinical trial we could use the marginal effects expected for the respective treatments and consequently the effect sizes anticipated if the trial was a parallel group investigation. These effects could then be used in the parallel group formula—taking the one arm sample size to be the total sample size. Working with the marginal totals may make it easier to formulate effects, and consequently trials should be easier to design.

In the rest of this chapter the approach of using the sample size formula for one arm of a parallel group trial as the total sample for a cross-over trial is the approach applied.

Note also that the conditional odds ratio is not the same as the marginal odds ratio but can be an approximation to "all things being equal".

10.2.2.1 *Worked Example 10.3*

In Worked Example 10.2 a sample size was calculated for a study based on the marginal totals. The sample size was estimated to be 203 patients in total. If instead we had used (10.5) the total sample size would be 200 patients.

Note that there is a little rounding here as $91/0.45 = 203$ while $90.36/0.45 = 201$. Either way, we can see that the two approaches give quite similar sample sizes.

If we wished to base the sample size purely on the discordant sample size, recruiting until the discordant sample size is reached, then the sample size would be (using the result of 200 per arm) $200 \times (0.30 + 0.15)$ or 90 patients.

10.2.2.2 Worked Example 10.4

An investigator wishes to design a study in which the anticipated response on the control therapy is 50%. The effect of interest is an odds ratio of 1.5 in favour of the investigative therapy, and the investigator wishes to design the study with Types I and II errors fixed at 5% and 10%, respectively. From Table 10.6 (taken from Chapter 9) we can see that the total sample size required would be 518 patients.

With a response rate of 50% anticipated on the control an odds ratio of 1.5 would equate to an investigative response rate of 60% or a 10% increase.

TABLE 10.6

Total Sample Size Estimates for a Cross-over Trial Using Parallel Group Methodology for Various Expected Outcome Responses for a Given Treatment π_A and Odds Ratios for a Two-Sided Type I Error Rate of 5% and 90% Power

	Odds Ratio					
π_A	1.25	1.50	1.75	2.00	3.00	4.00
0.05	8,002	2,212	1,072	650	208	110
0.10	4,278	1,200	588	362	122	68
0.15	3,058	868	432	268	94	56
0.20	2,468	710	356	224	82	50
0.25	2,132	620	316	200	76	46
0.30	1,926	566	290	186	72	44
0.35	1,800	534	276	180	70	44
0.40	1,726	518	270	176	70	46
0.45	1,692	512	270	176	72	46
0.50	1,694	518	274	180	76	50
0.55	1,730	532	284	188	80	52
0.60	1,804	560	300	200	86	56
0.65	1,924	602	326	218	94	62
0.70	2,106	664	360	242	106	70
0.75	2,382	756	412	278	122	80
0.80	2,820	900	494	334	146	98
0.85	3,574	1,150	632	430	190	126
0.90	5,112	1,654	914	622	276	184
0.95	9,780	3,182	1,766	1,202	536	360

If we had used (10.3), then we would have estimated the discordant sample size to be 258.6 or 259 subjects. The total sample size by (10.4) would be 259/0.55 = 471 subjects.

10.3 Analysis of a Trial Revisited

As well as ignoring concordant data, the McNemar test ignores the fact that subjects are assigned to different sequences, that is, either AB or BA for a two-period cross-over trial, and thus ignores any possible existing period effect. To allow for any possible period effect Table 10.1 can be re-written as sequence differences as in Table 10.7. The numbers in Table 10.7 can, in turn, be rewritten in terms of Table 10.8 as $a_1 + a_2 = n_{10}$, $b_1 + b_2 = n_{01}$ and $n_{AB} + n_{BA} = n_d$.

This approach is analogous to the period-adjusted t test (Senn, 1993). Sequence differences can be used to give a period-adjusted estimate of the odds ratio by taking the log odds ratio for sequence B-A away from A-B and dividing by 2

$$\text{Log } \psi = (\log \psi_{AB} - \log \psi_{BA})/2 =$$

$$(\log a_1/b_1 - \log b_2/a_2)/2 = 0.5 \log(a_1 a_2/b_1 b_2) = 0.5 \log OR_p, \qquad (10.12)$$

where OR_p is the period-adjusted odds ratio. From (10.12) it is therefore evident that the non-period odds ratio is equivalent to the square-rooted odds

TABLE 10.7

Summary of Period-Adjusted Analysis of Hypothetical Cross-over Trial

Sequence Difference	Treatment Difference		Total
	−1	1	
A-B	a_1	b_1	n_{AB}
B-A	b_2	a_2	n_{BA}

TABLE 10.8

Summary of Period-Adjusted Analysis of Hypothetical Cross-over Trial

Sequence Difference	Treatment Difference	
	−1	+1
A-B	p_{a_1}	p_{b_1}
B-A	p_{b_2}	p_{a_2}
	$\bar{p}_{-1}$	$\bar{p}_{+1}$

ratio from the period-adjusted analysis. Thus, $\psi = \sqrt{OR_p}$, and hence a test statistic for the period-adjusted test can be derived

$$\frac{\log(\psi)^2}{\text{var}(\log(\psi))} \sim \chi_1^2.$$

(10.13)

Therefore, (10.13) is asymptotically equivalent to the McNemar test as well as to alternative period-adjusted tests such as the Mainland-Gartt test and the Prescott test (Senn, 1993).

The period-adjusted approach described here is an extension of the two-group analysis described by Whitehead (1993) and McCullagh (1980). The period-adjusted analysis can be undertaken via logistic regression using the sequence difference as the outcome with sequence in the model. The log odds ratio derived from this analysis would be the same as (10.12), and the test statistic would be (10.13). To attain an estimate of the odds ratio and confidence interval equivalent to the McNemar test you must exponentiate and then square root the $\log(OR_p)$ from the analysis.

If a period-adjusted analysis were undertaken on data for which there is no period effect, then there would be no effect on the inference. The converse is not true. Imagine there are two treatment sequences AB and BA with the odds ratios for each treatment sequence defined, respectively, as

$$\psi_{AB} = \frac{ka_1}{b_1} = k\psi \quad \text{and} \quad \psi_{BA} = \frac{kb_2}{a_2} = \frac{k}{\psi},$$

where k ($k < 1.00$) is the known period effect. It is therefore evident that for the special case of $a_1 = a_2$ and $b_1 = b_2$ an unbiased estimate of the odds ratio is obtained no matter what the value of the odds ratio and k. However, if the period difference is ignored such that the data is simply pooled across the sequences, then the naïve estimate of the odds ratio, assuming k and ψ are known, is defined as

$$\psi_p = \frac{\psi k(\psi + k) + \psi(\psi k + 1)}{k(k\psi + 1) + (\psi + k)}.$$

(10.14)

The bias estimated from (10.14) is given in Table 10.9 for different values of k. It is evident therefore that by ignoring a possible period effect the results are becoming biased towards the null hypothesis, with the bias increasing with increasing effect size (in absolute terms but not relatively). Overall, though, except for large period differences, the bias is relatively small.

As with previous chapters how you plan to analyse a trial will influence how you calculate the sample size. If a period-adjusted analysis is planned, then an estimate of the odds ratio from a trial with such a trial would be optimal. However, the bias due to ignoring the possible effect of period is not great, so a recommendation is to ignore the effect of period and stick to the relatively straightforward sample size calculations described using (10.3) and (10.5).

TABLE 10.9

Bias in Estimated Odds Ratio through Ignoring Possible Period Effects

	Odds Ratio						
k	1.00	1.25	1.50	1.75	2.00	3.00	4.00
0.50	1.000	1.220	1.435	1.647	1.857	2.684	3.500
0.60	1.000	1.233	1.463	1.691	1.918	2.818	3.711
0.70	1.000	1.241	1.481	1.721	1.959	2.908	3.853
0.80	1.000	1.247	1.493	1.738	1.984	2.963	3.941
0.90	1.000	1.249	1.498	1.747	1.996	2.992	3.987
1.00	1.000	1.250	1.500	1.750	2.000	3.000	4.000

We do not mention period-adjusted sample size calculations again in this book.

10.4 Sensitivity Analysis about the Estimates of the Population Effects Used in the Sample Size Calculations

Following from the arguments on equating the one-arm sample size of a parallel trial with that of the total sample size of a cross-over study, the methodology described in Chapter 9 for parallel group studies can be adapted to assess the sensitivity of a cross-over trial.

To investigate sensitivity of the study design to the imprecision of the estimate of control marginal response rate a range of plausible values could be constructed through a 95% confidence interval. The power could then be assessed for the two tails of this confidence interval, with the effect size fixed, by using the following, which is (10.5) rewritten in terms of power

$$1 - \beta = \Phi \left(\sqrt{n(\log OR)^2 \left[1 - \sum_{i=0}^{1} \bar{p}_i^3 \right] / 6} - Z_{1-\alpha/2} \right). \tag{10.15}$$

10.5 Calculations Taking Account of the Imprecision of the Estimates of the Population Effects Used in the Sample Size Calculations

As with assessing the sensitivity of a study to calculate the total sample size of a cross-over study to account for the imprecision in the variance estimate used in the sample size calculations, the results from the parallel group case

can be extended to give

$$1-\beta = \frac{1}{0.998} \sum_{perc=0.001}^{0.998} 0.5 \left[\begin{array}{l} \Phi\left(\sqrt{n(\log OR)^2\left[1-\sum_{i=0}^{1}\bar{p}_{perc_i}^3\right]}/6 - Z_{1-\alpha/2}\right) \\ +\Phi\left(\sqrt{n(\log OR)^2\left[1-\sum_{i=0}^{1}\bar{p}_{(perc+0.001)_i}^3\right]}/6 - Z_{1-\alpha/2}\right) \end{array} \right],$$

(10.16)

which can be iterated on n until the appropriate power has been reached.

10.6 Calculations Taking Account of the Imprecision of the Estimates Used in the Sample Size Calculations: Bayesian Methods

Bayesian methods described for parallel group trials in Chapter 9 can also be extended to studies with a cross-over design. A posterior distribution for a control response can be estimated, and (10.16) can be used for sample size estimation.

Key Messages

- Marginal totals can be used to estimate the responses in a crossover trial to assist in the sample size calculations.
- Sample size calculations for one arm of a parallel group trial can be used as an estimate of the total sample size for a cross-over study.

11

Sample Size Calculations for Non-inferiority Trials with Binary Data

11.1 Introduction

Before describing sample size calculations for non-inferiority trials we recall the definitions of the null (H_0) and alternative (H_1) hypotheses:

H_0: A given treatment is inferior with respect to the risk response ($\pi_A \geq \pi_B$).

H_1: The given treatment is non-inferior with respect to the risk response ($\pi_A < \pi_B$).

These hypotheses can be written in terms of a clinical difference d (Committee for Proprietary Medicinal Products [CPMP], 2000; Chen, Tsong and Kang, 2000; Chan, 2003)

$$H_0: \pi_A - \pi_B \geq d$$

$$H_1: \pi_A - \pi_B < d$$

where d is the non-inferiority margin (Julious, 2004d; Chen, Tsong and Kang, 2000; Committee for Medicinal Products for Human Use [CHMP], 2005).

The standard approach is to test the null hypothesis using a one-sided test at the 2.5% level of significance (International Conference on Harmonisation [ICH] E9, 1998). Operationally non-inferiority is tested through constructing a 95% confidence interval and declaring non-inferiority if the appropriate (lower or upper) bound excludes the limit d; this is how most non-inferiority trials are actually analysed (Julious, 2004d).

The issue to highlight in the context of this chapter is that under both the null and alternative hypotheses there is a non-zero difference between treatments; this has implications in the estimation of the variance. For non-inferiority trials with a Normal response as discussed in Chapter 6 we also have non-zero difference under the null and alternative hypotheses, but we can assume the variance remains constant for both hypotheses. Similarly for superiority trials with binary data we have different variances under the null and alternative hypotheses, but the estimation of these variances is straightforward. For non-inferiority trials there are issues with variance estimation that are highlighted in the chapter.

11.2 Choice of Non-inferiority Limit

The choice of non-inferiority (and equivalence) limit was discussed generally in Chapters 1 and 2. However, it is worth reinterrogating this issue for binary data as it is one of the few areas in which there is regulatory guidance. The guidance is for the antimicrobial therapeutic area in which active controlled trials are the norm, although the issues raised are generic to other therapeutic areas.

Table 11.1 gives the non-inferiority margins for different response rates as recommended by CPMP (2004a) and the Food and Drug Administration (FDA; 1992). The FDA guidelines are redundant now, but they do raise interesting points.

What is evident from Table 11.1 is that whilst the CPMP recommends a flat equivalence margin the FDA margins are a step function according to the anticipated control response rate. Table 11.1 is also figuratively described in Figure 11.1.

It is when considering non-inferiority trials (and equivalence trials in Chapter 12) that we can see an advantage of working on the odds ratio scale as working with a step function does present problems when working with absolute differences. Suppose we designed a trial based on an anticipated active response rate of 78% and a margin of 20%, but we actually observed 82%. This brings us over into the next margin level of 15%.

Working on the odds ratio scale avoids the problems associated with a stepped non-inferiority margin. This is because on the odds ratio scale a fixed margin would equate to different margins on the absolute risk scale. This has been recognised by a number of authors. Garrett (2003) recommended using a margin of 0.5 on the odds ratio scale, whilst Senn (1997) recommended a margin of 0.55 and Tu (1998) a margin of 0.43. However, a

TABLE 11.1

Non-inferiority Margins for Different
Control Response Rates

Response Rate (%)	Non-inferiority Margin (%)	
	FDA	**CPMP**
≥90	−10	10
80–89	−15	10
70–79	−20	10

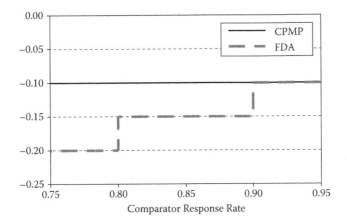

FIGURE 11.1 Graphical illustration of CPMP and FDA non-inferiority limits.

margin of 0.47 would be one that seems to perform best. The relative merits of these margins can be seen in Table 11.2 and Figure 11.2.

Table 11.2 gives the equivalent difference on the proportional scale for different odds ratios and control response rates. The margin of 0.55 is the most conservative and would guarantee that the difference is no greater than 15% no matter what the control prevalence is, while that of 0.50 although less conservative has the advantage of being a round number. Figure 11.2 figuratively demonstrates these points as a repeat of Figure 11.1 with the margins of 0.50 and 0.43 now included.

TABLE 11.2

Differences on the Proportional Scale That Are Equivalent to Different Odds Ratios for Various Anticipated Expected Responses on One Treatment Arm

p_A	Odds Ratio					
	0.40	0.45	0.47	0.50	0.55	0.60
0.95	0.066	0.054	0.051	0.045	0.037	0.031
0.90	0.117	0.098	0.091	0.082	0.068	0.056
0.85	0.156	0.132	0.123	0.111	0.093	0.077
0.80	0.185	0.157	0.147	0.133	0.113	0.094
0.75	0.205	0.176	0.165	0.150	0.127	0.107
0.70	0.217	0.188	0.177	0.162	0.138	0.117
0.65	0.224	0.195	0.184	0.169	0.145	0.123
0.60	0.225	0.197	0.187	0.171	0.148	0.126
0.55	0.222	0.195	0.185	0.171	0.148	0.127
0.50	0.214	0.190	0.180	0.167	0.145	0.125

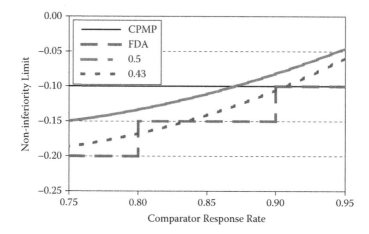

FIGURE 11.2 Graphic illustration of CPMP and FDA non-inferiority limits on the proportional scale for fixed odds ratios.

11.3 Parallel Group Trials Sample Size with the Population Effects Assumed Known

11.3.1 Absolute Risk Difference

The issue in calculating the sample is that under both the null and alternative hypotheses there is a non-zero difference between treatments. Generally, the sample size can be thought of in terms

$$n_A = \frac{(Z_{1-\alpha}\sqrt{\text{Variance under Null}} + Z_{1-\beta}\sqrt{\text{Variance under the Alternative}})^2}{((\pi_A - \pi_B) - d)^2},$$

$$(11.1)$$

where $Z_{1-\alpha}$ is multiplied by the variance under the null hypothesis, and $Z_{1-\beta}$ is multiplied by the variance under the alternative hypothesis. Now (11.1) can be thought of in terms of

$$n_A = \frac{(Z_{1-\alpha}\sqrt{\pi_A(1-\pi_A) + \pi_B(1-\pi_B)} + Z_{1-\beta}\sqrt{\pi_A(1-\pi_A) + \pi_B(1-\pi_B)})^2}{((\pi_A - \pi_B) - d)^2}, \quad (11.2)$$

where π_A and π_B are estimates of the responses on treatment under the null hypothesis used to estimate the variance under this hypothesis, that is,

$$\frac{\pi_A(1-\pi_A)}{n_A} + \frac{\pi_B(1-\pi_B)}{n_B}. \quad (11.3)$$

Now, for non-inferiority trials we can have that $\pi_A \neq \pi_B$; that is, the two treatments do not have an equal response. As the estimates of π_A and π_B affect the estimate of the variance the definition of the null hypothesis hence influences the variance under this hypothesis. There are a number of ways of estimating (11.3); three are now discussed.

11.3.1.1   Method 1: Using Anticipated Responses

The first method of estimating the variance under the null hypothesis is simply to replace π_A and π_B with anticipated estimates of the response, π_A and π_B, respectively (Dunnett and Gent, 1977; Farrington and Manning, 1990). Hence, the variance under the null hypothesis becomes

$$\frac{\pi_A(1-\pi_A)}{n_A} + \frac{\pi_B(1-\pi_B)}{n_B}. \tag{11.4}$$

Hence, for the special case of an equal sample size between groups (i.e. $n_A = n_B$) a direct estimate of the sample size can be obtained from (Dunnett and Gent, 1977)

$$n_A = \frac{(\pi_A(1-\pi_A)+\pi_B(1-\pi_B))(Z_{1-\beta}+Z_{1-\alpha})^2}{((\pi_A-\pi_B)-d)^2}, \tag{11.5}$$

where π_A is the assumed proportion of responses expected in subjects on treatment A, and π_B is the assumed proportion of responses in subjects on treatment B.

11.3.1.2   Method 2: Using Anticipated Responses in Conjunction with the Non-inferiority Limit

The second method is to estimate π_A and π_B from (Dunnett and Gent, 1977)

$$\tilde{\pi}_A = (\pi_A+\pi_B+d)/2 \quad \text{and} \quad \tilde{\pi}_B = (\pi_A+\pi_B-d)/2, \tag{11.6}$$

where d is the non-inferiority limit. Hence, (11.6) can be applied to the estimate of the variance (11.3), and an estimate of the sample size can be obtained from (11.2).

For (11.2) to be used the following inequality must hold (Farrington and Manning, 1990):

$$\max\{-d,d\} < \pi_A + \pi_B < 2 + \min\{-d,d\}. \tag{11.7}$$

The equation (11.7) can be violated, but it holds for all sensible values for d, π_A and π_B; that is, if we set $d = 0.20$ when we expected a response rate of 0.90 for both regiment A and B it will be violated, but this is not a logical limit for such a high response rate. For $d = 0.10$, a more sensible limit, (11.7) would not be violated.

11.3.1.3 Method 3: Using Maximum Likelihood Estimates

The third method is to use maximum likelihood estimates for p_A and p_B (Farrington and Manning, 1990; Miettinen and Nurminen, 1985; Koopman, 1984) defined, respectively, as

$$\pi_A = 2u\cos(w) - \frac{b}{3a} \quad \text{and} \quad \pi_B = \pi_A + d_1 \tag{11.8}$$

to enter into (11.3) where $d_1 = \pi_A(1-d)d$, $c = d^2 - 2d(\pi_A + 1) + \pi_A + \pi_B$, $b = -(2 + \pi_A + \pi_B - 3d)$, $a = 2$, $u = \text{sign}(v)\sqrt{(b^2)/(9a^2) - c/(3a)}$, $w = [\pi + \cos^{-1}(v/u^3)]/3$ and $v = b^3/(27a^3) - (bc)/(6a^2) + d_1/(2a)$. With (11.8) and (11.3) an estimate of the sample size can be estimated from (11.2).

11.3.1.4 Comparison of the Three Methods of Sample Size Estimation

As evidenced by their descriptions the three methods for estimating the variances under the null hypothesis are markedly different, and as a consequence they give different estimates for the sample size. The differences are not marked except for high response rates—greater than 85%. Method 3 is the most conservative approach, while Method 1 is the least conservative.

This book concentrates on using Method 1 as it is consistent with the approach described for superiority trials in Chapter 9. As discussed in this chapter if there are question marks with respect to the assumptions in the sample size calculations, then these would need to be investigated.

Table 11.3 gives sample sizes for Method 1 for a finite range of responses for reference.

11.3.2 Odds Ratio

For non-inferiority studies the variance of the measure of effect must satisfy

$$Var(S) = \frac{(d - \Delta)^2}{(Z_{1-\alpha} + Z_{1-\beta})^2}, \tag{11.9}$$

and the variance about the log odds ratio can be approximated by (Whitehead, 1993)

$$Var(S) = \frac{6}{n_A \left(1 - \sum_{i=0}^{1} \bar{\pi}_i^3 \right)}, \tag{11.10}$$

TABLE 11.3

Sample Sizes for a Non-inferiority Study Estimated from Method 1 for 90% Power and a Type I Error Rate of 2.5%

π_A	π_B	Limit	Sample Size	π_A	π_B	Limit	Sample Size
0.70	0.70	0.05	1,766	0.80	0.70	0.15	1,556
		0.10	442		0.75	0.10	1,461
		0.15	197			0.15	366
		0.20	111		0.80	0.05	1,344
	0.75	0.05	418			0.10	337
		0.10	186			0.15	150
		0.15	105		0.85	0.05	303
		0.20	67			0.10	135
	0.80	0.05	173			0.15	76
		0.10	98		0.90	0.05	117
		0.15	63			0.10	66
		0.20	44			0.15	43
	0.85	0.05	89				
		0.10	57	0.85	0.75	0.15	1,324
		0.15	40		0.80	0.10	1,209
		0.20	29			0.15	303
	0.90	0.05	51		0.85	0.05	1,072
		0.10	36			0.10	268
		0.15	26			0.15	120
		0.20	20		0.90	0.05	229
0.75	0.70	0.10	1,671			0.10	102
		0.15	418			0.15	58
		0.20	186	0.90	0.85	0.10	915
	0.75	0.05	1,577		0.90	0.05	757
		0.10	395			0.10	190
		0.15	176				
		0.20	99				
	0.80	0.05	366				
		0.10	163				
		0.15	92				
		0.20	59				
	0.85	0.05	148				
		0.10	83				
		0.15	54				
		0.20	37				
	0.90	0.05	73				
		0.10	47				
		0.15	33				
		0.20	24				

TABLE 11.4

Sample Sizes for Different Non-inferiority Limits on the Odds Ratio Scale and Anticipated Responses for 90% Power and Type I Error of 2.5%

π_A	Odds Ratio	Margin			
		0.43	0.47	0.50	0.55
0.80	0.7	498	745	1,044	2,031
	0.8	319	435	557	876
	0.9	234	302	369	525
	1.0	185	231	274	368
	1.1	154	187	218	282
	1.2	132	158	181	228
	1.4	105	122	137	167
0.85	0.7	612	915	1,282	2,496
	0.8	396	539	690	1085
	0.9	292	377	460	655
	1.0	232	290	344	462
	1.1	194	236	275	355
	1.2	167	200	230	289
	1.4	133	156	175	212
0.9	0.7	848	1,268	1,778	3,460
	0.8	553	753	965	1518
	0.9	411	531	648	923
	1.0	328	410	487	654
	1.1	275	336	391	505
	1.2	239	286	328	412
	1.4	191	223	251	304

where $\bar{\pi}_i$ is the average response across each outcome category [$\bar{\pi}_1 = (\pi_A + \pi_B)/2$ and $\bar{\pi}_1 = 1 - \bar{\pi}_0$]. By equating (11.9) with (11.10) the sample size can be estimated from

$$n_A = \frac{6[Z_{1-\beta} + Z_{1-\alpha}]^2}{\left[1 - \sum_{i=0}^{1} \bar{\pi}_i^3\right](\log(OR) - d)^2},$$

(11.11)

where d in this instance is the non-inferiority limit on the log odds ratio scale. In this chapter appropriate values were mentioned as $\log(0.43)$, $\log(0.50)$ or $\log(0.55)$ as well as $\log(0.47)$; Table 11.4 gives sample sizes from (11.11) for these.

11.3.2.1 Worked Example 11.1

An investigator wishes to design a trial in which the anticipated response rate on the active control is 85%. The investigator also expects an 85%

response rate on the investigative therapy. Using an odds ratio of 0.50 for the non-inferiority limit (11.11) gives the sample size as 344 patients per arm. In comparison working on the absolute risk scale, with the same anticipated responses but with a non-inferiority limit of 15%, we require just 120 patients per arm.

Note here that although the sample sizes seem quite disparate for the odds ratio scale compared to the proportional scale, we must bear in mind that we are not comparing like with like. For an anticipated control response of 85%, an odds ratio of 0.5 equates to an 11.1% difference, a little short of 15%.

If we used a 10% non-inferiority limit then the sample size would increase to 268 patients per arm.

11.3.3 Superiority Trials Revisited

In Chapter 6 it was discussed how, instead of setting up a non-inferiority study, we could set up a superiority study but with a significance level greater than the nominal 2.5%. This would have the benefit of ensuring that the observed active response rate is greater than the control $(\pi_B > \pi_A)$ even if a lower bound of a 95% confidence interval passes zero.

If a study was being set up as a superiority study the sample size for a given power and one-tailed level of significance can be estimated from

$$n_A = \frac{(Z_{1-\alpha}\sqrt{2\bar{\pi}(1-\bar{\pi})} + Z_{1-\beta}\sqrt{\pi_A(1-\pi_A) + \pi_B(1-\pi_B)})^2}{(\pi_A - \pi_B)^2}, \qquad (11.12)$$

where $\bar{\pi} = (\pi_A + \pi_B)/2$. Note that under the superiority null hypothesis $\pi_A = \pi_B$, so we use $\bar{\pi}$ (a common response) to estimate the variance under the null hypothesis. Sample sizes using (11.12) are given in Table 11.5. The sample sizes are given for different control response rates and different improvements on the investigative treatment, assuming $\pi_B > \pi_A$.

11.3.4 Sensitivity Analysis about the Estimates of the Population Effects Used in the Sample Size Calculations

As highlighted in Chapter 9 for superiority trials, it is the response rate on control p_A, an estimate of π_A, to which the study design is sensitive. This response rate in turn feeds into the estimate of variance used in the calculations.

Non-inferiority studies may be particularly sensitive to assumptions about the control response both as the control response is often anticipated to be quite high (which has an impact on the variance estimate) and because a high control response rate may make showing non-inferiority more difficult (it may narrow the effect the investigative treatment has over the control).

TABLE 11.5

Sample Sizes for a Superiority Study for Different Significance Levels for 90% Power for Various Anticipated and Control Response Rates

π_A	$\pi_B - \pi_A$	Significance Level							
		0.025	0.050	0.075	0.100	0.125	0.150	0.175	0.200
0.50	0.025	8,402	6,848	5,920	5,254	4730	4296	3928	3606
	0.050	2,096	1,708	1,476	1,310	1180	1072	980	900
	0.075	928	756	654	580	522	474	434	398
	0.100	520	424	366	324	292	266	242	222
0.55	0.025	8,276	6,746	5,832	5,174	4658	4232	3868	3552
	0.050	2,054	1,674	1,448	1,284	1156	1050	960	882
	0.075	904	738	638	566	510	462	422	388
	0.100	504	410	354	314	284	258	236	216
0.60	0.025	7,982	6,506	5,624	4,990	4492	4082	3732	3424
	0.050	1,970	1,606	1,388	1,232	1108	1008	920	846
	0.075	862	704	608	540	486	442	404	370
	0.100	478	388	336	298	268	244	224	204
0.65	0.025	7,520	6,128	5,298	4,702	4232	3846	3516	3226
	0.050	1,844	1,502	1,300	1,152	1038	942	862	792
	0.075	802	654	566	502	452	410	374	344
	0.100	440	358	310	276	248	226	206	190
0.70	0.025	6,888	5614	4854	4,308	3878	3522	3220	2956
	0.050	1,676	1,366	1,180	1,048	944	856	784	718
	0.075	722	588	510	452	406	370	338	310
	0.100	394	320	278	246	222	202	184	168
0.75	0.025	6,090	4,964	4,292	3,808	3428	3114	2846	2614
	0.050	1,466	1,194	1,032	916	824	750	684	628
	0.075	624	508	440	390	352	320	292	268
	0.100	336	274	236	210	188	172	156	144
0.80	0.025	5,122	4,176	3,610	3,204	2884	2620	2394	2198
	0.050	1,212	988	854	758	682	620	568	520
	0.075	508	414	358	318	286	260	238	218
	0.100	266	218	188	166	150	136	124	114
0.85	0.025	3,988	3,250	2,810	2,494	2244	2040	1864	1712
	0.050	918	748	648	574	518	470	430	394
	0.075	372	304	262	232	210	190	174	160
	0.100	188	154	132	118	106	96	88	80
0.90	0.025	2,684	2,188	1,892	1,678	1512	1372	1254	1152
	0.050	582	474	410	364	328	298	272	250

As with superiority trials the sensitivity of the non-inferiority study design to the control response rate can be investigated through construction of a 95% confidence interval. The power could then be assessed at the two tails of the confidence interval.

The following result for the absolute difference could be used to investigate the sensitivity of a study. Note that in this formula the study design will be sensitive to both the control response rate and the variance,

$$1 - \beta = \Phi\left(\sqrt{\frac{n_A((p_A - p_B) - d)^2}{(p_A(1 - p_A) + p_B(1 - p_B))}} - Z_{1-\alpha}\right). \tag{11.13}$$

The equivalent result to investigate the sensitivity of study about an odds ratio is

$$1 - \beta = \Phi\left(\sqrt{n_A(\log(OR) - d)^2\left[1 - \sum_{i=1}^{2} \bar{p}^3\right]/6} - Z_{1-\alpha}\right). \tag{11.14}$$

11.3.4.1 Worked Example 11.2

Suppose that in Worked Example 11.1 the control response rate was assessed from a previous study in 100 patients. It was assumed that the investigative response rate is correct at 85% with a confidence interval that indicates that a plausible range for the control response is between 78% and 92%.

Table 11.6 gives a breakdown of the sensitivity of the study design to the estimate of the control response rate. For this example it is the upper point of the confidence interval to which the study is sensitive.

TABLE 11.6

Sensitivity Analysis for Non-inferiority

a. Absolute Difference

	Observed	95% Confidence Interval Lower	Upper
Control response	0.85	0.78	0.92
Non-inferiority margin	0.15	0.15	0.15
Investigative response	0.85	0.85	0.85
Power	90%	>90%	11%

b. Odds Ratio Scale

	Observed	95% Confidence Interval Lower	Upper
Control response	0.85	0.78	0.92
Investigative response	0.85	0.850	0.850
Power	90%	>90%	3%

For this worked example therefore we have designed a study with 90% power based on a previously observed control response rate of 85%. If the true control response rate is nearer to 78% (which is plausible based on the confidence interval), then we would have greater than the nominal power set *a priori*. However, if the control response was truly 92%, then our power could be as low as 3%.

Note in this example when assessing the sensitivity it was assumed that if we observed a control response rate lower or higher than expected, then the original non-inferiority would still be used. However, if a higher-than-expected control response rate was observed, then this may not be appropriate.

11.3.5   Absolute Risk Difference versus Odds Ratios Revisited

Calculations on the odds ratio scale are overly sensitive, compared to the absolute difference, to assumptions around the variance. In fact this is a function of the properties of the odds ratio—the fact that a fixed odds ratio would equate to smaller and smaller differences as the control response gets greater. In comparison on the absolute difference scale the margins are relatively fixed (albeit stepped) such that the same margin could be used, 10%, independent of the anticipated response.

Which statistical analysis, and consequent sample size calculation, to use depends on the robustness of our assumptions. If it is reasonable to have relatively fixed margins, then we can work completely on the absolute risk scale. If we wish to have more flexible margins then we should work on the odds ratio scale.

In truth, however, there is no generic answer regarding which scale to use. For example an anticipated response of 90% raises far greater questions (should the margin narrow if a response rate greater than 90% is observed?) than one of 80%. Thus, the decision regarding most calculations must be undertaken on a case-by-case basis with a thorough investigation made of the sensitivity of one's calculations to the assumptions inherent in them.

11.3.6   Calculations Taking Account of the Imprecision of the Estimates of the Population Effects Used in the Sample Size Calculations

As described in Chapter 9 for superiority trials, using appropriate confidence interval methodology around the observed control response rate p_A, the power and, hence iteratively, the sample size can be calculated using numerical methods. By extending this methodology the power for a non-inferiority trial, in which the absolute risk difference is of interest, can be estimated from the result

$$
1-\beta = \frac{1}{0.998} \sum_{perc=0.001}^{0.998} 0.5 \left[\begin{array}{c} \Phi\left(\sqrt{\dfrac{n_A((p_A-p_B)-d)^2}{(p_{perc_A}(1-p_{perc_A})+p_B(1-p_B))}} - Z_{1-\alpha} \right) + \\[2em] \Phi\left(\sqrt{\dfrac{n_A((p_A-p_B)-d)^2}{(p_{(perc+0.001)_A}(1-p_{(perc+0.001)_A})+p_B(1-p_B))}} - Z_{1-\alpha} \right) \end{array} \right].
$$

(11.15)

The equivalent calculation for a non-inferiority study design around the odds ratio would be estimation from

$$
1-\beta = \frac{1}{0.998} \sum_{perc=0.001}^{0.998} 0.5 \left[\begin{array}{c} \Phi\left(\sqrt{n_A(\log(OR)-d)^2 \left[1-\sum_{i=1}^{2}\bar{p}_{perc}^3\right]/6} - Z_{1-\alpha} \right) \\[2em] +\Phi\left(\sqrt{n_A(\log(OR)-d)^2 \left[1-\sum_{i=1}^{2}\bar{p}_{(perc+0.001)}^3\right]/6} - Z_{1-\alpha} \right) \end{array} \right].
$$

(11.16)

Consequently the sample can be estimated through iteration; that is, for each sample size we can estimate the power of the study, and we iterate on the sample size until the requisite power is reached.

11.3.6.1 Worked Example 11.3

Suppose that the investigator wishes to revisit the calculation from Worked Example 11.1 to allow for the fact that the control response rate was estimated from 100 patients. Repeating the sample calculations on the absolute difference scale decreases the size to 122 patients per arm. This is a sample size two greater than the original calculation.

11.3.7 Calculations Taking Account of the Imprecision of the Estimates Used in the Calculation of Sample Sizes: Bayesian Methods

The percentiles for a posterior control response can be calculated as described in Chapter 9. From these percentiles (11.15) and (11.16) could be used to estimate the sample size allowing for the imprecision in the estimate of the control response rate (Julious, 2004c).

It is best to highlight the points through a worked example.

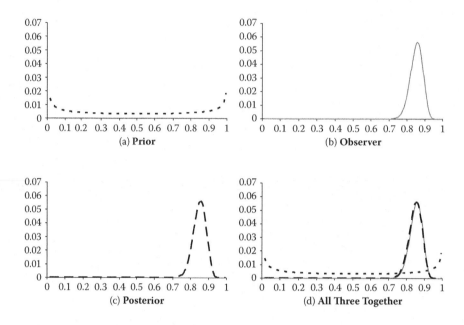

FIGURE 11.3 Prior, observed and posterior responses for a non-informative prior.

11.3.7.1 Worked Example 11.4

With a non-informative prior, $a_1 = 85$, $b_1 = 15$ and $a_0 = 0.5$ and $b_0 = 0.5$. The distributions of the different responses are given in Figure 11.3. The sample size is estimated to be 122 patients per arm. This is the same as calculated in Worked Example 11.3.

With a more pessimistic prior, the most likely response is 80% with 90% certainty that it is greater than 75%, $a_1 = 85$, $b_1 = 15$ and $a_0 = 106.304$ and $b_0 = 27.326$. The distributions for the different responses are given in Figure 11.4. The sample size as a result is increased to 139 patients per arm.

With a prior that the control response rate observed is about right, the most likely response is 85% with 90% certainty that it is greater than 80%, $a_1 = 85$, $b_1 = 15$ and $a_0 = 98.716$ and $b_0 = 18.244$. The distributions for the responses are given in Figure 11.5. The sample size is estimated to be 122 patients per arm—the same as with a non-informative prior.

11.3.8 Calculations Taking Account of the Imprecision of the Estimates of the Population Effects with Respect to the Assumptions about the Mean Difference and the Variance Used in the Sample Size Calculations

When we are designing a non-inferiority study the imprecision in the risk difference as well as the variance may be of importance. This is particularly so for non-inferiority studies (and equivalence studies described in Chapter 12)

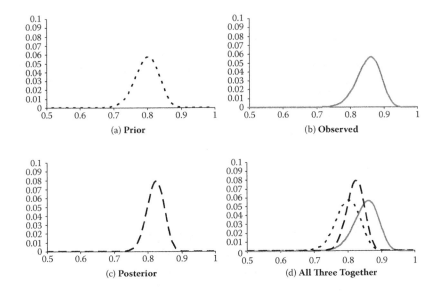

FIGURE 11.4 Prior, observed and posterior responses for a pessimistic prior.

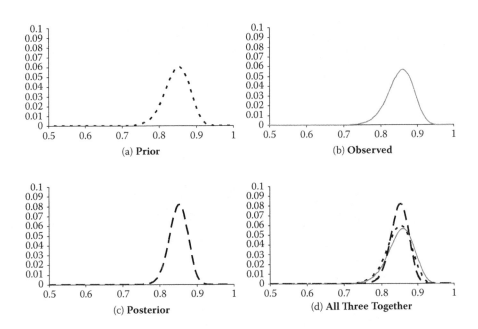

FIGURE 11.5 Prior, observed and posterior responses for an optimistic prior.

in which the mean response, assessed by p_A, feeds into the assumptions about both the risk difference and the variance.

To allow for the imprecision in the risk difference and variance we could use numerical methods to calculate the sample size on the absolute difference scale and obtain

$$1 - \beta = \frac{1}{0.998} \sum_{perc=0.001}^{0.998} 0.5 \left[\begin{array}{c} \Phi\left(\sqrt{\dfrac{n_A((p_{perc_A} - p_B) - d)^2}{(p_{perc_A}(1 - p_{perc_A}) + p_B(1 - p_B))}} - Z_{1-\alpha} \right) + \\[3ex] \Phi\left(\sqrt{\dfrac{n_A((p_{perc_A} - p_B) - d)^2}{(p_{(perc+0.001)_A}(1 - p_{(perc+0.001)_A}) + p_B(1 - p_B))}} - Z_{1-\alpha} \right) \end{array} \right].$$

(11.17)

Note that in this instance, in contrast to non-inferiority calculations already discussed, a number of issues also need to be considered:

1. The investigative response rate p_B remains assumed fixed, calculated from the initial p_A but not from individual p_{perc_A}.
2. Following from issue 1, for instance when $p_{perc_A} - p_B$ exceeds the non-inferiority bound, then the power for this percentile (to be averaged across for power calculation) is set to 0.

The equivalent calculation for a non-inferiority study designed around the odds ratio would be

$$1 - \beta = \frac{1}{0.998} \sum_{perc=0.001}^{0.998} 0.5 \left[\begin{array}{c} \Phi\left(\sqrt{n_A(\log OR_{perc} - d)^2 \left[1 - \sum_{i=1}^{2} \bar{p}_{perc}^3 \right] / 6} - Z_{1-\alpha} \right) \\[3ex] + \Phi\left(\sqrt{n_A(\log OR_{perc} - d)^2 \left[1 - \sum_{i=1}^{2} \bar{p}_{(perc+0.001)}^3 \right] / 6} - Z_{1-\alpha} \right) \end{array} \right].$$

(11.18)

As the odds ratio does not suffer from the issues of stepped non-inferiority bounds, the calculations are relatively more straightforward. However, the following two points should be considered similar to the proportional difference:

1. The investigative response rate p_B remains assumed fixed calculated from the initial p_A but not from individual p_{perc_A}.
2. Following from point 1, for instance when $OR_{perc} = (p_{perc_A}(1 - p_B))/(p_B(1 - p_{perc_A}))$ exceeds the non-inferiority bound,

then the power for this percentile (to be averaged across for power calculation) is set to 0.

11.3.8.1   Worked Example 11.5

Repeating the sample calculations from Worked Example 11.1 on the absolute risk difference scale increases the sample size to 134 patients per arm.

11.3.9   Calculations That Take Account of the Imprecision of the Estimate Effects with Respect to the Assumptions about the Mean Difference and the Variance Used in the Sample Size Calculations: Bayesian Methods

As discussed the percentiles for a posterior control response can be calculated as in Worked Example 11.4, and from these percentiles (11.7) and (11.8) can be used to give an estimate of the sample size (Julious, 2004c). Again it is best to highlight the points through a worked example.

11.3.9.1   Worked Example 11.6

For the absolute difference scale with a non-informative prior the sample size is estimated to be 134 patients per arm. This is the same as the sample size calculated. With a more pessimistic prior (the most likely response being 90% with 90% certainty that it is greater than 85%), the sample size estimate is increased to 166 patients per arm.

Note that this is more of a pessimistic prior than when just looking at variability. Here a higher control response could equate to a narrowing of the effect of the investigative treatment over the control. This will adversely affect the sample size.

With a prior that the control response rate observed is about right (the most likely response being 85% with 90% certainty it is greater than 80%) the sample size estimate is increased to 124 patients per arm.

11.3.10   Cross-over Trials

There are a number of articles that have dealt specifically with the topic of cross-over equivalence trials (Lu and Bean, 1995; Tango, 1998, 1999; Nam, 1997; Tang, 2003; Tang, Tang and Chan, 2003). However, these methodologies are simply extensions of methodologies for superiority cross-over trials and parallel group non-inferiority trials.

In Chapter 10 it was highlighted how to estimate the sample size for a superiority trial; you could simply use the sample sizes for parallel group superiority trials and take the sample size per arm to be the total sample size for a cross-over trial. This argument can be extended now to non-inferiority trials. It is therefore recommended to use the parallel group methodologies described in this chapter to estimate the total sample size for a non-inferiority cross-over trial.

11.4   As-Good-as-or-Better Trials

As discussed in Chapter 6, to calculate the sample size required for an as-good-as-or-better trial we should apply the methodologies described for superiority (Chapter 9) and non-inferiority trials.

Other issues with as-good-as-or-better trials are either the same as described for Normal data in Chapter 6 or generic and described in Chapter 1. Hence, this chapter does not go into detail on these types of trial.

 Key Messages

- For non-inferiority trials with high anticipated response rates the studies may be quite sensitive to assumptions about the anticipated response rates.
- Simple Bayesian methods should be considered to calculate the sample size.

12

Sample Size Calculations for Equivalence Trials with Binary Data

12.1 Introduction

For equivalence trials, the null H_0 and alternative H_1 hypotheses are defined as follows:

H_0: A given treatment is inferior with respect to the mean response $(\pi_A \neq \pi_B)$.

H_1: The given treatment is equivalent with respect to the mean response $(\pi_A = \pi_B)$.

Formally, these hypotheses can be written in terms of a clinical difference d (Committee for Proprietary Medicinal Products [CPMP], 2000)

H_0: $\pi_A - \pi_B \geq d$ or $\pi_A - \pi_B \leq -d$.

H_1: $-d < \pi_A - \pi_B < d$.

The issue to highlight here is that like non-inferiority trials under both the null and alternative hypotheses there is a non-zero difference between treatments. The implications are similar to those for non-inferiority trials discussed in Chapter 11 as there will be consequences with respect to the variance estimates under the null and alternative hypotheses.

12.2 Parallel Group Trials

12.2.1 Sample Sizes with the Population Effects Assumed Known: General Case

12.2.1.1 Absolute Risk Difference

Recall from Chapter 1 that the total Type II error (defined as $\beta = \beta_1 + \beta_2$) is calculated from the result

$$Z_{1-\beta_1} = \frac{-d-\Delta}{\sqrt{Var(S)}} - Z_{1-\alpha} \quad \text{and} \quad Z_{1-\beta_2} = \frac{d-\Delta}{\sqrt{Var(S)}} - Z_{1-\alpha}. \qquad (12.1)$$

As with trials in which the primary response is anticipated to take a Normal form discussed in Chapter 5, for equivalence trials for the general case in which the expected true mean difference is not fixed to be zero the sample size cannot be derived directly as the total Type II error is the sum of the Type II errors associated with each one-tailed test.

In addition as with non-inferiority trials described in Chapter 11 there are a number of approaches for the derivation of the variance under the null and alternative hypotheses. The generic solution to estimation of the power for a given sample size is thus

$$
1 - \beta = \Phi\left(\sqrt{\frac{n_A((\pi_A - \pi_B) - d)^2}{\pi_A(1 - \pi_A) + \pi_B(1 - \pi_B)}} - \frac{Z_{1-\alpha}\sqrt{\tilde{\pi}_A(1 - \tilde{\pi}_A) + \tilde{\pi}_B(1 - \tilde{\pi}_B)}}{\sqrt{\pi_A(1 - \pi_A) + \pi_B(1 - \pi_B)}} \right)
$$

$$
+ \Phi\left(\sqrt{\frac{n_A((\pi_A - \pi_B) + d)^2}{\pi_A(1 - \pi_A) + \pi_B(1 - \pi_B)}} - \frac{Z_{1-\alpha}\sqrt{\tilde{\pi}_A(1 - \tilde{\pi}_A) + \tilde{\pi}_B(1 - \tilde{\pi}_B)}}{\sqrt{\pi_A(1 - \pi_A) + \pi_B(1 - \pi_B)}} \right) - 1.
$$

(12.2)

This chapter now discusses the different methods for estimation of the variances.

12.2.1.1.1 *Method 1: Using Anticipated Responses*

The first method of estimating the variance under the null hypothesis is simply to replace π_A and π_B with anticipated estimates of the response, π_A and π_B, respectively. Hence, the variance under the null hypothesis becomes

$$
\frac{\pi_A(1 - \pi_A)}{n_A} + \frac{\pi_B(1 - \pi_B)}{n_B},
$$

(12.3)

and the power for a given sample size can hence be estimated from

$$
1 - \beta = \Phi\left(\sqrt{\frac{n_A((\pi_A - \pi_B) - d)^2}{\pi_A(1 - \pi_A) + \pi_B(1 - \pi_B)}} - Z_{1-\alpha} \right)
$$

$$
+ \Phi\left(\sqrt{\frac{n_A((\pi_A - \pi_B) + d)^2}{\pi_A(1 - \pi_A) + \pi_B(1 - \pi_B)}} - Z_{1-\alpha} \right) - 1.
$$

(12.4)

To estimate the sample size you iterate (12.4) on the sample size until the nominal power is reached.

*12.2.1.1.2   Method 2: Using Anticipated Responses
                in Conjunction with the Equivalence Limit*

The second method is to estimate π_A and π_B from (Dunnett and Gent, 1977)

$$\pi_A = (\pi_A + \pi_B + d)/2 \quad \text{and} \quad \pi_B = (\pi_A + \pi_B - d)/2, \tag{12.5}$$

where d indicates symmetric equivalence limits. Applying (12.5) to (12.2), an estimate of the power for a given sample size can be obtained.

We use this result to iterate to find the required sample size. For this method the following inequality must hold (Farrington and Manning, 1990):

$$\max\{-d, d\} < \pi_A + \pi_B < 2 + \min\{-d, d\}.$$

12.2.1.1.3   Method 3: Using Maximum Likelihood Estimates

The third method is to use maximum likelihood estimates for π_A and π_B (Farrington and Manning, 1990; Miettinen and Nurminen, 1985; Koopman, 1984), defined as

$$\pi_A = 2u\cos(w) - \frac{b}{3a},$$

$$\pi_B = \pi_A + d_1,$$

to enter into (12.2), where $d_1 = \pi_A(1 - d)d$, $c = d^2 - 2d(\pi_A + 1) + \pi_A + \pi_B$, $b = -(2 + \pi_A + \pi_B - 3d)$, $w = [\pi + \cos^{-1}(v/u^3)]/3$, $u = \text{sign}(v)\sqrt{b^2/9a^2 - c/3a}$, $a = 2$, and $v = b^3/27a^3 - bc/6a^2 + d_1/2a$.

12.2.1.1.4   Comparison of the Three Methods

The three methods give quite different estimates for the sample size. The greatest difference is when there is a high (or low) response rate (>0.85). Through the remainder of the chapter Method 1 is described, and Table 12.1 gives sample sizes for this method for a finite range of responses.

12.2.1.2   Odds Ratio

Remember that the variance about the log odds ratio can be approximated as (Whitehead, 1993)

$$Var(S) = \frac{6}{n_A\left(1 - \Sigma_{i=0}^1 \bar{\pi}_i^3\right)}, \tag{12.6}$$

where $\bar{\pi}_i$ is the average response on each outcome category [$\bar{\pi}_1 = (\pi_A + \pi_B)/2$ and $\bar{\pi}_1 = 1 - \bar{\pi}_0$]. Consequently the sample size for a given power can be

TABLE 12.1

Sample Sizes for an Equivalence Study Estimated by Method 1 and Alternative Methods for 90% Power and a Type I Error Rate of 2.5%

π_A	π_B	Limit	Sample Size	π_A	π_B	Limit	Sample Size
0.70	0.70	0.05	2,184	0.80	0.70	0.15	1,556
		0.10	546		0.75	0.10	1,461
		0.15	243			0.15	366
		0.20	137		0.80	0.05	1,664
	0.75	0.10	1,671			0.10	416
		0.15	418			0.15	185
		0.20	186		0.85	0.10	1,209
	0.80	0.15	1,556			0.15	303
		0.20	389		0.90	0.15	1051
	0.85	0.20	1,419				
				0.85	0.75	0.15	1,324
0.75	0.70	0.10	1,671		0.80	0.10	1209
		0.15	418			0.15	303
		0.20	186		0.85	0.05	1,326
	0.75	0.05	1,950			0.10	332
		0.10	488			0.15	148
		0.15	217		0.90	0.10	915
		0.20	122			0.15	229
	0.80	0.10	1,461				
		0.15	366	0.90	0.85	0.10	915
		0.20	163		0.90	0.05	936
	0.85	0.15	1,324			0.10	234
		0.20	331				
	0.90	0.20	1,167				

estimated from

$$1-\beta = \Phi\left(\sqrt{n_A\left[1-\Sigma_{i=0}^{1}\,\bar{\pi}_i^3\right](\log(OR)-d)^2/6} - Z_{1-\alpha}\right)$$

$$+\,\Phi\left(\sqrt{n_A\left[1-\Sigma_{i=0}^{1}\,\bar{\pi}_i^3\right](\log(OR)+d)^2/6} - Z_{1-\alpha}\right)-1, \tag{12.7}$$

where d in this instance is the symmetric equivalence limit on the log scale. For non-inferiority trials described in Chapter 11 suggested values for d were given as $\log(0.43)$, $\log(0.47)$, $\log(0.50)$ or $\log(0.55)$. The rationale for their use in non-inferiority trials can be generalised o equivalence trials.

Table 12.2 gives sample sizes for a finite range of responses.

12.2.2　Sample Sizes with the Population Effects Assumed Known: No Treatment Difference

As with equivalence trials discussed for Normal data in Chapter 5 when the assumption is made of no true difference between treatments the calculations are greatly simplified, with a direct estimate of the sample size now possible.

TABLE 12.2

Sample Sizes for Different Equivalence Limits on the Odds Ratio Scale and Anticipated Responses for 90% Power and Type I Error of 2.5%

		Equivalence Limit			
π_A	Odds Ratio	0.43	0.47	0.50	0.55
0.80	0.70	498	745	1,044	2031
	0.80	319	435	557	876
	0.90	243	311	377	532
	1.00	229	285	339	455
	1.10	254	323	391	546
	1.20	318	424	532	804
	1.40	564	829	1,141	2124
0.85	0.70	612	915	1,282	2496
	0.80	396	539	690	1085
	0.90	303	388	471	663
	1.00	287	358	425	571
	1.10	320	407	492	688
	1.20	403	536	673	1017
	1.40	717	1,054	1,452	2703
0.90	0.70	848	1,268	1,778	3460
	0.80	553	754	965	1518
	0.90	427	547	663	934
	1.00	406	507	602	808
	1.10	455	580	700	979
	1.20	575	766	962	1452
	1.40	1030	1,514	2,085	3883

12.2.2.1 Absolute Risk Difference

12.2.2.1.1 Method 1: Using Anticipated Responses

For the special case of no anticipated treatment difference the power can be estimated from

$$1-\beta = 2\Phi\left(\sqrt{\frac{n_A d^2}{\pi_A(1-\pi_A)+\pi_B(1-\pi_B)}} - Z_{1-\alpha}\right) - 1. \qquad (12.8)$$

However, as $\pi_A = \pi_B$ (12.8) can be rewritten as

$$1-\beta = 2\Phi\left(\sqrt{\frac{n_A d^2}{2\bar{\pi}(1-\bar{\pi})}} - Z_{1-\alpha}\right) - 1, \qquad (12.9)$$

where $\bar{\pi} = (\pi_A + \pi_B)/2$ is interpreted in this instance as the anticipated overall response. Consequently (12.9) can in turn be rewritten to give a direct estimate of the sample size

$$n_A = \frac{2(Z_{1-\beta/2} + Z_{1-\alpha})^2 \bar{\pi}(1-\bar{\pi})}{d^2}. \tag{12.10}$$

12.2.2.1.2   Method 2: Using Anticipated Responses in Conjunction with the Equivalence Limit

Following from the arguments for Method 1 the power is estimated from

$$1-\beta = 2\Phi\left(\sqrt{\frac{n_A d^2}{\bar{\pi}(1-\bar{\pi})}} - \frac{Z_{1-\alpha}\sqrt{\pi_A(1-\pi_A) + \pi_B(1-\pi_B)}}{\sqrt{\bar{\pi}(1-\bar{\pi})}}\right) - 1, \tag{12.11}$$

where $\pi_A = \bar{\pi} + d/2$ and $\pi_B = \bar{\pi} - d/2$ and the inequality hence now become $\max\{-d, d\} < 2\bar{\pi} < 2 + \min\{-d, d\}$. From (12.11) for a direct estimate of the sample size we get

$$n_A = \frac{\left(Z_{1-\alpha}\sqrt{\pi_A(1-\pi_A) + \pi_B(1-\pi_B)} + Z_{1-\beta/2}\sqrt{2\bar{\pi}(1-\bar{\pi})}\right)^2}{d^2}. \tag{12.12}$$

12.2.2.1.3   Method 3: Using Maximum Likelihood Estimates

For Method 3 π_A and π_B for use in (12.11) and (12.12) are now a little different

$$\pi_A = 2u\cos(w) - \frac{b}{3a},$$

$$\pi_B = \pi_A + d_1,$$

where

$d_1 = \bar{\pi}(1-d)d$, $c = d^2 - 2(d(\bar{\pi}+1) + \hat{\pi})$, $b = -(2(1+\bar{p}) - 3d)$, $a = 2$, $v = b^3/27a^3 - bc/6a^2 + d_1/2a$, $u = \text{sign}(v)\sqrt{b^2/9a^2 - c/3a}$ and $w = [\pi + \cos^{-1}(v/u^3)]/3$.

12.2.2.2   Odds Ratio

With the assumption of no true difference between treatments (equivalent to $OR = 1$) the power can be estimated from

$$1-\beta = 2\Phi\left(\sqrt{n_A\left[1 - \sum_{i=0}^{1} \bar{\pi}_i^3\right] d^2/6} - Z_{1-\alpha}\right) - 1, \tag{12.13}$$

whilst a direct estimate of the sample size can be obtained from

$$n_A = \frac{6[Z_{1-\beta} + Z_{1-\alpha}]^2}{\left[1 - \Sigma_{i=0}^1 \pi_i^3\right] d^2}. \tag{12.14}$$

12.2.2.3 Worked Example 12.1

An investigator wishes to design an equivalence trial in which the anticipated response rate on the active control is 85%. The investigator also expects an 85% response rate on the investigative therapy. Using an odds ratio of 0.50, Table 12.2 gives the sample size as 425 patients per arm.

In comparison, working on the proportional scale, with the same anticipated responses but with an equivalence limit of 15%, we would require (from Table 12.1) just 148 patients per arm. With a 10% equivalence limit the sample size is 335 patients per arm.

12.2.3 Sensitivity Analysis about the Estimates of the Population Effects Used in the Sample Size Calculations

As with superiority and non-inferiority trials described in Chapters 10 and 11 the sensitivity of an equivalence study design to the control response rate can be investigated through construction of a 95% confidence interval. The power could then be assessed at the two tails of the confidence interval.

This confidence interval could then be used with (12.4) for an absolute risk difference and (12.7) for an odds ratio to interrogate the sensitivity of the study to the control response rate.

12.2.3.1 Worked Example 12.2

Suppose the control response rate was assessed from a previous study in 100 patients, and it is assumed that the investigative response rate is fixed at 85%. The confidence interval indicates that a plausible range for the control response is between 78% and 92%.

Table 12.3 gives a breakdown of the sensitivity of the study design to the estimate of the control response rate. As evidenced from this table this equivalence study is sensitive to both the lower and upper points of the confidence interval as these both bring the point estimate closer to the equivalence boundary.

For the odds ratio calculation the lower and upper tails of the confidence interval have powers of 24% and 3%, respectively. For the absolute difference the lower and upper tails have 43% and 59% power, respectively.

12.2.4 Calculations Taking Account of the Imprecision of the Estimates of the Population Effects Used in the Sample Size Calculations

By using appropriate confidence interval methodology around the control response rate p_A, the power and hence the sample size can be calculated

TABLE 12.3

Sensitivity Analysis for Equivalence Worked Example

a. Odds Ratio Scale

		95% Confidence Interval	
	Observed	Lower	Upper
Control response	0.85	0.78	0.92
Investigative response	0.85	0.850	0.850
Power	90%	24%	3%

b. Absolute Risk Difference Scale

		95% Confidence Interval	
	Observed	Lower	Upper
Control Response	0.85	0.78	0.92
Non-inferiority margin	0.15	0.15	0.15
Investigative response	0.85	0.85	0.85
Power	90%	43%	59%

using numerical methods for equivalence trials. Hence, if the absolute risk difference is of interest, the sample size can be estimated from

$$1-\beta = \frac{1}{0.998} \sum_{perc=0.001}^{0.998} \frac{\lambda_1 + \lambda_2}{2}, \qquad (12.15)$$

where λ_A and λ_B are defined, respectively, as

$$\lambda_1 = \Phi\left(\sqrt{\frac{n_A((p_A - p_B) - d)^2}{(p_{perc_A}(1 - p_{perc_A}) + p_B(1 - p_B))}} - Z_{1-\alpha}\right)$$

$$+ \Phi\left(\sqrt{\frac{n_A((p_A - p_B) - d)^2}{(p_{perc_A}(1 - p_{perc_A}) + p_B(1 - p_B))}} - Z_{1-\alpha}\right) - 1,$$

$$\lambda_2 = \Phi\left(\sqrt{\frac{n_A((p_A - p_B) - d)^2}{(p_{(perc+0.001)_A}(1 - p_{(perc+0.001)_A}) + p_B(1 - p_B))}} - Z_{1-\alpha}\right)$$

$$+ \Phi\left(\sqrt{\frac{n_A((p_A - p_B) - d)^2}{(p_{(perc+0.001)_A}(1 - p_{(perc+0.001)_A}) + p_B(1 - p_B))}} - Z_{1-\alpha}\right) - 1.$$

The equivalent calculation for an equivalence study designed around the odds ratio would be

$$1 - \beta = \frac{1}{0.998} \sum_{perc=0.001}^{0.998} \frac{\eta_1 + \eta_2}{2}, \tag{12.16}$$

where η_1 and η_2 are defined, respectively, as

$$\eta_1 = \Phi\left(\sqrt{n_A(\log(OR) - d)^2 \left[1 - \sum_{i=1}^{2} \bar{p}_{perc_i}^3\right] / 6} - Z_{1-\alpha} \right)$$

$$+ \Phi\left(\sqrt{n_A(\log(OR) + d)^2 \left[1 - \sum_{i=1}^{2} \bar{p}_{perc_i}^3\right] / 6} - Z_{1-\alpha} \right) - 1$$

$$\eta_2 = \Phi\left(\sqrt{n_A(\log(OR) - d)^2 \left[1 - \sum_{i=1}^{2} \bar{p}_{(perc+0.001)_A}^3\right] / 6} - Z_{1-\alpha} \right)$$

$$+ \Phi\left(\sqrt{n_A(\log(OR) + d)^2 \left[1 - \sum_{i=1}^{2} \bar{p}_{(perc+0.001)_A}^3\right] / 6} - Z_{1-\alpha} \right) - 1.$$

12.2.4.1 Worked Example 12.3

Suppose the control response rate was estimated from 100 patients. Repeating the same calculations obtained for the same equivalence limit of $OR = 0.5$ the sample size should be increased to 449 patients per arm, around a 6% increase in the sample size compared to Worked Example 12.1 to account for the imprecision in the estimate of the control response.

With respect to estimating the sample size on the absolute risk difference scale increases the same size to 156 patients per arm. This is an increase in the sample size of 5% compared to Worked Example 12.1.

12.2.5 Calculations That Take Account of the Imprecision in the Estimates of the Effects Used in the Sample Size Calculations: Bayesian Methods

As described in Chapters 10 and 11 the percentiles for a posterior control response can be calculated to give an estimate of the sample size, which we now discuss through a worked example.

12.2.5.1   Worked Example 12.4

For the absolute difference scale with a non-informative prior the sample size is estimated as 153 patients per arm. This is three less than the sample size calculated in Worked Example 12.3. With a more pessimistic prior (the most likely response being 80% with 90% certainty that it is greater than 75%), the sample size estimate is increased to 173 patients per arm. With a prior that the control response rate observed is about right (the most likely response being 85% with 90% certainty that it is greater than 80%) the sample size estimate is 152 patients per arm.

Similar calculations could be done if equivalence is defined in terms of an odds ratio.

12.2.6   Calculations Taking Account of the Imprecision of the Population Effects with Respect to the Assumptions about the Mean Difference and the Variance Used in the Sample Size Calculations

To allow for the imprecision in the assumptions about both the mean difference and variance numerical methods could be used to calculate the sample size on the absolute difference scale from

$$1-\beta = \frac{1}{0.998} \sum_{perc=0.001}^{0.998} \frac{\lambda_1 + \lambda_2}{2}, \tag{12.17}$$

where λ_1 and λ_2 are defined, respectively, as

$$\lambda_1 = \Phi\left(\sqrt{\frac{n_A((p_{perc_A} - p_B) - d)^2}{(p_{perc_A}(1 - p_{perc_A}) + p_B(1 - p_B))}} - Z_{1-\alpha}\right)$$

$$+ \Phi\left(\sqrt{\frac{n_A((p_{perc_A} - p_B) - d)^2}{(p_{perc_A}(1 - p_{perc_A}) + p_B(1 - p_B))}} - Z_{1-\alpha}\right) - 1$$

$$\lambda_2 = \Phi\left(\sqrt{\frac{n_A((p_{perc_A} - p_B) - d)^2}{(p_{(perc+0.001)_A}(1 - p_{(perc+0.001)_A}) + p_B(1 - p_B))}} - Z_{1-\alpha}\right)$$

$$+ \Phi\left(\sqrt{\frac{n_A((p_{perc_A} - p_B) - d)^2}{(p_{(perc+0.001)_A}(1 - p_{(perc+0.001)_A}) + p_B(1 - p_B))}} - Z_{1-\alpha}\right) - 1.$$

A number of issues also need to be considered:

1. The investigative response rate p_B remains assumed fixed, calculated from the initial p_A and not from individual p_{perc_A}.
2. Following from issue 1, for instance when $p_{perc_A} - p_B$ exceeds an equivalence bound, then the power for this percentile (to be averaged across for power calculation) is set to 0.

The equivalent calculation to estimate the sample size for an equivalence study design based around the odds ratio would be

$$1 - \beta = \frac{1}{0.998} \sum_{perc=0.001}^{0.998} \frac{\eta_1 + \eta_2}{2} \tag{12.18}$$

where η_1 and η_2 are defined, respectively, as

$$\eta_1 = \Phi\left(\sqrt{n_A(\log(OR_{perc}) - d)^2 \left[1 - \sum_{i=1}^{2} \bar{p}^3_{perc_A}\right]/6} - Z_{1-\alpha}\right)$$

$$+ \Phi\left(\sqrt{n_A(\log(OR_{perc}) + d)^2 \left[1 - \sum_{i=1}^{2} \bar{p}^3_{perc_A}\right]/6} - Z_{1-\alpha}\right) - 1$$

$$\eta_2 = \Phi\left(\sqrt{n_A(\log(OR_{perc}) - d)^2 \left[1 - \sum_{i=1}^{2} \bar{p}^3_{(perc+0.001)_A}\right]/6} - Z_{1-\alpha}\right)$$

$$+ \Phi\left(\sqrt{n_A(\log(OR_{perc}) + d)^2 \left[1 - \sum_{i=1}^{2} \bar{p}^3_{perc+0.001)_A}\right]/6} - Z_{1-\alpha}\right) - 1.$$

The following two points should be considered, however:

1. The investigative response rate p_B remains fixed and is estimated from the initial p_A.
2. Following from point 2, for instances when $OR_{perc} = (p_{perc_A}(1 - p_B))/(p_B(1 - p_{perc_A}))$ exceeds an equivalence bound then the power for this percentile (to be averaged across for power calculation) is set to 0.

12.2.6.1   Worked Example 12.5

Repeating the worked example in which the control response rate was estimated from 100 patients the sample calculations on the absolute difference scale increase the sample size to 194 patients per arm.

12.2.7   Calculations That Take Account of the Imprecision of the Population Effects with Respect to the Assumptions about the Mean Difference and the Variance Used in the Sample Size Calculations: Bayesian Methods

In the following worked example the calculations are repeated using Bayesian methods to estimate posterior percentiles for use in (12.17).

12.2.7.1   Worked Example 12.6

For the absolute difference scale with a non-informative prior the sample size is estimated to be 202 patients per arm. This is eight greater than the sample size previously calculated in Worked Example 12.5. With a prior (the most likely response being 90% with 90% certainty that it is greater than 85%), the sample size estimate is 177 patients per arm. With a prior for which the control response rate observed is correct (the most likely response being 85% with 90% certainty it is greater than 80%) the sample size estimate is 172 patients per arm.

12.3   Cross-over Trials

The arguments for superiority and non-inferiority trials can be extended to equivalence trials. Although there are a number of articles that dealt specifically with this topic (Tango 1998, 1999; Nam, 1997; Tang, Tang and Chan, 2003), it is recommended to use the parallel group sample size methodologies per arm to estimate the total sample size for an equivalence cross-over trial.

 Key Message

- For equivalence trials with high anticipated response rates the studies may be quite sensitive to assumptions about the anticipated responses.

13

Sample Size Calculations for Precision-Based Trials with Binary Data

13.1 Introduction

Chapter 1 introduced the concept of trials based on precision about the estimates, while Chapter 8 discussed the sample size calculations for Normal data. For binary data what we are designing is a trial to obtain an estimate for the possible treatment effect with respect to a binary response rate.

For binary data we only need an estimate of a response rate to estimate the sample size. This response rate need not be broken down by treatment but could be an anticipated response overall—across treatments.

13.2 Parallel Group Trials

13.2.1 Absolute Risk Difference

In a two-arm trial in which the primary outcome is binary, the objective is to estimate a possible population difference

$$p_A - p_B,$$

where p_A and p_B are sample proportional responses on treatment groups A and B, respectively. As discussed in Chapter 9 a $(1 - \alpha)100\%$ Normal approximation confidence interval for $p_A - p_B$ has a half-width

$$w = Z_{\alpha/2}\sqrt{Var(S)}, \tag{13.1}$$

where $Var(S)$, assuming $n_A = n_B$ is defined as

$$Var(S) = \frac{p_A(1-p_A)+p_B(1-p_B)}{n_A}, \tag{13.2}$$

which can in turn be approximated from

$$Var(S) \approx \frac{2\bar{p}(1-\bar{p})}{n_A}, \tag{13.3}$$

TABLE 13.1

Sample Sizes Required per Group for Two-Sided 95%
Confidence Intervals for Different Values of Width w
for Various Expected Mean Absolute Responses

			w		
$\bar{p}$	5	10	15	20	25
0.05	146	37	17	10	6
0.10	277	70	31	18	12
0.15	392	98	44	25	16
0.20	492	123	55	31	20
0.25	577	145	65	37	24
0.30	646	162	72	41	26
0.35	700	175	78	44	28
0.40	738	185	82	47	30
0.45	761	191	85	48	31
0.50	769	193	84	49	31

where $\bar{p} = (p_A + p_B)/2$, that is the mean risk response expected across both treatments. In Chapter 9 it was highlighted that this approximate variance formula holds for absolute risks (p_A and p_B) that are within ±0.30 of each other and thus cover most practical situations. For trials based on precision considerations, therefore, it may be optimal to use an estimate of the mean overall response for the variance and subsequent sample size calculations. Given that an objective of a precision-based study may be to estimate possible individual treatment responses, having a sample size calculation that does not require responses to be specified in each group may be the best approach. However, if we have reasonable estimates for each treatment response, then these should be used in calculations.

A conservative approach would be to set $\bar{p} = 0.5$ as if we do not have any idea of the overall response; this would give us a maximum estimate of the variance for the $\bar{p}$ absolute risk difference and would not be too conservative provided that $\bar{p}$ is within the range (0.3, 0.7). Therefore, for a given half confidence interval width w the following condition must be met to obtain the sample size per group

$$n_A = \frac{2\bar{p}(1 - \bar{p})Z_{1-\alpha/2}^2}{w^2}. \tag{13.4}$$

Table 13.1 is derived from (13.4). Table 13.1 gives the sample size required for different values of the expected mean response across treatment groups $\bar{p}$ and widths w. Two-sided 95% confidence intervals are assumed to be calculated in the final analysis. The mean responses $\bar{p}$ given in the table vary from 0.05 to 0.50. Values greater than 0.50 are not given as the sample size required for $\bar{p} = 0.60$ is equivalent to $\bar{p} = 0.40$, the sample size for $\bar{p} = 0.70$ is the same as $\bar{p} = 0.30$, and so on.

13.2.2 Odds Ratio

For binary data the treatment response rate may also be expressed in terms of an odds ratio OR

$$OR = \frac{p_A(1-p_B)}{p_B(1-p_A)}. \tag{13.5}$$

A $(1-\alpha)100\%$ confidence interval for $\log(d)$ can be derived using the following variance estimate (Whitehead, 1993):

$$Var(\log(S)) = \frac{6}{n_A\left[1-\Sigma_{i=0}^1 \bar{p}_i^3\right]}. \tag{13.6}$$

where $\bar{p}_i$ are the expected mean responses. Remember that for binary data $\bar{p}_1 = (p_A + p_B)/2 = \bar{p}$, say, and $\bar{p}_2 = 1 - \bar{p}_1 = 1 - \bar{p}$ and thus correspond to $\bar{p}$ given previously in this chapter. Therefore, as for binary data for a given half confidence interval width w around the odds ratio, the following condition must be met to obtain the sample size per group:

$$n_A = \frac{6\,Z_{1-\alpha/2}^2}{(-\log(1-w))^2\left[1-\Sigma_{i=0}^1 \bar{p}_i^3\right]}. \tag{13.7}$$

Note that in this instance w is on the log scale, so $w = 0.60$ would equate to a confidence interval for a given odds ratio being within $(1-w) \times OR$ to $OR/(1-w)$, that is, $0.40 \times OR$ to $2.5 \times OR$. Also note that $\log(1-w)$ is on the arithmetic scale, that is, $\log(1-w) = -\log[1/(1-w)]$.

Table 13.2 gives sample sizes required for different values of the mean response across treatment groups $\bar{p}$ and widths w estimated using (13.7). Two-sided 95% confidence intervals are again assumed to be calculated in the final analysis. As with Table 13.1 the mean responses $\bar{p}$ given in the table vary from 0.05 to 0.50. To obtain a sample size for $\bar{p} > 0.5$ look up $1 - \bar{p}$.

13.2.3 Equating Odds Ratios with Proportions

As with superiority trials discussed in Chapter 9 (13.4) and (13.7) can be approximately equated if we redefine the half-widths around the confidence intervals of the odds ratios w_{or} and proportional differences w_p. Furthermore, if $(p_A - p_B)$ is an estimate of the treatment response and $(p_{A_L} - p_{B_L})$ is the lower bound for a 95% confidence interval for this response, then w_p would be defined as

$$w_p = (p_A - p_B) - (p_{A_L} - p_{B_L}). \tag{13.8}$$

Likewise, using the same arguments, for w_{or} we would have

$$1 - w_{or} = OR/OR_L = \frac{p_A(1-p_B)}{p_B(1-p_A)} \bigg/ \frac{p_{A_L}(1-p_{B_L})}{p_{B_L}(1-p_{A_L})}. \tag{13.9}$$

TABLE 13.2

Sample Sizes Required per Group for Two-Sided 95% Confidence Intervals for Different Values of Width w around the Odds Ratio for Various Expected Mean Proportional Responses

$\bar{p}$	\multicolumn{11}{c}{w}										
	0.25	0.30	0.35	0.40	0.45	0.50	0.55	0.60	0.65	0.70	0.75
0.05	1,955	1,272	872	620	453	337	254	193	147	112	85
0.10	1,032	672	461	328	239	178	134	102	78	59	45
0.15	729	474	325	231	169	126	95	72	55	42	32
0.20	581	378	259	185	135	100	76	58	44	34	25
0.25	496	323	221	158	115	86	65	49	38	29	22
0.30	443	288	198	141	103	77	58	44	34	26	20
0.35	409	266	182	130	95	71	53	41	31	24	18
0.40	387	252	173	123	90	67	51	39	30	23	17
0.45	376	245	168	119	87	65	49	37	29	23	17
0.50	372	242	166	118	86	64	49	37	28	23	16

Thus, (13.4) and (13.7) can be rewritten, respectively, as

$$n_A = \frac{2\bar{p}(1-\bar{p})Z^2_{1-\alpha/2}}{[(p_A - p_B)-(p_{A_L} - p_{B_L})]^2},$$ (13.10)

$$n_A = \frac{6Z^2_{1-\alpha/2}/(\log OR - \log OR_L)^2}{1-\sum_{i=0}^{1}\bar{p}_i^3}.$$ (13.11)

Remembering that,

$$\frac{6}{\left(1-\sum_{i=0}^{1}\bar{p}_i^3\right)} = \frac{2}{\bar{p}(1-\bar{p})},$$ (13.12)

and $\log OR \approx 2(OR-1)/(OR+1)$, which holds for odds ratios within $0.33 \le OR \le 3.00$, hence

$$\frac{2(OR-1)}{OR+1} \approx \frac{p_A - p_B}{\bar{p}(1-\bar{p})},$$ (13.13)

and

$$\log OR_L \approx \frac{p_{A_L} - p_{B_L}}{\bar{p}(1-\bar{p})}.$$ (13.14)

Assuming $\bar{p}(1-\bar{p}) \approx \bar{p}_L(1-\bar{p}_L)$ where $\bar{p}_L = (p_{A_L} + p_{B_L})/2$ and substituting (13.12), (13.13) and (13.14) into (13.7) we obtain

$$n_A = Z^2_{1-\alpha/2}\frac{2}{\bar{p}(1-\bar{p})}\left(\frac{\bar{p}(1-\bar{p})}{(p_A - p_B)-(p_{A_L} - p_{B_L})}\right)^2 = \frac{2\bar{p}(1-\bar{p})Z^2_{1-\alpha/2}}{[(p_A - p_B)-(p_{A_L} - p_{B_L})]^2}.$$ (13.15)

Thus, similar to superiority trials, (13.4) and (13.7) can be used interchangeably depending on preference. Due to this property we therefore have

$$\frac{2\bar{p}(1-\bar{p})Z_{1-\alpha/2}^2}{(w_p)^2} \approx \frac{2\,Z_{1-\alpha/2}^2}{(\log(1-w_{OR}))^2\,\bar{p}(1-\bar{p})}, \tag{13.16}$$

and hence

$$w_p \approx |\log(1-w_{OR})|\,(\bar{p}(1-\bar{p})). \tag{13.17}$$

Using (13.17) Table 13.3 can be derived.

13.2.4   Worked Example 13.1

A pilot study is planned to estimate the odds ratio between comparator and control regimens. The expected mean response rate is 50% across the two treatments, and the wish is to quantify the odds ratio within ±55% (i.e. $w = 55\%$). This means that if an odds ratio of 0.70 was observed, we would be able to say that the true odds ratio is likely to be between 0.32 and 1.56. Therefore, from Table 13.2 the sample size required is 49 per group.

Following from the example from Table 13.3 $w = 0.55$ on the odds ratio scale is equivalent to proportional half confidence width of 20% for a mean response rate of 50%. From Table 13.2 a width of 20% and a mean proportional response of 50% gives 49 subjects per group again.

13.2.5   Sensitivity Analysis about the Estimates of the Population Effects Used in the Sample Size Calculations

Extending the arguments for other types of trial discussed in this book the sensitivity of a precision-based analysis can be investigated through

TABLE 13.3

Widths on the Absolute Difference Scale That Are Equivalent to the Widths w around the Odds Ratio for Various Anticipated Expected Mean Proportions

						w					
$\bar{p}$	0.25	0.30	0.35	0.40	0.45	0.50	0.55	0.60	0.65	0.70	0.75
0.05	0.014	0.017	0.020	0.024	0.028	0.033	0.038	0.044	0.050	0.057	0.066
0.10	0.026	0.032	0.039	0.046	0.054	0.062	0.072	0.082	0.094	0.108	0.125
0.15	0.037	0.045	0.055	0.065	0.076	0.088	0.102	0.117	0.134	0.154	0.177
0.20	0.046	0.057	0.069	0.082	0.096	0.111	0.128	0.147	0.168	0.193	0.222
0.25	0.054	0.067	0.081	0.096	0.112	0.130	0.150	0.172	0.197	0.226	0.260
0.30	0.060	0.075	0.090	0.107	0.126	0.146	0.168	0.192	0.220	0.253	0.291
0.35	0.065	0.081	0.098	0.116	0.136	0.158	0.182	0.208	0.239	0.274	0.315
0.40	0.069	0.086	0.103	0.123	0.143	0.166	0.192	0.220	0.252	0.289	0.333
0.45	0.071	0.088	0.107	0.126	0.148	0.172	0.198	0.227	0.260	0.298	0.343
0.50	0.072	0.089	0.108	0.128	0.149	0.173	0.200	0.229	0.262	0.301	0.347

construction of a 95% confidence interval around the anticipated overall response rate. For each tail of this confidence interval we can reinvestigate the precision of the trial to give a quantification of its sensitivity.

13.2.5.1 Worked Example 13.2

Suppose the expected response rate of 50% for Worked Example 13.1 was estimated from a trial with 50 patients. The 95% confidence interval for this would be between 36% and 64%. On the absolute risk difference scale these lower and upper tails would give a precision of 19%, which is a slight improvement over the previous calculations due to 50% giving the maximum variance estimate. On the odds ratio scale the precision for each tail would be 56%, which is a little worse than previously.

13.3 Cross-over Trials

As with the other types of trial discussed in this book it is recommended that the total sample size for a cross-over precision-based trial be taken from the one-arm sample size for a parallel group trial.

 Key Message

- For precision-based studies with a binary outcome there is no need to have an estimate of the response in each treatment group to estimate the sample size.

14

Sample Size Calculations for Clinical Trials with Ordinal Data

14.1 Introduction

If there is one type of sample size calculation on which I have concentrated a lot of research energies it has been the calculation of sample sizes for ordinal data. However, a realisation dawned when first I gave a sample size course I wrote. I had put together a detailed slide presentation and long practical but noticed a stirring in the class when they became aware that after the lecture, which I had just given, they were now expected to work on the practical.

I asked for a show of hands and asked if anyone had done, or could see themselves doing in the foreseeable future, a sample size calculation for ordinal data. No hands came up. In fact in subsequent presentations of the course a hand has yet to go up. Despite this it was agreed that it is useful to know how to do the sample size calculations for ordinal outcomes and have the reference material for future use.

This got me thinking due as to why I had determined the need so incorrectly, which brought the realisation that as someone seen as an 'expert' in the field of sample size calculation people approach me when they have a problem. The vast majority of the time people are planning a trial with a standard analysis and for which a standard sample size calculation is required that they are perfectly able to do themselves. They come to see me only when there is need for a non-standard solution—such as for an ordinal response. I had picked up a pattern from this and falsely interpolated the level of learning need.

This is not to say that reading this chapter is a waste of time. Much of the detail in the chapter comes from hands-on real-world experience; hence the recommendations made are done in light of practical experience. The methodologies applied also have applications in other types of sample size calculation, and in Chapter 15 on survival analysis the methods in this chapter are revisited.

This chapter therefore describes the calculations for clinical trials in which the expectation is that the outcome data will take an ordinal form. To highlight the issues of designing a trial with an ordinal this chapter uses data on quality-of-life (QoL) outcome scores from a palliative clinical trial in lung cancer patients (Medical Research Council Lung Cancer Working Party, 1996).

14.2 The Quality-of-Life Data

The data in this chapter were taken from a randomised parallel group controlled trial of a standard treatment against a less-intensive treatment in 310 patients with small-cell lung cancer and poor prognosis (Medical Research Council Lung Cancer Working Party, 1996). The standard treatment (*A*) consisted of a four-drug regime (etoposide, cyclophosphamide, methotrexate and vincristine), while the new less-intensive treatment (*B*) under investigation contained just two of these compounds (etoposide and vincristine). The two treatment schedules were the same, comprising three cycles of chemotherapy at the same dosage. Each cycle was given on 3 consecutive days at 3-week intervals.

The QoL questionnaire used in the trial was the Hospital Anxiety and Depression Scale (HADS). The HADS was developed by Zigmond and Snaith (1983). It is a self-rating questionnaire that a patient completes in the waiting room in order to reflect how they have felt during the past week before meeting a doctor. It has 14 items that split equally into the two subscales and provides scores in the range 0–21 in two dimensions: anxiety and depression. The HADS has three clinically predefined categories for each dimension: a total score 0–7 is defined as a 'Normal', 8–10 as a 'borderline case' and 11–21 as a 'case' suggesting significant anxiety or depression. In the clinical trial case study in this chapter the 310 patients' baseline scores prior to randomisation are used for expository purposes as the outcome for the control therapy. There were 266 patients who completed a baseline response which we will use for expository purposes.

Figure 14.1 displays the distribution of the HADS anxiety scores at baseline. It is negatively skewed. The scores do not seem to take an approximate Normal distributional form, although not alarmingly so. It therefore seems that the usual mean and standard deviation may not be adequate to summarise the distributions. As a consequence, for the purposes of this chapter

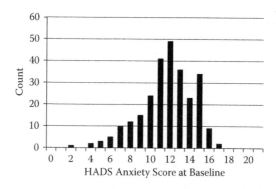

FIGURE 14.1 Distribution of HADS anxiety scores at baseline (*n* = 266).

it is recommended that distribution-free techniques should be considered for testing treatment differences.

Note that in practice transformations such as a log transformation may be considered for such data with inference then made on the transformed scale. For the purposes of this chapter, however, transformations are not considered.

14.3   Superiority Trials

14.3.1   Parallel Group Trials

The calculation of sample sizes for ordinal data is not immediately straightforward. Two methods are described in detail in this chapter: one proposed by Whitehead (1993) and a second proposed by Noether (1987). Unlike for previous chapters in which sample size tables could be provided, this is not possible for ordinal data. However, the steps required for the calculations are not that difficult and are now described through means of worked examples.

14.3.2   Sample Sizes That Are Estimated Assuming That the Population Effects Are Known

14.3.2.1   Whitehead's Method

Most QoL scales have categories that can be ordered, but the scores should not be treated as meaningful numbers; for example, a change in HADS from 5 to 10 is not the same as a change from 10 to 15. However, methods have been developed for sample size calculations for ordinal data (Whitehead, 1993).

As discussed in Chapter 1, in general terms for a two-tailed, α-level test we require the following for the variance if the test is going to have the correct power

$$Var(S) = \frac{d^2}{(Z_{1-\beta} + Z_{1-\alpha/2})^2}. \tag{14.1}$$

Here d is the effect size of interest (assessed through a log odds ratio) with the sample variance $Var(S)$ about the log odds ratio for an ordinal response estimated from (Whitehead, 1993; McCullagh, 1980; Jones and Whitehead, 1979, Campbell, Julious and Altman, 1995)

$$Var(S) = \frac{6}{n_A \left(1 - \Sigma_{i=1}^k \bar{\pi}_i^3\right)}. \tag{14.2}$$

Here k is the number of categories on the QoL instrument, $\bar{\pi}_i$ is the mean proportion expected in category i, that is, $\bar{\pi}_i = (\pi_{Ai} + \pi_{Bi})/2$, where π_{Ai} and π_{Bi}

are the proportions anticipated in category i for the two treatment groups A and B, respectively, and α and β are the overall Type I and Type II errors, respectively, with $Z_{1-\alpha/2}$ and $Z_{1-\beta}$ denoting the percentage points of a standard Normal distribution for these two errors. Here n_A is the sample size in one group assuming $n_A = n_B$. Note that in this chapter, as for binary data, the issue of allocation ratios between treatments is ignored.

Now by equating (14.1) with (14.2) we have (Julious, George and Campbell, 1995; Julious et al., 1997, 2000; Campbell, Julious, et al., 2001; Whitehead, 1993)

$$n_A = \frac{6[Z_{1-\beta} + Z_{1-\alpha/2}]^2/(\log OR)^2}{\left[1 - \Sigma_{i=1}^{k} \bar{\pi}_i^3\right]}. \tag{14.3}$$

The result (14.3) is based on the Mann-Whitney U test for ordered categorical data. It estimates the sample size based on the odds ratio (OR) of a patient being in a given category or less in one treatment group compared to the other group.

A form of this equation was used in Chapter 9 for binary data—a binary response being a special case of (14.3). For an analysis under the assumption of proportion odds the anticipated effect size is expressed as an odds ratio defined as

$$OR = \frac{\pi_{Ai}(1 - \pi_{Bi})}{\pi_{Bi}(1 - \pi_{Ai})}.$$

This is a measure that is not immediately straightforward to interpret for binary data and, as a consequence, is more difficult for an ordinal response. It is best to discuss the application of (14.3) through a worked example.

14.3.2.1.1   *Worked Example 14.1: Full Ordinal Scale*

When designing a clinical trial to estimate the odds ratio we can utilise the predefined clinical cut points of the HADS. For example, 27.1% of patients at baseline are defined as clinical cases on the HADS Anxiety dimension score at baseline (see Table 14.1), that is, 27.1% record values resulting in a score of 10 or less. This we could take, for expository purposes, as what we would expect on standard therapy (A). The odds with A are thus $0.271/(1 - 0.271) = 0.372$. Suppose a new therapy (B) is to be studied and the investigator decides that a clinically meaning effect is one that would increase the proportion of non-cases to 40.0% or a postulated odds of $0.40/(1 - 0.40) = 0.67$. The ratio of these odds gives $OR = 0.372/0.667 = 0.56$ in favour of B. This value can then be used as the basis for the sample size calculation.

The result (14.3) makes no assumption about the distribution of the data, but it does assume proportional odds between the treatments across the QoL dimension. This implies that the odds ratios are identical for each pair of adjacent categories throughout the scale. What this means practically can be highlighted by extending the example given. When using the predefined clinical cut point for

TABLE 14.1

Frequency of Responses on the HADS Anxiety Scores as Baseline for Patients with Small-Cell Lung Cancer

Category	Score	Number of Patients
Normal	0	0
	1	0
	2	1
	3	0
	4	2
	5	3
	6	5
	7	10
Borderline	8	12
	9	15
	10	24
Clinical case	11	41
	12	49
	13	36
	14	23
	15	34
	16	9
	17	2
	18	0
	19	0
	20	0
	21	0
	Total	266
Normal	0–8	21 (7.9%)
Borderline	9–103	51 (19.2%)
Clinical case	11–21	194 (72.9%)
Mean		11.70
SD (σ)		2.66
Median		12

non-cases the investigator anticipated the *OR* would be 0.56. The assumption of proportional odds implies that, if instead of using 10 or less as the definition of a non-case, 9 or less had been used, we would nevertheless obtain $OR_9 = 0.56$, and so on for OR_8, OR_7, and so on. Thus, although the actual observed odds ratios might differ from each other across the scale, the corresponding population values are assumed all equal, which implies that $OR_1 = OR_2 = OR_3 = \cdots = OR_{21} = 0.56$. However, the calculation of sample size using (14.3) are robust to departure from this ideal, provided all the odds ratios indicate an advantage to the same treatment (Julious, George, Machin et al., 1995; Julious et al., 2000).

Using the odds ratio of 0.56 the anticipated new therapy responses can be derived as per Table 14.2. From these anticipated responses an estimate of the variance can be made from (14.2) that when placed in (14.3) with the odds

TABLE 14.2

Anticipated Percentages of Response on the HADS Anxiety Scores for Standard Treatment and New Treatment for Patients with Small-Cell Lung Cancer

Category	Score[a]	Standard Therapy S		New Therapy T	
		Percentage P_{Si}	Cumulative Percentage Q_{Si}	Percentage P_{Ti}	Cumulative Percentage Q_{Ti}
Normal	0–3	0.4	0.4	0.7	0.7
	4	0.8	1.2	1.4	2.1
	5	1.1	2.3	1.9	4.1
	6	1.9	4.2	3.2	7.3
	7	3.8	8.0	6.2	13.5
Borderline	8	4.5	12.5	6.9	20.4
	9	5.6	18.1	8.0	28.4
	10	9.0	27.1	11.6	40.0
Clinical case	11	15.4	42.5	17.0	57.0
	12	18.4	60.9	16.6	73.6
	13	13.5	74.4	10.3	83.9
	14	8.6	83.0	5.8	89.8
	15	12.8	95.8	7.8	97.6
	16	3.4	99.2	1.9	99.6
	17–21	0.8	100.0	0.4	100.0

[a] The 22 categories of Table 14.1 are reduced to $k = 15$.

ratio gives an estimate of the sample size of 188 patients per arm (for 90% power and two-sided Type I error rate of 5%).

Each cell for the new therapy is derived using the standard therapy's anticipated response and the odds ratio, for example,

$$Q_{T10} = 1/(1 + 0.56 \times (1 - 0.271)/0.271) = 0.40$$

$$Q_{T11} = 1/(1 + 0.56 \times (1 - 0.425)/0.425) = 0.57$$

$$Q_{T12} = 1/(1 + 0.56 \times (1 - 0.609)/0.609) = 0.74$$

(there is a little rounding when done by hand).

The application of proportional odds therefore allows that, if the distribution of one of the treatment groups can be specified, then the anticipated cumulative proportions for the other treatment can be directly derived. Hence, with prior knowledge of the distribution of just one treatment group and an effect size assessed by an *OR*, an estimate of the sample size can be obtained.

14.3.2.1.2 Worked Example 14.2: Effects of Dichotomisation

An advantage of the HADS instrument is that for the process of anticipating the effect size, and consequent sample size, it has a predefined definition of what constitutes a case that can then be used to obtain a value of a readily interpretable effect size. This effect size, here expressed as an odds ratio, can then be extended across the full QoL scale and an estimate of the sample size made.

These cut-offs, however, can encourage some researchers to dichotomise QoL scales to calculate sample sizes. For example, with the HADS Anxiety dimension, one of the cut-offs can classify subjects as either a clinical case or borderline or better. For this, now binary, situation, (14.3) can still be used to estimate a sample size but ignoring the full ordered categorical nature of the data, may result in a substantial overestimation of the sample size. For example, if a clinically meaningful difference was set again at 0.56 around the cut-off of non-cases/clinical cases on the HADS Anxiety score, then by dichotomising (14.3) gives an estimate of the sample size of 277 compared to only 188 when all $k = 22$ categories are used in the calculations. This is a potential overestimate of 47% in the necessary sample size if the data were analysed using all 22 categories.

Obviously, if the intention is to analyse the scale as a dichotomous endpoint then the binary sample size calculated may be appropriate, although this approach may be questioned also as wasting patients. Dichotomising the QoL scale to estimate a sample size, and consequently to analyse the data as ordinal, should be avoided if possible as sample sizes could be unnecessarily inflated.

14.3.2.1.3   *Worked Example 14.3: Additional Categories*

It may not be essential to use the full categorical scale. For example, with HADS there is an additional category of 'Normal' for subjects with a score of 8 or less, and just less than 8% of patients are classified as such on the anxiety dimension. If we then calculated the sample size using the $k = 3$ groups of Normal, borderline case and clinical case as the categories, the estimated sample size, from (14.3), is 267 subjects—only a marginally closer estimate. However, if we identified an additional category of 'severe clinical case' for subjects with a HADS score 14 or above (Julious et al., 1997, 2000) and based the sample size calculations on the four categories, the estimated sample size of 210 patients is now quite close to the optimal 188. Therefore, knowledge of anticipated responses in only a handful of categories can give sample size estimates that are more precise for only a modest increase in the complexity of the calculations.

The reason why ignoring the ordinal scale substantially increases the sample size is due to the increase in variance estimated from (14.2). Table 14.3 illustrates this point. The minimum the variance can be for any number of categories on a scale is for the special case in which the anticipated mean responses for each category are equal, that is, $\bar{\pi}_1 = \bar{\pi}_2 = \bar{\pi}_3 = \ \bar{\pi}_{k-1} = \bar{\pi}_k$. If this result is placed into (14.2) we can obtain the anticipated relative variances for different numbers of categories for the most optimal responses. The ratio of these variances can in turn give inflation factors for the sample size for

TABLE 14.3

Correction Factor to Be Used When the Number
of Categories Is Less Than 5

Number of Categories	Mean Proportions Anticipated	Correction Factor
2	$\bar{\pi}_1 = \bar{\pi}_2 = 0.500$	1.333
3	$\bar{\pi}_1 = \bar{\pi}_2 = \bar{\pi}_3 = 0.333$	1.125
4	$\bar{\pi}_1 = \bar{\pi}_2 = \bar{\pi}_3 = \bar{\pi}_4 = 0.250$	1.067
5	$\bar{\pi}_1 = \bar{\pi}_2 = \bar{\pi}_3 = \bar{\pi}_4 = \bar{\pi}_5 = 0.200$	1.042

different numbers of categories relative to the optimum number of categories, that is, a continuous scale by which

$$1 - \sum_{i=1}^{k} \bar{\pi}_i^3 = 1.$$

From Table 14.3 we can see that for the optimum mean responses we would anticipate a 33% increase compared to a continuous response as opposed to just 5% for five categories (Campbell, Julious and Altman, 1995). Thus, what these results show is that although dichotomising could lead to a serious inflation of the sample size, even using only a little extra information (from extra categories) can substantially improve a sample size estimate.

From Table 14.3 we can therefore derive a quick sample size formula for the case when we have a large number of categories assuming the distribution of responses is evenly spread and one category does not dominate

$$n_A = \frac{6[Z_{1-\beta} + Z_{1-\alpha/2}]^2}{[\log OR\,]^2}, \qquad (14.4)$$

which for 90% power and a two-sided significance level becomes

$$n_A = \frac{63}{[\log OR\,]^2}. \qquad (14.5)$$

14.3.2.1.4   *Worked Example 14.4: Quick Result*

For the same worked example as for a two-sided Type I error rate of 5% and 90% power for an odds ratio of 0.56 both results (14.4) and (14.5) give a sample size of 188 patients per arm, which is the same as calculated using all categories.

14.3.2.2　Noether's Method

An alternative ordinal method for sample size calculation is that of Noether (1987) by which the sample size per group is calculated from

$$n_A = \frac{(Z_{1-\alpha/2} + Z_{1-\beta})^2}{6(P-0.5)^2}. \tag{14.6}$$

Here P is defined for two treatment groups A and B as the probability of A being greater than B (or vice versa), that is, $P = P(A > B)$. Indeed the methodology of Noether (1987) is of particular interest as it is so simply written. The method itself makes no assumption about the distributional form of the data. The main requirement (not assumption) is that the data are (relatively) continuous.

For quick calculations to detect a difference with 90% power at the two-sided 5% level of significance we could use

$$n_A = \frac{1.75}{(P-0.5)^2}. \tag{14.7}$$

As with the method of Whitehead the calculations are not immediately straightforward and are best described through a worked example.

14.3.2.2.1　*Worked Example 14.5: Illustrative Example*

Worked Example 14.5, although using real data, is a little artificial but allows a detailed description of the steps for calculating the sample size using Noether's approach. The following data show the age at diagnosis of Type 2 diabetes in young adults:

Males (A):	19	22	16	29	24
Females (B):	20	11	17	12	

To calculate the probability that $P(A > B)$ we calculate the Mann-Whitney U statistic as described in Table 14.4.

Now to find $P(A > B)$ you take 17 and divide it by the multiple of the two sample sizes (here 5 and 4) and hence $P(A > B) = 17/20 = 0.85$. Similarly for $P(B > A)$ we have 0.15.

An odds ratio can be derived by taking the ratio of these two numbers, that is, $OR = P(A > B)/P(B > A) = 5.66$

If we wished to design a study with 90% power and a two-sided significance level of 5% to assess the difference between males and females taking the effect size as what we have observed before, $P = 0.85$, then the sample size required is 15 subjects per arm.

If we had used the quick result, (14.1), we would again have estimated the sample size to be 15 subjects per arm.

TABLE 14.4

Worked Example of Calculation of U for a Mann-Whitney U Statistic

Step 1	Arrange the observations in order of magnitude:

Males (A)   16   19   22   24   29
Females (B)   11   12   17   20

Step 2	Affix either A or B to each observation:

          B   B   A   B   A   B   A   A   A

Step 3	Under each A, write down the number of B's to the left of it:

          B   B   A   B   A   B   A   A   A
                       2   3   4   4   4

Under each B, write down the number of A's to the left of it:

          B   B   A   B   A   B   A   A   A
          0   0   1   2

Step 4	Sum the A scores $U_A = 2 + 3 + 4 + 4 + 4 = 17$ (i.e. $A > B$ 17 times)
	Sum the B scores $U_B = 0 + 0 + 1 + 2 = 3$ (i.e. $B > A$ 3 times)

To avoid doing the steps in the table we could use

$$P(A > B) = \Phi\left(\frac{\bar{x}_A - \bar{x}_B}{\sqrt{s_A^2 + s_B^2}} \right).$$ (14.8)

Strictly speaking this result assumes that the data are Normally distributed to obtain an estimate for $P(A > B)$. For these data $\bar{x}_A = 22$, $s_A = 4.95$, $\bar{x}_B = 15$ and $s_A = 4.95$, and $P(A > B)$ is estimated as 0.86, which is quite similar to the previous estimate and would lead to an estimate of the sample size of 14 subjects per arm.

14.3.2.2.2   Worked Example 14.6: Worked Example 14.1 Revisited—Full Ordinal Scale

The calculations undertaken in the illustrative example are now undertaken on the data set given in Table 14.1. The anticipated responses are as in Table 14.2. The counts in Table 14.5 for the new treatment arm were derived through multiplying the cell frequencies in Table 14.2. by 266. There is a little rounding error as these new counts add to 264.

To do the calculations as described in Table 14.5 the derivation is a little more complicated due to the fact there are non-unique values. Table 14.5 uses Noether's method for the data in Table 14.2.

The U value is calculated as 38,096. This is usually divided by the multiple of two sample sizes. However, we have ties, so the final column is calculated to work out the instances that would need to be accounted for by ties. These instances were accounted for by allocating them equally to the U's for both A and B, that is,

$P(A > B) = (38{,}096 + 7{,}584 \times 0.5)/(266 \times 264) = 41{,}888/70{,}224 = 0.596.$

TABLE 14.5

Worked Example Using the Method of Noether

Cells	Standard (1)	New (2)	Step 3 from Table 14.4 (3)	Columns (1) × (3)	Columns (1) × (2)
0–3	1	2			2
4	2	4	2	4	8
5	3	5	6	18	15
6	5	9	11	55	45
7	10	16	20	200	160
8	12	18	36	432	216
9	15	21	54	810	315
10	24	31	75	1,800	744
11	41	45	106	4,346	1,845
12	49	44	151	7,399	2,156
13	36	27	195	7,020	972
14	23	15	222	5,106	345
15	34	21	237	8,058	714
16	9	5	258	2,322	45
17–21	2	1	263	526	2
266	266	264		38,096	7,584

The result from Noether's method therefore gives a sample size of 190 patients per arm. This compares to 188 calculated using Whitehead's method.

For these data we have $\bar{x}_{Standard} = 11.70$ and $s_{Standard} = 2.66$; from Table 14.4 we anticipated $\bar{x}_{New} = 10.80$ and $s_{New} = 2.67$, and $P(X > Y)$ is estimated as 0.595 from (14.8), which would return a sample size of 194.

14.3.2.2.3   *Worked Example 14.7: Four Categories*

The calculations for a finite number of categories are given in Table 14.6. For this table we have

$$P(A > B) = (30{,}356 + 21{,}992 \times 0.5)/(266 \times 266) = 0.584,$$

which gives a sample size of 249 patients per arm. This result is conservative compared to the Whitehead approach estimated with four categories (which

TABLE 14.6

Worked Example Using the Method of Noether

Cells	Score	Standard (1)	New (2)	Step 3 from Table 14.4 (3)	Columns (1) × (3)	Columns (1) × (2)
Normal	0–7	21	36			756
Borderline	8–10	51	70	36	1,836	3,570
Clinical case	11–13	126	117	106	133,356	14,742
Severe clinical	14+	68	43	223	15,164	2,924
					30,356	21,992

estimated the sample size as 210). This is probably because of the number of
ties in this sample size calculation with the approach of Noether requiring
(relatively) continuous data. The calculations are therefore, with Noether's
method, less straightforward with ties.

14.3.3   Comparison of Methods

Although quite time consuming, both the calculations to estimate the sample
size using the approaches of Noether and Whitehead are relatively straightforward. The Noether approach is probably more complex in that defining
$P(A > B)$ is not straightforward. For the comparisons here we used the hypoth-
esised responses for the investigative treatment estimated using the effect size of
the Whitehead approach to use with the Noether approach. Reassuringly in this
instance, for the same effect sizes, the two approaches were not too different.

To assist in using the approach of Noether (14.8) can be adapted, assuming
a common variance across treatments, to give the effect sizes for different
standardised differences ($\delta = d/\sigma$); we have

$$P(A > B) = \Phi\left(\frac{\delta}{\sqrt{2}}\right), \tag{14.9}$$

from which Table 14.7 can be derived. Again it should be noted that this result
assumes that the data are Normally distributed, but it could be used to help interpret $P(A > B)$ or to provide an estimate for $P(A > B)$ for sample size calculations.

Given the easier interpretation of effect sizes this chapter concentrates on
the Whitehead approach as it has the advantage of being thought of as generalised from binary methodology and as a result (as highlighted in another
section) has a measure of effect that can be interpreted in terms of the binary
response while of course not having the penalty of inflating the sample size
like the binary approaches would.

Note also that another common way to calculate sample sizes for ordinal
responses is to use the Normal data methodology described in Chapter 3.
Julious et al. demonstrated that assuming the data take a Normal form might
give suboptimal results (Julious, George and Campbell, 1995; Julious et al.,
2000).

Assuming the data take a Normal form, Table 14.8 gives a comparison of the
sample sizes using Noether's method (and (14.9)) and using the Normal approximation approach described in Chapter 4. What this table suggests is that if you
have data that are anticipated to take a Normal form, using the Noether approach
to estimate the sample size would give a conservative sample size estimate.

14.3.4   Sensitivity Analysis about the Estimates of the Population
             Effects Used in the Sample Size Calculations

In the chapters describing calculations for data anticipated to take a Normal
form it was described how the sensitivity of a trial design to the variance

TABLE 14.7

$P(A > B)$ for Different Standardised Differences Assuming the Outcome Is Normally Distributed

δ	$P(A > B)$
0.05	0.514
0.10	0.528
0.15	0.542
0.20	0.556
0.25	0.570
0.30	0.584
0.35	0.598
0.40	0.611
0.45	0.625
0.50	0.638
0.55	0.651
0.60	0.664
0.65	0.677
0.70	0.690
0.75	0.702
0.80	0.714
0.85	0.726
0.90	0.738
0.95	0.749
1.00	0.760
1.05	0.771
1.10	0.782
1.15	0.792
1.20	0.802
1.25	0.812
1.30	0.821
1.35	0.830
1.40	0.839
1.45	0.847
1.50	0.856

could be investigated using highly plausible values for the variance. The same principle could be applied to ordinal data for which for a given sample size calculation the sensitivity could be assessed through evaluating the loss of power due to a highly plausible variance from

$$1 - \beta = \Phi\left(\sqrt{n_A \left[1 - \sum_{i=1}^{k} \bar{p}_i^3 \right] (\log OR)^2 / 6} - Z_{1-\alpha/2} \right). \tag{14.10}$$

For Normal data, as discussed in Chapter 3, we can obtain a highly plausible value for the variance by assuming the variance is sampled from a

TABLE 14.8

Sample Sizes Estimated Using the Standardised
Difference and Normal Methodology and Using
$P(A > B)$ and Noether's Method Assuming the
Outcome Is Normally Distributed

δ	$P(A > B)$	Noether	Normal
0.05	0.514	8808	8406
0.10	0.528	2206	2102
0.15	0.542	982	934
0.20	0.556	554	526
0.25	0.570	356	338
0.30	0.584	250	234
0.35	0.598	184	172
0.40	0.611	142	132
0.45	0.625	114	104
0.50	0.638	92	86
0.55	0.651	78	70
0.60	0.664	66	60
0.65	0.677	56	50
0.70	0.690	50	44
0.75	0.702	44	38
0.80	0.714	40	34
0.85	0.726	36	30
0.90	0.738	32	26
0.95	0.749	30	24
1.00	0.760	26	22

chi-squared distribution. This assumption about the variance probably could
not hold for an ordinal response. A solution to the problem is to form a bootstrap distribution for the sample variance for a particular example and from
this take a 95th percentile. We can estimate this bootstrap distribution by
sampling with replacement from the trial on which the sample size calculation was based. For each sample we can estimate the variance. If we repeated
the sampling a large number of times we would form a bootstrap distribution. The upper 95th percentile from this bootstrap distribution could then
be used to investigate the sensitivity of a study.

14.3.4.1 Worked Example 14.8: Full Ordinal Scale

Revisiting Worked Example 14.1 in which the sample size was estimated
to be 188 patients per arm, the estimate of the variance used in the sample size calculation was 6.089. Through a bootstrap sample of 10,000 drawn
with replacement from the original data used for the sample size calculation
(based on 266 patients) the 95th percentile was estimated as 6.119, which if
put into (14.10) would give power of 89.9%, hardly a decrease at all.

TABLE 14.9

Sensitivity Analysis for Worked Example
Superiority Study Assuming All Categories
Are Used in the Calculations

Sample Size	95th Percentile	Power
50	6.296	0.891
100	6.156	0.898
266	6.125	0.899
1,000	6.101	0.900

Note: The estimated 95th percentiles for the variance
were calculated through bootstrapping.

Table 14.9 gives a summary of the sensitivity assessment along with repeated calculations assuming the same distribution of responses was observed but drawn from studies with sample sizes of 50, 100, 266 (the actual sample size) and 1000.

14.3.4.2 Worked Example 14.9: Four-Point Scale

In Worked Example 14.3 for the same effect size as in Worked Example 14.2 the 22-point scale was reduced to 4 points (using clinical cut-offs) for ease of calculations. The estimated variance as a result was increased to 6.796, which increased the sample size to 210 patients. A bootstrap 95th percentile for the variance is estimated as 7.041, which if it was nearer the true variance would mean the power was closer to 89.1%.

Table 14.10 gives a summary of the sensitivity assessment along with repeated calculations for different sample sizes. A point worth highlighting from this table is that although, in terms of the initial sample size calculation, discarding categories does not have a major effect, by comparing Table 14.10

TABLE 14.10

Sensitivity Analysis for Worked Example
Superiority Study Assuming Four Categories
Are Used in the Calculations

Sample Size	95th Percentile	Power
50	8.522	0.826
100	7.251	0.882
266	7.041	0.891
1,000	6.911	0.896

Note: The estimated 95th percentiles for the variance
were calculated through bootstrapping.

with Table 14.9 it does seem that calculations can be sensitive to the assumptions about the variance.

14.3.5 Calculations Taking Account of the Imprecision of the Estimates of the Population Effects Used in the Sample Size Calculations

If there is a wish to account for the imprecision in the sample variance in the calculations, then the following result,

$$1 - \beta = \frac{1}{0.998} \sum_{perc=0.001}^{0.998} 0.5 \left[\begin{array}{c} \Phi\left(\sqrt{n_A (\log (OR))^2 / [Var(\log(OR))]_{perc}} - Z_{1-\alpha/2} \right) \\ + \Phi\left(\sqrt{n_A (\log (OR))^2 / [Var(\log(OR))]_{perc}} - Z_{1-\alpha/2} \right) \end{array} \right],$$

(14.11)

can be applied, and the sample size can be estimated through numerical methods. Remember that for binary data in previous chapters values for $[Var(\log(OR))]_{perc}$ were estimated through the percentiles from the control prevalence—from which the variance and sample size were based.

To assess sensitivity it was recommended that a bootstrap distribution be built around the variance and a 95th percentile taken from this. It is now recommended that the same arguments be extended to provide values for $[Var(\log(OR))]_{perc}$ to be put into (14.11). To do this, carry out the following steps:

1. Generate an empirical bootstrap distribution for $[Var(\log(OR))]_{perc}$ through sampling with replacement from the original distribution.
2. Rank the empirical distribution of $[Var(\log(OR))]_{perc}$ in order of size.
3. Take the smallest value as the first percentile, second smallest as the second percentile, and so on.
4. Use these empirical percentiles in (14.11) and calculate the average power across these for a given sample size.
5. Iterate the sample size until the required power is reached.

It is again easy to highlight the calculations through a worked example.

14.3.5.1 Worked Example 14.10: Full Ordinal Scale

Remember the worked example in which a trial was designed with a calculated sample size of 188 patients per arm. The variance of 6.089 was estimated from a trial of 266 evaluable patients. Forming an empirical bootstrap distribution of 10,000 drawn with replacement from the original data for the

TABLE 14.11

Sample Sizes for Worked Example Superiority Study
Assuming All Categories Are Used in the Calculations

Original Sample Size	Calculated Sample Size
10	196
25	191
50	189
100	189
266	188

Note: The sample sizes were estimated taking percentiles for
the variance calculated through bootstrapping.

percentiles for the variance (14.11) also gives 188 patients per arm. Table 14.11
gives a summary of the sample size calculations along with repeated calculations assuming the same distribution of responses observed was drawn
from sample sizes of 10, 15, 50, 100 and 266 (the actual sample size).

14.3.5.2 Worked Example 14.11: Four-Point Scale

Reducing the scale to four points increases the sample size estimate to 210
patients. Taking into account the original variance was estimated from 266
patients, through bootstrapping, and (14.11) also gives a sample size of 210.

Table 14.12 gives a summary of the sample calculations along with
repeated calculations assuming the bootstrap sample was taken from different sample sizes. It is worth noting that in comparison to Table 14.11 the
imprecision of the variance estimate (assessed through the original sample
size from which the estimate was drawn) has greater effect on the four-point
scale. When using all the categories, accounting for the imprecision has little effect on the sample size calculations (for the case study described), so
this chapter uses the four-point scale in worked examples in the remainder
of the chapter.

TABLE 14.12

Sample Sizes for Worked Example Superiority Study
Assuming Four Categories Are Used in the Calculations

Original Sample Size	Calculated Sample Size
10	234
25	218
50	214
100	212
266	210

Note: The sample sizes were estimated taking percentiles for the
variance calculated through bootstrapping.

TABLE 14.13

Summary of Hypothetical Cross-over Trial

		Treatment B				
		1	**2**	**3**	**4**	
Treatment A	1	λ_{11}	λ_{12}	λ_{13}	λ_{14}	π_{A1}
	2	λ_{21}	λ_{22}	λ_{23}	λ_{24}	π_{A2}
	3	λ_{31}	λ_{32}	λ_{33}	λ_{34}	π_{A3}
	4	λ_{41}	λ_{42}	λ_{43}	λ_{44}	π_{A4}
		π_{B1}	π_{B2}	π_{B3}	π_{B4}	1

14.3.6   Cross-over Trials

14.3.6.1   *Sample Sizes That Are Estimated Assuming That the Population Effects Are Known*

Remember from Chapter 10 how the methodology for parallel group trials for a binary response could be generalised to that for cross-over trials when the data are binary. The practical consequence was that equivalent effect sizes could be used, and the sample size for one arm of a parallel group trial could be taken as the total sample size for a cross-over.

The same principles as applied to binary data can be extended to ordinal data through applying the results of Agresti (1993, 1999). Table 14.13 gives a table of hypothetical cross-over data with each cell of the 4×4 table derived from the marginal totals.

Table 14.14 gives the 2×2 tables around each cut-off on the ordinal scale corresponding to Table 14.13. Under the assumption of proportional odds the odds ratios from each of these tables should equal each other. Also extending the work from Chapter 10 the odds ratios from each of these tables will also approximately equal the equivalent odds ratios calculated from the marginal totals, that is, the odds ratio from a parallel group trial.

To obtain an overall estimate of the odds ratio Agresti (1993, 1999) gave the following result:

$$OR = \frac{\sum_{i<j}(j-i)\lambda_{ij}}{\sum_{j<i}(i-j)\lambda_{ij}}, \tag{14.12}$$

where i and j are the row and column numbers, respectively, and λ_{ij} corresponds to the cell counts (see Table 14.13). The variance for (14.12) is defined as

$$Var[\log(OR)] = \left(\frac{\sum_{i<j}(j-i)^2\lambda_{ij}}{[\sum_{i<j}(i-j)\lambda_{ij}]^2} + \frac{\sum_{i>j}(j-i)^2\lambda_{ij}}{[\sum_{i>j}(j-i)\lambda_{ij}]^2} \right), \tag{14.13}$$

which can be rewritten in terms of the cell probabilities p_{ij} as

$$Var[\log(OR)] = \frac{1}{n} \left(\frac{\sum_{i<j}(j-i)^2 p_{ij}}{[\sum_{i<j}(i-j)p_{ij}]^2} + \frac{\sum_{i>j}(j-i)^2 p_{ij}}{[\sum_{i>j}(j-i)p_{ij}]^2} \right). \tag{14.14}$$

TABLE 14.14

Summary of Hypothetical Cross-over Trial Revisited

a. First Cut-off

		Treatment B		
		1	2 + 3 + 4	
Treatment A	1	P_{11}	$P_{12} + P_{13} + P_{14}$	Q_{A1}
	2 + 3 + 4	$P_{21} + P_{31} + P_{41}$	$P_{22} + P_{23} + P_{24} + P_{32} + P_{43}$ $+ P_{44} + P_{42} + P_{43} + P_{44}$	$1 - Q_{A1}$
		Q_{B1}	$1 - Q_{B2}$	1

b. Second Cut-off

		Treatment B		
		1 + 2	3 + 4	
Treatment A	1 + 2	$P_{11} + P_{12} + P_{21} + P_{22}$	$P_{13} + P_{14} + P_{23} + P_{24}$	Q_{A2}
	3 + 4	$P_{31} + P_{32} + P_{41} + P_{42}$	$P_{33} + P_{34} + P_{43} + P_{44}$	$1 - Q_{A2}$
		Q_{B2}	$1 - Q_{B2}$	1

c. Third Cut-off

		Treatment B		
		1 + 2 + 3	4	
Treatment A	1 + 2 + 3	$P_{11} + P_{12} + P_{13} + P_{21} + P_{22}$ $+ P_{23} + P_{31} + P_{32} + P_{33}$	$P_{41} + P_{42} + P_{43}$	Q_{A3}
	4	$P_{41} + P_{42} + P_{43}$	P_{44}	$1 - Q_{A3}$
		Q_{B3}	$1 - Q_{B3}$	1

By definition this odds ratio would equate to that we would expect from a parallel group study, which is a useful result. To calculate the required sample size we could equate (14.14) and (14.12) with (14.1) to give a sample size estimate for the total sample size of the form

$$n = \frac{[Z_{1-\beta} + Z_{1-\alpha/2}]^2 Var(\log(OR))}{[\log(OR)]^2}.$$ (14.15)

Again it is best to highlight the calculations through a worked example.

14.3.6.2 Worked Example 14.12: Full Ordinal Scale

Suppose an investigator wishes to design a trial in which the outcome is a four-point ordinal response. The anticipated responses on the control treatment (treatment A) are given in the final "overall" column of Table 14.15. The effect size of interest is an odds ratio of 0.56. From this odds ratio the anticipated responses for the investigative treatment are given in the final row, assuming proportional odds of the marginal responses. The Type I and Type II errors are set at 5% and 10%, respectively.

TABLE 14.15

Summary of Cross-over Trial for Worked Example

		Treatment B				
		1	2	3	4	Overall
Treatment A	1	0.011	0.021	0.035	0.013	0.080
	2	0.026	0.051	0.084	0.031	0.191
	3	0.064	0.125	0.208	0.076	0.473
	4	0.034	0.068	0.113	0.041	0.256
	Overall	0.134	0.265	0.439	0.162	1

The individual cells are derived through multiplying the marginal totals. From these individual cells and through using (14.15) the total sample size is estimated as 229 patients. There are anticipated to be 31.1% concordant responses (from the diagonal), so from this the discordant sample size could be estimated as 161 patients.

14.3.6.3   *Worked Example 14.13: Applying Parallel Group Methodology*

In Chapter 10, for binary data the methodology for a parallel group trial was extended to that for cross-over trials in which the sample size per arm calculated for a parallel group study was taken as the total sample for a cross-over study. Applying the same arguments to the ordinal case, using the marginal totals as the basis for the sample size calculation and (14.3) the total sample size is estimated to be 213 patients or 149 discordant patients. This approach gives a sample size around 7% lower than using (14.15).

14.3.6.4   *Worked Example 14.14: Applying Binary Methodology*

Julious and Campbell (1998) highlighted that we can simplify our calculations by ignoring the ordinal nature of the data, dichotomising the overall responses around the direction that subjects are discordant (i.e. either just −1 or 1) and then using a discordant sample size formula from Chapter 10

$$n_d = \frac{(Z_{1-\alpha/2}(\psi+1)+2Z_{1-\beta}\sqrt{\psi})^2}{(\psi-1)^2}. \tag{14.16}$$

Here, the odds ratio ψ is the ratio of positive to negative responses.

Before applying (14.16) we must first estimate ψ. For 43% of the patients the responses on the control therapy are expected to be higher than on the investigative therapy, whilst for 26% of patients the responses are expected to be lower on the control. Thus, ψ could be estimated as 0.60 (approximately the same as 0.56, the treatment effect from the initial calculations), and an estimate of the discordant sample size from (14.16) is 164 patients, a little higher than from (14.15).

14.3.7   Sensitivity Analysis about the Estimates of the Population Effects Used in the Sample Size Calculations

Similar to parallel group data to assess the sensitivity of a trial to the estimate of the variance bootstrapping can be applied to get an estimate of an upper percentile for the sample variance. This plausibly high value for the variance can be put into (14.15) written in terms of power,

$$1 - \beta = \Phi(\sqrt{n(\log OR)^2/Var(\log(OR))} - Z_{1-\alpha/2}), \tag{14.17}$$

to get an assessment of the sensitivity of the study.

14.3.7.1   Worked Example 14.15

In Worked Example 14.12 suppose that the original data, which produced a variance estimate of 7.30, had been estimated from a trial with 100 patients. Bootstrapping on the observed data produced a bootstrap 95th percentile estimate of 7.90, a plausible high estimate of the variance, 8.2% higher than used in the sample size calculation. If this value were applied to (14.17), then the power would be reduced 87.7%. Hence, the study seems reasonably robust to assumptions about the variance used in the calculations.

14.3.8   Calculations Taking Account of the Imprecision of the Estimates of the Population Effects Used in the Sample Size Calculations

To account for the imprecision of the sample variance in the estimate of the sample size, similar to parallel group trials, the following result can be applied:

$$1 - \beta = \frac{1}{0.998} \sum_{perc=0.001}^{0.998} 0.5 \left[\begin{array}{c} \Phi\left(\sqrt{n(\log(OR))^2/[Var(\log(OR))]_{perc}} - Z_{1-\alpha/2} \right) \\ + \Phi\left(\sqrt{n(\log(OR))^2/[Var(\log(OR))]_{perc}} - Z_{1-\alpha/2} \right) \end{array} \right], \tag{14.18}$$

where the percentiles for the $Var(\log(OR))$ are estimated from an empirical bootstrap distribution derived from the original data on which the variance estimate was based.

14.3.8.1   Worked Example 14.16

For Worked Example 14.12, to allow for the fact that the variance was estimated from 100 subjects the sample size would need to be increased by 2 to 231 patients total.

14.4   Non-inferiority Trials

Although this chapter discusses sample size calculations for non-inferiority trials, and equivalence in a separate discussion trials, for ordinal data for such trials these calculations are not recommended. The reason for this is that although the data, as collected, are ordinal in form, in many ways for non-inferiority and equivalence trials this is the wrong scale on which to base our inference. The rationale for this is due to the objective of the trial.

For a superiority trial the objective is to assess whether two populations differ. This assessment is done primarily through a P-value. When analysing ordinal data there are a number of ways of determining this P-value. In this chapter the concentration has been on methodologies based on the assumption of proportional odds. Remember here we assume that that the odds ratio for each cumulative 2×2 is equal across all k categories, that is, $OR_1 = OR_2 = OR_3 = \cdots = OR_k$. In practice the individual observed odds ratios will deviate slightly around the overall odds ratio. However, the overall estimate, and inference, will hold.

For non-inferiority, and equivalence, trials we wish to determine whether two populations do not differ. This assessment is primarily done through a confidence interval by which, for a non-inferiority trial, we wish to determine whether the lower bound is greater than some prespecified non-inferiority margin. As discussed in previous chapters, this is operationally the same as doing a one-sided test. However, it is the determination and interpretation of this non-inferiority margin that is the issue here. In previous chapters the issues with determining non-inferiority margins were highlighted; in this chapter it is also highlighted how prespecified cut-offs could be used to determine a treatment effect for designing a superiority trial.

Extending these arguments we can determine non-inferiority limits for ordinal data. This is when the crux of the problem is encountered because for a non-inferiority trial if a cut-off is used to determine the non-inferiority limit then it is about this that interpretation it could be argued would need to be made. Obviously we can assume proportional odds, and that $OR_1 = OR_2 = OR_3 = \cdots = OR_k$. However, as highlighted previously in practice individual observed odds ratios will deviate at different cumulative cut-offs around an overall effect. This could be suboptimal if the observed odds ratio around the clinically meaningful cut-off is approaching the non-inferiority limit.

The HADS highlights this point as a score of 0–7 would, for example, indicate that a patient is assessed as 'Normal.' Hence, there would be no point demonstrating non-inferiority with an overall assessment of the odds ratio if it cannot be proven at the clinically meaningful cut-offs of 'Normal' if this cut-off is important.

To resolve such a problem obviously we could do some form of step-down procedure. First test the overall odds ratio and if non-inferior test the odds ratio around a cut-off for non-inferiority. However, such an approach would be driven by the least-efficient comparison (i.e. the one on the dichotomous cut-off).

In a roundabout way, therefore, what we are saying is that for non-inferiority trials it is operationally easier to design and analyse them as if they were binary, using the methods described in Chapter 11, about the clinically meaningful cut-offs (or several dichotomous cut-offs simultaneously as for HADS). This has an obvious adverse effect on the sample size, as highlighted in the discussions on superiority trials earlier in this chapter; however, non-inferiority trials are conservative by nature, and our approach should reflect this. The remainder of this section briefly describes the calculations as if the trial will be designed and analysed on the ordinal scale.

14.4.1 Parallel Group Trials

14.4.1.1 Sample Sizes That Are Estimated Assuming That the Population Effects Are Known

Remember the result for non-inferiority studies from Chapter 1

$$Var(S) = \frac{(d - \Delta)^2}{(Z_{1-\alpha} + Z_{1-\beta})^2}. \tag{14.19}$$

Here d here is the non-inferiority limit of interest, Δ is the anticipated mean difference and $Var(S)$ is the estimated sample variance for the log odds ratio for an ordinal response.

An estimate of the variance for the log odds ratio can be made from (Whitehead, 1993),

$$Var(S) = \frac{6}{n_A \left(1 - \Sigma_{i=1}^k \bar{\pi}_i^3 \right)}, \tag{14.20}$$

where $\bar{\pi}_i$ is the average response for each outcome category. By equating (14.19) with (14.20) we require

$$n_A = \frac{6[Z_{1-\beta} + Z_{1-\alpha}]^2}{\left[1 - \Sigma_{i=1}^k \bar{\pi}_i^3 \right] (\log(OR) - d)^2}, \tag{14.21}$$

where d is the non-inferiority limit, k is the number of categories and $\log(OR)$ is an estimate of the difference between treatments.

14.4.1.2 Sensitivity Analysis about the Variance That Is Used in the Sample Size Calculations

To assess the sensitivity of the study to the variance used in the calculations (14.21) could be rewritten in terms of power as

$$1-\beta = \Phi\left(\sqrt{n_A\left[1-\sum_{i=1}^{k}\bar{\pi}_i^3\right](\log OR - d)^2/6} - Z_{1-\alpha}\right). \qquad (14.22)$$

The power could then be assessed *a priori* to a highly plausible value of the variance, determined through bootstrapping, to determine the study's sensitivity to the assumptions about the sample variance.

14.4.1.3 Calculations Taking Account of the Imprecision of the Variance Used in the Sample Size Calculations

To account for the imprecision in the variance estimate used in the sample size calculations the following result could be used:

$$1-\beta = \frac{1}{0.998}\sum_{perc=0.001}^{0.998} 0.5\left[\begin{array}{c}\Phi\left(\sqrt{n_A(\log(OR)-d)^2/[Var(\log(OR))]_{perc}} - Z_{1-\alpha}\right) \\ +\Phi\left(\sqrt{n_A(\log(OR)-d)^2/[Var(\log(OR))]_{perc}} - Z_{1-\alpha}\right)\end{array}\right]. $$

$$(14.23)$$

The percentiles for $Var(\log(OR))$ are estimated through bootstrapping.

14.4.2 Cross-over Trials

The arguments for superiority trials could be extended and parallel methodologies extended to calculate sample sizes for cross-over trials. For completeness, cross-over methodologies are presented.

14.4.2.1 Sample Sizes That Are Estimated Assuming That the Population Effects Are Known

To calculate the sample size for a cross-over non-inferiority trial for ordinal data the following result could be used:

$$n = \frac{[Z_{1-\beta}+Z_{1-\alpha}]^2 Var(\log(OR))}{[\log(OR)-d]^2}, \qquad (14.24)$$

where OR and $Var(\log(OR))$ are as defined by (14.12) and (14.14), respectively.

14.4.2.2 Sensitivity Analysis About the Variance That Is Used in the Sample Size Calculations

To assess the sensitivity of the study to the variance used in the calculations (14.24) could be rewritten in terms of power as

$$1 - \beta = \Phi\left(\sqrt{n(\log OR - d)^2 / Var(\log(OR))} - Z_{1-\alpha}\right), \tag{14.25}$$

with a plausibly high value used, estimating from bootstrapping, to assess the study's sensitivity.

14.4.2.3 Calculations Taking Account of the Imprecision of the Variance Used in the Sample Size Calculations

To account for the imprecision in the variance estimate used in the sample size calculations use this result

$$1 - \beta = \frac{1}{0.998} \sum_{perc=0.001}^{0.998} 0.5 \left[\begin{array}{c} \Phi\left(\sqrt{n(\log(OR)-d)^2/[Var(\log(OR))]_{perc}} - Z_{1-\alpha}\right) \\ + \Phi\left(\sqrt{n(\log(OR)-d)^2/[Var(\log(OR))]_{perc}} - Z_{1-\alpha}\right) \end{array} \right], \tag{14.26}$$

where the percentiles for $Var(\log(OR))$ are estimated through bootstrapping.

14.5 As-Good-as-or-Better Trials

The issues of as-good-as-or-better trials were discussed in detail in previous chapters, and these arguments can be extended to ordinal data. The one issue to highlight is that in designing such trials we may be undertaking two different types of sample size calculation, one assuming the data are binary for the non-inferiority calculation and one assuming they are ordinal for superiority calculations. Obviously it would be the non-inferiority calculation that would drive the sample size if there is a dichotomisation for this assessment.

14.6 Equivalence Trials

The same issues for non-inferiority trials discussed in this chapter generalise to sample size calculations for equivalence trials with ordinal responses. If practical it is recommended that the data be treated as a binary response around an ordinal cut-off (such as for HADS as discussed), and the methodologies described in Chapter 12 for binary data can be used.

14.6.1   Parallel Group Trials

14.6.1.1   *Sample Sizes That Are Estimated Assuming That the Population Variance Is Known*

14.6.1.1.1   *General Case*

Remember again that the variance about the log odds ratio can be defined as (Whitehead, 1993)

$$Var(S) = \frac{6}{n_A\left(1 - \Sigma_{i=1}^k \bar{\pi}_i^3\right)},\tag{14.27}$$

where $\bar{\pi}_i$ is the average response on each outcome category, and k is the number of categories. Consequently an estimate of the sample size for a given power can be estimated from

$$1 - \beta = \Phi\left(\sqrt{n_A\left[1 - \sum_{i=1}^k \bar{\pi}_i^3\right](\log(OR) - d)^2 \bigg/ 6} - Z_{1-\alpha}\right)$$

$$+ \Phi\left(\sqrt{n_A\left[1 - \sum_{i=1}^k \bar{\pi}_i^3\right](\log(OR) + d)^2 \bigg/ 6} - Z_{1-\alpha}\right) - 1,\tag{14.28}$$

where d is the equivalence limit, k is the number of categories and $\log(OR)$ is an estimate of the difference between treatments.

14.6.1.1.2   *Special Case of No Treatment Difference*

As with equivalence trials discussed in previous chapters when an assumption is made of no true difference between treatments the calculations are simplified—with a direct estimate of the sample size possible. With the assumption of no true difference between treatments (equivalent to $OR = 1$) the power can be estimated from

$$1 - \beta = 2\Phi\left(\sqrt{n_A\left[1 - \sum_{i=1}^k \bar{\pi}_i^3\right]d^2 \bigg/ 6} - Z_{1-\alpha}\right) - 1,\tag{14.29}$$

whilst a direct estimate of the sample size can be obtained from

$$n_A = \frac{6[Z_{1-\beta/2} + Z_{1-\alpha}]^2}{\left[1 - \Sigma_{i=1}^k \bar{\pi}_i^3\right]d^2}.\tag{14.30}$$

14.6.1.2   *Sensitivity Analysis about the Variance That Is Used in the Sample Size Calculations*

As with superiority and non-inferiority trials discussed in the chapter, to assess the sensitivity of a study to assumptions about the sample variance the power, for the same sample size, could be assessed from (14.28) using a plausibly high value of the variance. This highly plausible value for the variance could be taken as a 95th percentile from a bootstrap sample.

14.6.1.3 Calculations Taking Account of the Imprecision of the Variances Used in the Sample Size Calculations

The sample size for an equivalence study accounting for the imprecision of the sample variance can be estimated from

$$1 - \beta = \frac{1}{0.998} \sum_{perc=0.001}^{0.998} \frac{\eta_1 + \eta_2}{2}, \tag{14.31}$$

where η_1 and η_2 are defined, respectively, as

$$\eta_1 = \Phi\left(\sqrt{n_A (\log (OR_{perc}) - d)^2 / [Var(\log(OR))]_{perc}} - Z_{1-\alpha} \right)$$

$$+ \Phi\left(\sqrt{n_A (\log (OR_{perc}) + d)^2 / [Var(\log(OR))]_{perc}} - Z_{1-\alpha} \right) - 1$$

$$\eta_2 = \Phi\left(\sqrt{n_A (\log (OR_{perc}) - d)^2 / [Var(\log(OR))]_{perc+0.001}} - Z_{1-\alpha} \right)$$

$$+ \Phi\left(\sqrt{n_A (\log (OR_{perc}) + d)^2 / [Var(\log(OR))]_{perc+0.001}} - Z_{1-\alpha} \right) - 1$$

As discussed in this chapter the percentiles for the variance used in the calculation are estimated through bootstrapping.

14.6.2 Cross-over Trials

The arguments for superiority and non-inferiority trials can be extended to equivalence trials and parallel group methodologies applied. Cross-over results are presented for completeness.

14.6.2.1 Sample Sizes That Are Estimated Assuming That the Population Variance Is Known

14.6.2.1.1 General Case

An estimate of the sample size for a given power can be estimated from

$$1 - \beta = \Phi\left(\sqrt{n(\log(OR) - d)^2 / [Var(\log(OR))]} - Z_{1-\alpha} \right)$$

$$+ \Phi\left(\sqrt{n(\log(OR) + d)^2 / [Var(\log(OR))]} - Z_{1-\alpha} \right) - 1, \tag{14.32}$$

where OR and $Var(\log(OR))$ are as defined by (14.12) and (14.14), respectively.

14.6.2.1.2   Special Case of No Treatment Difference

For the special case of no true difference between treatments (equivalent to $OR = 1$) the power can be estimated from

$$1 - \beta = 2\Phi\left(\sqrt{nd^2/[Var(\log(OR))]} - Z_{1-\alpha} \right) - 1, \qquad (14.33)$$

whilst a direct estimate of the sample size can be obtained from

$$n = \frac{6[Z_{1-\beta} + Z_{1-\alpha}]^2}{[Var(\log(OR))]d^2}. \qquad (14.34)$$

14.6.2.2   Sensitivity Analysis about the Variance That Is Used in the Sample Size Calculations

As described in this chapter the sensitivity of a study to its variance estimate can be determined through bootstrapping (from the original data from which the variance is estimated) to calculate a highly plausible value for the variance. This power of the study could then be determined through (14.32) to assess the sensitivity of the study.

14.6.2.3   Calculations Taking Account of the Imprecision of the Variances Used in the Sample Size Calculations

The sample size for an equivalence study accounting for the imprecision in the sample variance can be estimated from

$$1 - \beta = \frac{1}{0.998} \sum_{perc=0.001}^{0.998} \frac{\eta_1 + \eta_2}{2}, \qquad (14.35)$$

where η_1 and η_2 are defined, respectively, as

$$\eta_1 = \Phi\left(\sqrt{n(\log(OR_{perc}) - d)^2/[Var(\log(OR))]_{perc}} - Z_{1-\alpha} \right)$$

$$+ \Phi\left(\sqrt{n(\log(OR_{perc}) + d)^2/[Var(\log(OR))]_{perc}} - Z_{1-\alpha} \right) - 1,$$

$$\eta_2 = \Phi\left(\sqrt{n(\log(OR_{perc}) - d)^2/[Var(\log OR)]_{perc+0.001}} - Z_{1-\alpha} \right)$$

$$+ \Phi\left(\sqrt{n(\log(OR_{perc}) + d)^2/[Var(\log(OR))]_{perc+0.001}} - Z_{1-\alpha} \right) - 1,$$

where the percentiles for $[Var(\log(OR))]$ are estimated through bootstrapping.

14.7 Estimation to a Given Precision

14.7.1 Parallel Group Trials

14.7.1.1 Sample Sizes That Are Estimated Assuming That the Population Variance Is Known

In this chapter detailed sample size derivation for efficacy trials with ordered categorical endpoints have been given. This work can be extended to trials based on precision. For ordered categorical data the difference between two regimens may also be expressed in terms of an odds ratio

$$d = OR = \frac{p_{A_i}(1-p_{B_i})}{p_{B_i}(1-p_{A_i})}. \tag{14.36}$$

A $(1-\alpha)\,100\%$ confidence interval for $\log(d)$ can be estimated using the variance (Whitehead, 1993)

$$Var(\log(d)) = \frac{6}{n_A\left[1 - \Sigma_{i=1}^k \bar{p}_i^3\right]}. \tag{14.37}$$

Therefore, for a given half confidence interval width w around the odds ratio this condition must be met to obtain the sample size per group

$$n_A = \frac{6\,Z_{1-\alpha/2}^2}{(\log(1-w))^2\left[1 - \Sigma_{i=1}^k \bar{p}_i^3\right]}, \tag{14.38}$$

where $\bar{p}_i$ are the expected mean responses for each of the categories on the scale. In fact it is an advantage to have the variance estimated from the mean responses here. This is because for estimation trials the objective is to estimate possible differences between treatment, and as such *a priori* it is reasonable to assume that the response on each treatment is unknown. What is more likely to be known is the anticipated mean response.

14.7.1.2 Worked Example 14.17

A pilot study is being planned to estimate the odds ratio between comparator and control regimens in which the primary endpoint is an ordered categorical outcome with four points on the scale. The wish is to quantify the odds ratio within ±55% (i.e. $w = 55\%$). It is anticipated that the mean responses across the scale are equal, that is, $\bar{p}_1 = \bar{p}_2 = \bar{p}_3 = \bar{p}_4 = 0.25$. Thus, the sample size required is 39 patients per arm.

14.7.1.3 Sensitivity Analysis about the Variance That Is Used in the Sample Size Calculations

In assessing sensitivity of a precision-based trial instead of interrogating the power of the study to highly plausible values for the variance we instead interrogate the loss in precision. This could be done through rewriting (14.38) in terms of precision (assuming $w < 1$):

$$\log(1 - w) = -\sqrt{\frac{Z_{1-\alpha/2}^2 [Var(\log(OR))]}{n_A}}.$$

(14.39)

As with other calculations in this chapter the highly plausible value for the variance is calculated through bootstrapping.

14.7.1.4 Worked Example 14.18

The estimated variance used in Worked Example 14.17 was 6.4. Suppose that this was based on data from just 25 patients. Bootstrapping produces an estimate for the 95th percentile for the variance of 6.87, a 7.4% increase. This will equate to the precision in the point estimates reducing to 56.1%.

14.7.1.5 Calculations Taking Account of the Imprecision of the Variance Used in the Sample Size Calculations

To account for the imprecision in the variance estimate for sample size calculations we could use

$$\frac{1}{0.998} \sum_{perc=0.001}^{0.998} 0.5 \left[\begin{array}{c} \Phi\left(\sqrt{n_A (\log(OR) - d)^2 / [Var(\log(OR))]_{perc}} - Z_{1-\alpha/2} \right) \cdot \\ + \Phi\left(\sqrt{n_A (\log(OR) - d)^2 / [Var(\log(OR))]_{perc}} - Z_{1-\alpha/2} \right) \end{array} \right] \geq 0.50,$$

(14.40)

where the percentiles for $Var(\log(OR))$ are estimated through bootstrapping.

14.7.1.6 Worked Example 14.19

Accounting for the fact that the original variance was estimated from 25 patients in the sample size calculation would increase the sample size to 40 patients from the 39 previously calculated.

14.7.2 Cross-over Trials

There is a big issue in the calculation of sample sizes for precision-based cross-over trials in that the results from (14.12) and (14.14) require information on individual cell counts, which *a priori* we would not be expected to know but would in fact be trying to estimate. In this chapter it was highlighted how to estimate the sample size for other types of trials (superiority, non-inferiority and equivalence); we could use the sample size for parallel group trials and take the sample size per arm to be the total sample size for a cross-over trial. This would potentially underestimate the sample size a little. However, as precision-based trials are quite small, in absolute terms the underestimation would be quite small. It is therefore recommended to use the parallel group methodologies described in this section of the chapter to estimate the total sample size for a precision-based trial.

 Key Messages

- Sample size calculations for trials in which the primary endpoint is ordinal responses are relatively straightforward.
- The approach of Whitehead makes no assumptions on the distributional form of the data but makes the assumption of proportional odds.
- The approach of Noether makes no assumptions about the distributional form of the data but requires the data to be (relatively) continuous with few ties.

15

Sample Size Calculations for Clinical Trials with Survival Data

15.1 Introduction

In this book methodologies have been described by which the primary endpoint was anticipated to take a Normal form, to be binary or to be ordinal. In clinical trials survival-type data are common primary endpoints if the trial is concerned with investigating the survival experience of the patients. Usually this survival experience is expressed in terms of survival status (e.g. alive or dead; recurred or recurrence free) and survival time (e.g. time to death; time to recurrence).

If the event of interest was observed in all subjects, then the analysis, and hence design, would be relatively straightforward as we would have a continuous primary endpoint with continuous methodologies applicable. However, most studies usually finish some fixed time after study start (e.g. 1 year) such that the event of interest is not observed in all subjects. The effect of this is that applying conventional methods for continuous endpoints would ignore subjects in whom the event was not observed.

Conversely if the data were treated as binary with the primary analysis based on a comparison of survival status by treatment, time would be ignored. A survival analysis therefore accounts for the survival experience of subjects not just by investigating whether the event of interest has been observed in subjects but also the time to this event. Subjects in whom the event has not been observed are treated as censored with the last follow-up time value used in the analysis. A *censored subject* is therefore defined as a subject for whom the event has not happened by the last follow-up time.

Figure 15.1 gives a graphical illustration of survival experience of subjects described through a Kaplan-Meier plot. The x axis is the follow-up time for the study, while the y axis is the cumulative survival experience of subjects in the trial. The two lines within the graph indicate the two illustrative treatment groups with the steps in each line being when an event occurred.

A planned survival analysis, and hence sample size calculation, depends on whether the event of interest is negative (e.g. death), for which a proportional hazards approach would be applied, or positive (e.g. cure), for which an accelerated failure time approach would be applied. For the former it is desirable to delay the time to when the event occurs, and a formal statistical

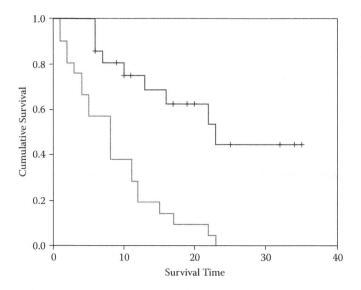

FIGURE 15.1 Graphical illustration of survival data.

test would be done through a Log-rank test. For the latter it is desirable to speed up the time to when the event occurs, and a formal statistical test would be through a Generalised Wilcoxon test.

This chapter describes sample size calculations for cases for which the event is negative and positive. The emphasis in this chapter is on parallel group trials.

15.2   Superiority Trials

15.2.1   Primary Endpoint Is Negative

Suppose the event of interest is a negative, for example, death or recurrence, such that the primary objective of the trial is to delay the event. The objective if the primary endpoint is negative would therefore be to delay the time to the primary event. The primary analysis for such a response would be a Log-rank test (Collett, 1994).

Now suppose the survival distributions for the two arms of the trial have instantaneous death rates of λ_A for treatment A and λ_B for treatment B. Now from this the hazard ratio (HR) is defined as

$$HR = \lambda_A/\lambda_B. \tag{15.1}$$

In terms of the hazard ratio the null H_0 and alternative H_1 hypotheses would be of the form

H_0: The survival experience for both treatment groups is the same ($HR = 1$).

H_1: The survival experience for both treatment groups differs ($HR \neq 1$).

If the hazard ratio does not change with time, then it can be estimated by

$$HR = \frac{\log \pi_A}{\log \pi_B}, \tag{15.2}$$

where π_A and π_B are two survival rates at some fixed time point. Assuming an exponential survival an alternative formula for the hazard ratio is to derive it in terms of the median survival terms for each treatment:

$$HR = \frac{M_B}{M_A}, \tag{15.3}$$

where M_A and M_B are the median survival times on A and B, respectively.

Note if the median cannot be estimated, then the hazard ratio could be defined in terms, say, of the 75th percentile for each treatment group.

15.2.1.1 Sample Size Calculations: Number of Events

15.2.1.1.1 Method 1: Assuming Exponential Survival

When calculating the sample sizes at the simplest level the calculations described for binary data in this book could be applied. However, this approach would ignore the survival times. A more plausible approach would be to use the methodologies for Normal data for the (probably logged) survival times. However, this approach would ignore the censored subjects, meaning that the sample size would be just for the number of events and not the total sample size.

Approaches that account for the overall survival experience were discussed by Machin et al. (1997). A common method is to assume that we have exponential survival. Under this assumption if we let T be the survival time random variable such that for treatment A we have

$$S(t) = P(T \geq t) = e^{-\lambda_A t}, \tag{15.4}$$

where λ_A is constant and does not change with t. From (15.4) we get

$$M_A = \log_e 2 / \lambda_A. \tag{15.5}$$

A similar result for M_B can be derived for λ_B; hence for a given hazard ratio the number of events E required in each patient group is approximately (Machin et al., 1997)

$$E = \frac{2(Z_{1-\alpha/2} + Z_{1-\beta})^2}{(\log HR)^2}. \tag{15.6}$$

TABLE 15.1

Number of Events for Different
Hazard Ratios for a Two-Sided 5%
Significance Level and 90% Power

Hazard Ratio	Number of Events
0.6	81
0.7	166
0.8	423
0.9	1,894
1.1	2,314
1.2	633
1.3	306
1.4	186
1.5	128
1.6	96
1.7	75
1.8	61
1.9	52
2.0	44

Note that (15.6) involves specifying the hazard ratio only. Sample sizes from (15.6) are given in Table 15.1 for different hazard ratios.

Note also that (15.6) estimates the number of events in each treatment arm.

For quick results for 90% power and a two-sided significance level of 5% we could use

$$E = \frac{21}{(\log HR)^2} .$$
(15.7)

15.2.1.1.2   Method 2: Proportional Hazards Only

An alternative method for sample size estimation is one that assumes neither that we have exponential survival or that $\lambda_A(t)$ and $\lambda_B(t)$ are constant over time t. However, it does assume that there is a constant hazards ratio, $HR = \lambda_A(t)/\lambda_B(t)$, over time t, such that the number of events E required in each patient group is approximately (Machin et al., 1997)

$$E = \frac{(HR+1)^2(Z_{1-\alpha/2} + Z_{1-\beta})^2}{2(HR-1)^2} .$$
(15.8)

Note that as with (15.6) this involves specifying hazard ratio only. As this approach makes fewer assumptions than (15.6) it will return slightly larger sample size estimates.

For quick results for 90% power and a two-sided significance level of 5% we could use

$$E = \frac{5.25(HR+1)^2}{(HR-1)^2}.\tag{15.9}$$

15.2.1.2 Worked Example 15.1

We wish to design a study investigating a new investigative treatment against a control; the primary endpoint is progression-free survival. It will be a 2-year study, and the effect size of interest is a hazard ratio of 1.5 against the control (or 0.67 in favour of investigative treatment). For a two-tailed level of significance of 5% and 90% power the sample size (in terms of number of events) assuming exponential survival would be 128 events per arm (from Table 15.1).

If we had used the quick result (15.7), which also assumes exponential survival, we also would have estimated the sample size to be 128 events per arm.

If we assumed proportional hazards only and not assumed exponential survival, the sample size estimate would be 132 events per arm (from Table 15.2), a little greater than by assuming an exponential survival.

If we had used the quick result (15.9), and also not assumed exponential survival, we also would have estimated the sample size to be 132 events per arm.

TABLE 15.2

Number of Events for Different Hazard Ratios for a Two-Sided 5% Significance Level and 90% Power

Hazard Ratio	Number of Events
0.6	85
0.7	169
0.8	426
0.9	1,897
1.1	2,317
1.2	636
1.3	309
1.4	190
1.5	132
1.6	99
1.7	79
1.8	65
1.9	55
2.0	48

15.2.1.3   Sample Size Calculations: Total Number of Subjects

The results (15.6) and (15.8) give sample sizes for the number of events that are independent of the anticipated event rates in the trial. If these results were applied, then the study would recruit so we have the specified number of observed events. There are obvious advantages to this approach. However, for planning purposes (for budgets, for timescales) an estimate of the total sample size would also be required.

To estimate the sample size in each group we need to have an estimate of the anticipated response rates at the end of the study, π_A and π_B for treatment groups A and B, respectively. Hence, the sample size n_A in each group, assuming $n_A = n_B$, can be approximated from (Machin et al., 1997)

$$n_A = \frac{2E}{2 - \pi_A - \pi_B},\tag{15.10}$$

which now as well as requiring the hazard ratio also requires the anticipated response rates π_A and π_B. From (15.2), (15.10) can be rewritten as

$$n_A = \frac{2E}{2 - e^{\log \pi_A / HR} - \pi_A}.\tag{15.11}$$

15.2.1.4   Loss to Follow-up

A proportion of subjects will be lost to follow-up during the follow-up period of the study. Such subjects will be classed as censored in the analysis but will have an impact on the total per group sample size. If we therefore anticipated a proportion w subjects to be lost to follow-up, then we would need to adjust the total sample size per group in (15.10) to be

$$n_{A_w} = \frac{n_A}{1 - w},\tag{15.12}$$

where w is the proportion lost to follow-up before the end of the study.

Note that this is quite a simple calculation. More sophisticated calculations are undertaken in another section.

15.2.1.5   Worked Example 15.2

Following Worked Example 15.1, 70% of patients are expected to survive in the control group. Using the result $HR = \log \pi_A / \log \pi_B$ we have $\log \pi_B = \log \pi_A / HR$ and hence an estimate of 79% of subjects expected to survive on the investigative treatment. Based on these data the anticipated total sample size per arm to ensure 132 evaluable is 517.6 or 518 patients total per arm.

If we had anticipated 10% of subjects would be lost to follow-up, then the total sample size would be 576 subjects.

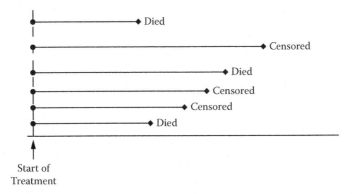

FIGURE 15.2 Survival endpoints for individual subjects.

15.2.1.6 Total Sample Size Revisited

So far in this chapter we have done quite simplistic calculations for studies with survival endpoints. We have based these calculations simply on the anticipated hazards ratio (for the number of events) and the anticipated number of events (for the total sample size). Due to the practical nature of clinical trials the total sample size calculation may be a little more complicated than this. We need to get back to basics to explain why.

Figure 15.2 pictorially describes the survival experience of subjects in a trial; from the start of treatment some subjects progress to the event (here death) or are censored. Actually Figure 15.2 is somewhat artificial as it assumes everyone arrives at the same time to be randomised simultaneously and then is followed up for observation of whether the event has occurred.

In actuality Figure 15.3 more accurately represents the time course of a trial because following the study start subjects are recruited for a period of time. This recruitment (accrual) period ends after a period of time, and then at a fixed point after this accrual period time the study ends, and subjects are analysed. Hence all subjects may be in for a minimum period of time, but the actual period of time subjects may have been in the trial may vary quite markedly.

Another complicating feature of course is that we have a study end at which we need to undertake a statistical analysis. Of course if we waited long enough all subjects would reach the survival endpoint (in terms of death) in particular, but as illustrated in Figure 15.3, at a given time point we undertake a statistical analysis.

Note that some studies actually have a fixed follow-up period during which all subjects are followed up for a fixed period of time; other studies have a variable follow-up such that, as illustrated in Figure 15.3, subjects have variable follow-up times depending on when in the recruitment window they were enrolled.

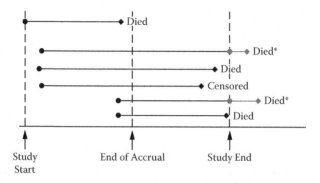

FIGURE 15.3 Survival endpoints for individual subjects accounting for actual time.

With respect to sample size calculations as discussed throughout Section 15.2.1, it is the number of events that is of important, and a sufficient number of subjects should be recruited to ensure a sufficient number of events. It is accrual world, however, and decisions need to be made regarding how to recruit a sufficient sample size to ensure a target number of events. As an extreme you could have a total sample size not much bigger than the number of events required and follow up subjects until most have the event, which may be a long period of time. The accrual period here may be relatively short. Another extreme would be to have a long accrual period such that the total sample size is large relative to the anticipated number of events but then a short period of follow-up. In practice a trial would be a balance of factors with an appropriate accrual period decided on depending on access to patients and budgetary considerations.

So the situation that we are in now is that we wish to estimate a sample size given that the total length of the study is T, and we will be accrualling patients for a period of time R. For this situation we need to multiply (15.6) or (15.8) by

$$\frac{\left(\frac{f(\lambda_A)}{\lambda_A^2} + \frac{f(\lambda_B)}{\lambda_B^2}\right)}{2}. \tag{15.13}$$

If we assumed a uniform recruitment rate, then we would have (Crisp and Curtis, 2008)

$$f(\lambda_A) = \lambda_A^2 \left(1 - \frac{e^{-(T-R)\lambda_A} - e^{-T\lambda_A}}{R\lambda_A}\right)^{-1} \tag{15.14}$$

$$f(\lambda_B) = \lambda_B^2 \left(1 - \frac{e^{-(T-R)\lambda_B} - e^{-T\lambda_B}}{R\lambda_B} \right)^{-1} \tag{15.15}$$

or to account for loss of follow-up

$$f(\lambda_A) = \lambda_A^2 \left[\left(\frac{\lambda_A}{v + \lambda_A} \right) \left(1 - \frac{e^{-(T-R)(\lambda_A + v)} - e^{-T(\lambda_A + v)}}{R(\lambda_A + v)} \right) \right]^{-1} \tag{15.16}$$

$$f(\lambda_B) = \lambda_B^2 \left[\left(\frac{\lambda_B}{v + \lambda_B} \right) \left(1 - \frac{e^{-(T-R)(\lambda_B + v)} - e^{-T(\lambda_B + v)}}{R(\lambda_B + v)} \right) \right]^{-1} \tag{15.17}$$

where

$$\lambda_A = (\log_e(\pi_A))/T \quad \text{and} \quad \lambda_B = (\log_e(\pi_B))/T \tag{15.18}$$

are the rates for the two treatments, and v is the rate of censoring. The results (15.16) and (15.17) can be simplified by using

$$\bar{\lambda} = (\log_e(\bar{\pi}))/T. \tag{15.19}$$

Although they do not look it these are quite simplistic expressions as a uniform recruitment rate may be unreasonable. A more realistic assumption for recruitment rate would be a truncated exponential, in which case (15.14) and (15.15) would, respectively, become (Crisp and Curtis, 2008; Lachin and Foulkes, 1986)

$$f(\lambda_A) = \lambda_A^2 \left(1 + \frac{\lambda_A \gamma e^{-T\lambda_A}[1 - e^{R(\lambda_A - \gamma)}]}{\lambda_A[1 - e^{-\gamma R}][\lambda_A - \gamma]} \right)^{-1} \tag{15.20}$$

$$f(\lambda_B) = \lambda_B^2 \left(1 + \frac{\lambda_B \gamma e^{-T\lambda_B}[1 - e^{R(\lambda_B - \gamma)}]}{\lambda_B[1 - e^{-\gamma R}][\lambda_B - \gamma]} \right)^{-1} \tag{15.21}$$

while (15.16) and (15.17) can be rewritten, respectively, as

$$f(\lambda_A) = \lambda_A^2 \left(\frac{\lambda_A}{v + \lambda_A} + \frac{\lambda_A \gamma e^{-T(\lambda_A + v)}[1 - e^{R(\lambda_A + v - \gamma)}]}{[\lambda_A + v][1 - e^{-\gamma R}][\lambda_A + v - \gamma]} \right)^{-1} \tag{15.22}$$

$$f(\lambda_B) = \lambda_B^2 \left(\frac{\lambda_B}{v + \lambda_B} + \frac{\lambda_B \gamma e^{-T(\lambda_B + v)}[1 - e^{R(\lambda_B + v - \gamma)}]}{[\lambda_B + v][1 - e^{-\gamma R}][\lambda_B + v - \gamma]} \right)^{-1}, \qquad (15.23)$$

where here γ is taken from the probability density (Crisp and Curtis, 2008)

$$f(t) = \frac{\gamma e^{-\gamma t}}{1 - e^{-\gamma R}}, \qquad 0 \leq t \leq R, \qquad (15.24)$$

which is used to model the recruitment rates into the study. If $\gamma < 0$, then the recruitment would be faster towards the end of the recruitment period; if $\gamma > 0$, recruitment would be faster towards the start ($\gamma \neq 0$). Here γ would be estimated from previous studies numerically through entering entry times into

$$L = \sum_{i=1}^{n} \log \left(\frac{\gamma e^{-\gamma t_i}}{1 - e^{-\gamma R}} \right), \qquad (15.25)$$

and finding the value for γ that minimises this. An alternative way to estimate γ from t and R is to use the cumulative density function defined as

$$F(t) = \frac{1 - e^{-\gamma t}}{1 - e^{-\gamma R}}. \qquad (15.26)$$

Hence, if you knew the time say that 50% of subjects are expected to be enrolled you could set $F(t)$ to be 0.5 and solve (15.26) for γ.

15.2.1.7   Worked Example 15.3: Uniform Recruitment

For uniform recruitment we repeat Worked Example 15.1 in which the sample size was calculated to be 132 events to detect a hazard ratio of 1.5. The study was 2 years long with a 3-month accrual phase. With π_A and π_B as the two survival proportions at the end of the study we have from (15.4) $\lambda_A = (\log_e 0.7)/-2 = 0.178$ and likewise $\lambda_B = 0.118$. From (15.13) using (15.14) and (15.15) we must multiply the evaluable sample size by 4.28, giving a sample size of 566 patients per group.

Previously we assumed 10% of subjects would be lost to follow-up, giving a rate of $v = (\log_e 0.9)/-2 = 0.053$. From (15.13) and using (15.16) and (15.17), we must multiply the evaluable sample size by 4.49 to give a sample size of 593 patients per group.

These sample sizes of 566 and 593 are a little conservative compared to previous estimates—518 and 576, respectively—but these sample sizes account for the fact that we have a 2-year study duration in which 3 months are spent on accrual.

TABLE 15.3

Sample Sizes for Different Study Durations for Uniform Enrollment

Study Duration (years)	Accrual Duration (years)	Estimation from (15.14) and (15.15)		Estimation from (15.16) and (15.17)	
		Multiplication Factor	Sample Size	Multiplication Factor	Sample Size
2.00	0.25	4.28	566	4.49	593
2.25	0.25	3.84	508	4.05	535
2.50	0.25	3.50	462	3.71	490
2.75	0.25	3.22	425	3.43	453
3.00	0.25	2.99	395	3.20	423
4.00	0.25	2.37	313	2.59	343

If we wished we could iterate (15.13) to find, say, a study duration that would achieve a sample size that may be consistent with a target sample size. For example from Table 15.3 we can see for the same accrual duration but with a 3-year study duration we would require 395 subjects or 423 accounting for those lost to follow-up. Thus, there is a balance to keep between study duration and sample size.

In truth the calculations do look relatively complicated but they are relatively easy to program. For this book Table 15.3 was calculated in Excel. Undertaking a range of calculations such as in Table 15.3 could add value to discussions within a team designing a trial as the trade-off can be observed between study duration and sample size.

15.2.1.8 Worked Example 15.4: Truncated Exponential Recruitment

As discussed in Section 15.2.1.6, the assumption of a uniform entry into the trial may be a little simplistic for many reasons, not least because it assumes that all centres are enrolling simultaneously into the trial at the start. Suppose here we have information from a previous trial on anticipated recruitment rates and from (15.25) we estimate γ to be -1.5. From (15.24) we can therefore produce Figure 15.4, which gives the percentage of subjects recruited into the trial for uniform and truncated exponential distributions. We can see from this that the truncated exponential distribution has fewer patients entering the trial initially with a greater proportion towards the end of accrual.

For the same assumptions for υ, λ_A and λ_B Table 15.4 gives the sample size estimates for the same scenarios as given in Table 15.3.

For this particular worked example there is no marked difference between the two approaches for estimating the total sample size, but recruitment was relatively short compared to the duration of the study.

An alternative way to estimate γ would be from t and R using (15.26). Suppose we were sure that by 11 weeks 50% of subjects would be recruited;

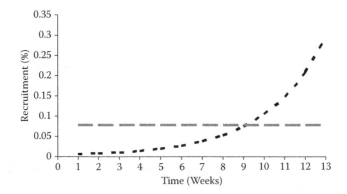

FIGURE 15.4 Entry of subjects into trial for worked example for uniform and truncated exponential distribution.

then we could solve for γ in (15.26) to obtain the result. Table 15.5 illustrates an extreme calculation.

15.2.1.9 Worked Example 15.5: Uniform and Truncated Exponential Recruitment Revisited

This example is a repeat of Worked Examples 15.3 and 15.4 with the same assumptions γ, υ, λ_A and λ_B. Here, however, the enrolment period and study durations are longer than before, with the accrual period being 2 years. Figure 15.5 gives an illustration of the enrolment rates for truncated exponential and uniform enrolment.

Table 15.6 and Table 15.7 give the sample sizes for the study using the enrolment patterns. It is evident from this example that the pattern of enrolment had a bigger effect on the total sample size than previously.

TABLE 15.4

Sample Sizes for Different Study Durations for Truncated Exponential Enrollment

Study Duration (years)	Accrual Duration (years)	Estimation from (15.20) and (15.21)		Estimation from (15.22) and (15.23)	
		Multiplication Factor	Sample Size	Multiplication Factor	Sample Size
2.00	0.25	4.30	568	4.50	595
2.25	0.25	3.85	509	4.06	537
2.50	0.25	3.51	463	3.72	491
2.75	0.25	3.22	426	3.44	454
3.00	0.25	2.99	396	3.21	424
4.00	0.25	2.37	313	2.59	343

TABLE 15.5

Cumulative Proportion Accrued at Different Weeks

Week	Cumulative Proportion
1	0.00
2	0.01
3	0.02
4	0.03
5	0.05
6	0.08
7	0.12
8	0.17
9	0.24
10	0.35
11	**0.49**
12	0.70
13	1.00

TABLE 15.6

Sample Sizes for Different Study Durations for Uniform Enrollment

Study Duration (years)	Accrual Duration (years)	Estimation from (15.14) and (15.15)		Estimation from (15.16) and (15.17)	
		Multiplication Factor	Sample Size	Multiplication Factor	Sample Size
3.0	2	4.09	540	4.31	570
3.5	2	3.38	446	3.60	477
4.0	2	2.90	384	3.13	413
4.5	2	2.57	340	2.80	370
5.0	2	2.32	307	2.55	337
10.0	2	1.39	184	1.66	220

TABLE 15.7

Sample Sizes for Different Study Durations for Truncated Exponential Enrollment

Study Duration (years)	Accrual Duration (years)	Estimation from (15.20) and (15.21)		Estimation from (15.22) and (15.23)	
		Multiplication Factor	Sample Size	Multiplication Factor	Sample Size
3.0	2	5.08	670	5.29	699
3.5	2	3.97	524	4.18	553
4.0	2	3.30	436	3.52	465
4.5	2	2.85	377	3.07	406
5.0	2	2.53	335	2.76	364
10.0	2	1.43	189	1.70	224

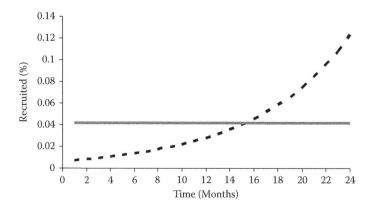

FIGURE 15.5 Entry of subjects into trial for worked example for uniform and truncated exponential distribution for a longer accrual period.

15.2.1.10 Comment on the Results

So far in this book sample size calculations have been investigated for their sensitivity to the assumptions made in the calculations. In this chapter we describe calculations for the total sample size that seemed to make a lot of assumptions in the calculations. The principles of sensitivity analysis still hold in this chapter but should be considered on a case-by-case basis.

For example for a study in which the events occur relatively quickly it may be appropriate to base recruitment on the number of events and the results (15.6) and (15.8) may be applied without consideration to accrual periods and so on.

Another extreme would be a study with a long accrual period and study duration. Here, the study maybe very sensitive to the assumptions made in the calculations, particularly if these are estimated imprecisely, and an assessment of study sensitivity, maybe through simulation, would be strongly recommended.

15.2.2 Primary Endpoint Is Positive

Simplistically we have split the two types of sample size calculation into trials in which the event is negative and, as now, sample size calculations in which the event is positive. A more formal distinction would be to separate the two types of study in terms of follow-up as studies in which incidence is the key primary driver (as discussed in Section 15.2.1) and studies in which time is the primary driver.

For example in a survival analysis sometimes the objective is to speed up the event (if the event is good). Positive events that could be investigated include time to cure, time to remission or time to target level of a biomarker.

The event could also be negative, however, with the objective to assess the speed to the particular event such as time to an adverse event.

In this section of the chapter the emphasis is on when the endpoint of interest is a positive one.

Keene (2002) described a trial in which the primary objective was time to alleviation of influenza symptoms. Figure 15.6 gives a Kaplan-Meier plot from this trial. For these data the actual event rate by the end of the trial was the same for both treatments, but one treatment had a faster onset of action.

Suppose the event of interest is a positive. The null H_0 and alternative H_1 hypotheses would be of the forms

H_0: The survival experience for both treatment groups is the same—the time to the event is the same in the two groups.

H_1: The survival experience for both treatment groups differs—the time to the event is different in the two groups.

For trials in which the objective is to speed up the time to the event the primary analysis would be a Generalised Wilcoxon test (Collett, 1994).

For the data summarised in Figure 15.6 Keene (2002) presented the results as median survival times, which were 6.0 days for placebo and 4.5 days for active treatment.

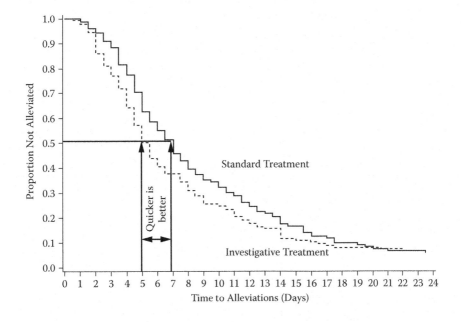

FIGURE 15.6 Time to alleviation of symptoms.

An alternative approach would be to model the data through an accelerated failure time model, an approach applied by different authors for similar data (Patel, Kay and Rowell, 2006). For data from Keene (2002) if they were summarised in terms of an 'acceleration factor', equivalent to a ratio of medians, then the estimate of effect would be $4.5/6.0 = 0.75$.

15.2.2.1   Sample Size Calculations: Number of Events and Total Sample Size

For data for which the objective is to speed time to event there is no unique solution. If we had pre-existing data we could remove the censored subjects and apply the following methods:

- The method of Whitehead (1993) as described in Chapter 14. The disadvantage of this approach is that the calculations depend on defining an odds ratio which does not reflect how the data will be analysed.

- The method of Noether (1987) as discussed in Chapter 14. For continuous data it has the advantage of being distribution free, although it does not have too easily interpretable estimates of treatment effect. For discrete data (which often include survival data in trials as subjects are assessed at fixed times) there can be limitations to the method.

- The simplest approach would be to log the survival times and assume the data take a log Normal form. The results from Chapters 3 to 8 could then be applied.

- If there is a need to account for censoring in the sample size calculation, then bootstrapping or simulation could be considered as an approach to calculate the sample size. The main advantage of this approach is that the sample size calculation may more accurately reflect the analysis.

On a case-by-case level it may be optimal to use one of the methods, depending on the study, and then use another approach or two to assess the robustness of the sample size estimate.

The same approaches as discussed in Section 15.2.1.6 could be used to calculate the total sample size.

15.2.2.2   Worked Example 15.6: Noether Approach

The data in Table 15.8 are from a pilot study for a new compound (B) to assess time (in weeks) to recovery against placebo (A). Assuming the difference observed here is the difference of interest, Noether's method is to be used to estimate the anticipated sample size for the main study assuming the two-sided Type I error is 5%, and Type II error is 10%.

The steps of the calculation are given in Table 15.9.

TABLE 15.8

Data from Pilot Study

Subject	Treatment	Time
1	A	13
2	A	21
3	A	14
4	A	28
5	A	23
6	A	7
7	A	15
8	A	26
9	B	19
10	B	10
11	B	17
12	B	11
13	B	6
14	B	24
15	B	12
16	B	18

Now to find $P(A > B)$ you take 43 and divide it by the multiple of the two sample sizes (here 8 and 8); hence $P(A > B) = 43/64 = 0.67$. Similarly for $P(B > A)$ we have 0.33.

Using the approach of Noether the sample size would 60.6 or 61 events on each arm.

15.2.2.3 Worked Example 15.7: Normal Approach

The mean difference and standard deviation on the log scale for the data in Table 15.8 are 0.23 and 0.452, respectively. Using the sample size approaches

TABLE 15.9

Steps for the Sample Size

Step 1	Arrange the observations in order of magnitude: (A) 7 13 14 15 21 23 26 28
	(B) 6 10 11 12 17 18 19 24
Step 2	Affix either A or B to each observation: B A B B B A A A B B B A A B A A

Step 3	Under each A, write down the number of B's to the left of it:
	B A B B B A A A B B B A A B A A
	   1 4 4 4 7 7 8 8
	Under each B, write down the number of A's to the left of it:
	B A B B B A A A B B B A A B A A
	     1 1 1 4 4 4 6

Step 4	Sum the A scores $U_A = 1 + 4 + 4 + 4 + 7 + 7 + 8 + 8 = 43$ (i.e. A > B 43 times) Sum the B scores $U_B = 1 + 1 + 1 + 4 + 4 + 4 + 6 = 21$ (i.e. B > A 21 times)

discussed in Chapter 3 the sample size estimate would be 82 events per arm.

15.3 Non-inferiority Trials

15.3.1 If Primary Endpoint Is Negative

The number of events E required in each patient group is approximately

$$E = \frac{2(Z_{1-\alpha} + Z_{1-\beta})^2}{(\log HR - \log(d))^2},$$ (15.27)

where d is the non-inferiority limit in terms of a hazard ratio. Sample sizes from (15.27) are given in Table 15.10 for different hazard ratios.

To estimate the total sample size the approaches described in this chapter for superiority trials could be applied.

The one reservation with this approach is that the non-inferiority limit is defined in relative terms, which can cause issues. Suppose we anticipate π_A subjects to survive to a given time. Then from (15.2) we have

$$\pi_B = \exp\left(\frac{\log \pi_A}{HR}\right),$$ (15.28)

and consequently

$$\pi_A - \pi_B = \pi_A - \exp\left(\frac{\log \pi_A}{HR}\right).$$ (15.29)

TABLE 15.10

Number of Events for Different Hazard Ratios for a One-Sided 2.5% Significance Level and 90% Power

Hazard Ratio	Percentage of log (HR)										
	−0.25	−0.20	−0.15	−0.10	−0.05	0.00	0.05	0.10	0.15	0.20	0.25
1.10	1,482	1,608	1,750	1,912	2,100	2,314	2,564	2,858	3,202	3,616	4,114
1.20	406	440	480	524	574	634	702	782	876	988	1,124
1.30	196	214	232	254	278	306	340	378	424	478	544
1.40	120	130	142	154	170	186	206	230	258	292	330
1.50	82	90	98	106	116	128	142	158	178	200	228
1.60	62	68	72	80	88	96	106	118	132	150	170
1.70	48	52	58	62	68	76	84	94	104	118	134
1.80	40	44	46	52	56	62	68	76	86	96	110
1.90	34	36	40	44	48	52	58	64	72	80	92
2.00	28	32	34	38	40	44	50	54	62	70	78

TABLE 15.11

Absolute Difference for Different Hazard Ratios and Survival Rates on π_A

	Hazard Ratio						
π_A	1.10	1.20	1.30	1.40	1.50	1.75	2.00
0.1	0.023	0.047	0.070	0.093	0.115	0.168	0.216
0.2	0.032	0.062	0.090	0.117	0.142	0.199	0.247
0.3	0.035	0.067	0.096	0.123	0.148	0.203	0.248
0.4	0.035	0.066	0.094	0.120	0.143	0.192	0.232
0.5	0.033	0.061	0.087	0.110	0.130	0.173	0.207
0.6	0.029	0.053	0.075	0.094	0.111	0.147	0.175
0.7	0.023	0.043	0.060	0.075	0.088	0.116	0.137
0.8	0.016	0.030	0.042	0.053	0.062	0.080	0.094
0.9	0.009	0.016	0.022	0.028	0.032	0.042	0.049

Hence on an absolute scale for a constant hazard ratio, the non-inferiority limit could be quite different (Table 15.11). Depending on the anticipated response rate for π_A there therefore may be an incentive to be optimistic or pessimistic in defining the non-inferiority limit to maximise it on the absolute scale.

If as discussed in Chapters 6 and 11 we set the study up as a superiority study to detect a small clinical difference but at greater than the nominal 2.5%, then Table 15.12 gives the sample sizes estimated from (15.6) while Table 15.13 gives the sample sizes estimated from (15.8).

TABLE 15.12

Number of Events for Different Hazard Ratios for Various One-Sided Significance Levels and 90% Power Assuming Exponential Survival

Hazard Ratio	Significance Level							
	0.025	0.500	0.075	0.100	0.125	0.150	0.175	0.200
1.02	53,590	8,378	37,764	33,506	30,164	27,404	25,050	22,992
1.04	13,662	2,136	9,628	8,542	7,690	6,986	6,386	5,862
1.06	6,190	968	4,362	3,870	3,484	3,166	2,894	2,656
1.08	3,550	556	2,502	2,220	1,998	1,816	1,660	1,524
1.10	2,314	362	1,632	1,448	1,304	1,184	1,082	994
1.12	1,638	256	1,154	1,024	922	838	766	702
1.14	1,226	192	864	766	690	626	574	526
1.16	954	150	674	598	538	488	446	410
1.18	768	120	542	480	432	394	360	330
1.20	634	100	446	396	356	324	296	272
1.22	532	84	376	334	300	272	250	230
1.24	456	72	322	284	256	234	214	196
1.26	394	62	278	246	222	202	184	170
1.28	346	54	244	216	196	178	162	148
1.30	306	48	216	192	172	158	144	132

TABLE 15.13

Number of Events for Different Hazard Ratios for Various One-Sided Levels of Significance and 90% Power Assuming Proportional Hazards

Hazard Ratio	Significance Level							
	0.025	0.050	0.075	0.100	0.125	0.150	0.175	0.200
1.02	53,594	43,680	37,766	33,508	30,166	27,406	25,050	22,994
1.04	13,666	11,138	9,630	8,544	7,692	6,988	6,388	5,864
1.06	6,194	5,048	4,366	3,872	34,86	3,168	2,896	2,658
1.08	3,552	2,896	2,504	2,222	2,000	1,818	1,662	1,524
1.10	2,318	1,890	1,634	1,450	1,306	1,186	1,084	994
1.12	1,640	1,338	1,156	1,026	924	840	768	704
1.14	1,228	1,002	866	768	692	628	574	528
1.16	958	782	676	600	540	490	448	412
1.18	772	630	544	482	434	396	362	332
1.20	636	520	448	398	358	326	298	274
1.22	536	438	378	336	302	274	252	230
1.24	458	374	324	288	258	236	214	198
1.26	398	324	280	250	224	204	186	172
1.28	350	284	246	218	198	180	164	150
1.30	310	252	218	194	174	158	146	134

15.3.2 If Primary Endpoint Is Positive

As with superiority trials there is no unique solution to the question of sample sizes if time to event is positive and speeding up to achieve the event is desirable. Sample size calculations would need to be done on a case-by-case basis. This also will be the case for equivalence and precision trials, so this will be the last mention of these types of trial in this chapter.

15.4 Equivalence Trials

15.4.1 If Primary Endpoint Is Negative

The number of events E required in each patient group could generally, assuming exponential survival, be estimated from

$$1 - \beta = \Phi\left(\sqrt{E} \left|\log HR - \log(d)\right|/\sqrt{2} - Z_{1-\alpha}\right)$$
$$+ \left(\sqrt{E} \left|\log HR - \log(d)\right|/\sqrt{2} - Z_{1-\alpha}\right) - 1, \tag{15.30}$$

where d is the equivalence limit in terms of a hazard ratio. To estimate the sample size you would need to iterate on E to obtain the required sample size.

For the special case of $HR = 1$ we can estimate the sample size from

$$E = \frac{2(Z_{1-\alpha} + Z_{1-\beta/2})^2}{(\log(d))^2}.$$ (15.31)

To estimate the total sample size the approaches described in this chapter for superiority trials could be applied.

15.5 Precision Trials

15.5.1 If Primary Endpoint Is Negative

The result (15.6) can be adapted by setting $\beta = 0.5$ to obtain a sample size to have the required precision w about the hazard ratio

$$E = \frac{2Z_{1-\alpha/2}^2}{(\log(1-w))^2}.$$ (15.32)

For the total sample size the approaches described in this chapter for superiority trials could be applied.

 Key Messages

- The key driver in the sample size calculation is the number of events.
- To estimate the total number of patients for each trial assumptions need to be made about accrual and censoring.
- The longer the follow-up period is, the fewer the subjects that may be required in the study.
- If the primary objective is to speed up the time to the event, then the calculations are not straightforward, and a number of methods may need to be applied.

References

Agresti, A. (1993). Distribution free fitting of logit models with random effects for repeated categorical responses. *Statistics in Medicine* **12**:1969–1987.

Agresti, A. (1999). Modelling ordered categorical data: recent advances and future challenges. *Statistics in Medicine* **18**:2191–2207.

Agresti, A., and Coull, B.A. (1998). Approximate is better than exact for interval estimation of binomial proportions. *The American Statistician* **52**:119–126.

Agresti, A., and Min, Y. (2001). On sample confidence intervals for parameters in discrete distributions. *Biometrics* **57**:963–971.

Altman, D.G. (1980). Statistics and ethics in medical research III—how large a sample? *British Medical Journal* **281**:1336–1338.

Armitage, P., and Berry, G. (1987). *Statistical Methods in Medical Research*, 2nd Ed. Blackwell Scientific, Oxford.

Bartlett, M.S. (1937). Properties of sufficiency and statistical tests. *Proceedings of the Royal Statistical Society Series A* **160**:268–282.

Bauer, P., and Kieser, M. (1996). A unifying approach for confidence intervals and testing equivalence difference. *Biometrika* **83**:934–937.

Berger, R.L., and Hsu, J.C. (1996). Bioequivalence trials, intersection-union tests and equivalence confidence sets. *Statistical Science* **11**:283–319.

Biomarkers Definitions Working Group. (2001). Biomarkers and surrogate endpoints: preferred definitions and conceptual framework. *Clinical Pharmacology and Therapeutics* **69**:89–95.

Brush, G.G. (1988). *How to Choose the Proper Sample Size*. American Society for Quality Control, Milwaukee, Wisconsin, USA.

Bunker, J.P., Frazier, H.W., and Mosteller, F. (1994). Improving health: measuring the effects of health care. *The Millbank Quarterly* **72**:225–258.

Campbell, M.J., Julious, S.A., and Altman, D.G. (1995). Estimating sample sizes for binary, ordered categorical, and continuous outcomes in two group comparisons. *British Medical Journal* **311**:1145–1148.

Campbell, M.J., Julious, S.A., Walker, S.J., George, S.L., and Machin, D. (2007). A review of the use of the main quality of life measures, and sample size determination for quality of life measures, particularly in cancer trials. In: *Advanced Handbook in Evidence-Based Healthcare*, Stevens, A., Abrams, K.R., Brazier, J., Fitzpatrick, R., and Lilford, R.J. (Eds.). Sage, London, 338–351.

Chalmers, I. (1998). Unbiased relevant and reliable assessments in health care. *British Medical Journal* **317**:1167–1168.

Chan, I.S.F. (2003). Proving non-inferiority or equivalence of two treatments with dichotomous endpoints using exact methods. *Statistical Methods in Medical Research* **12**:37–58.

Chen, J.J., Tsong, Y., and Kang, S.H. (2000). Tests for equivalence or non-inferiority between two proportions. *Drug Information Journal* **34**:569–578.

Chow, S.C., Shao, J., and Wang, H. (2002). A note on sample size calculations for mean comparisons based on noncentral t-statistics. *Journal of Pharmaceutical Statistics* **12**:441–456.

Collett, D. (1994). *Modelling Survival Data in Medical Research*. Chapman and Hall, London.

Committee for Medicinal Products for Human Use (CHMP). (2005). *Guideline on the Choice of Non-inferiority Margin*. Doc. CPMP/EWP/2158/99.

Committee for Proprietary Medicinal Products (CPMP). (1997). *Notes for Guidance on the Investigation of Drug Interactions*. Doc. CPMP/EWP/560/95.

Committee for Proprietary Medicinal Products (CPMP). (1998). *Notes for Guidance on the Investigation of Bioavailability and Bioequivalence*. Doc. CPMP/EWP/QWP1401/98.

Committee for Proprietary Medicinal Products (CPMP). (1999). *Concept Paper on the Development of a Committee for Proprietary Medicinal Products (CPMP) Points to Consider on Biostatistical Methodological Issues Arising from Recent CPMP Discussions on Licensing Applications: Choice of Delta*.

Committee for Proprietary Medicinal Products (CPMP). (2000). *Points to Consider on Switching between Superiority and Non-inferiority*. Doc. CPMP/EWP/482/99.

Committee for Proprietary Medicinal Products (CPMP). (2002). *Points to Consider on Multiplicity Issues in Clinical Trials*. Doc. CPMP/EWP/908/99.

Committee for Proprietary Medicinal Products (CPMP). (2003). *Points to Consider on Adjustment for Baseline Covariates*. Doc CPMP/EWP/2863/99.

Connett, J.E., Smith, J.A., and McHugh, R.B. (1987). Sample size and power for paired-matched case-control studies. *Statistics in Medicine* **6**:53–59.

Crisp, A., and Curtis, P. (2008). Sample size estimation for non-inferiority trials of time to event data. *Pharmaceutical Statistics* **7**:236–244.

D'Agostino, R.B., Massaro, J., and Sullivan, L.M. (2003). Non-inferiority trials: design concepts and issues—the encounters of academic consultants in statistics. *Statistics in Medicine* **22**:169–186.

Day, S. (1988). Clinical trial numbers and confidence intervals of pre-specified size. *The Lancet* **2**:1427.

Diletti, E., Hauschke, D., and Steinijans, V.W. (1991). Sample size determination for bioequivalence assessment by means of confidence intervals. *International Journal of Clinical Pharmacology, Therapy and Toxicology* **29**:1–8.

Donner, A., and Klar, N. (2000). *Design and Analysis of Cluster Randomization Trials in Health Research*. Arnold, London.

Dunnett, C.W., and Gent, M. (1977). Significance testing to establish equivalence between treatments, with special reference to data in the form of 2×2 tables. *Biometrics* **33**:593–602.

Farrington, C.P., and Manning, G. (1990). Test statistics and sample size formulae for comparative binomial trials with null hypothesis of non-zero risk difference or non-unity relative risk. *Statistics in Medicine* **9**:1447–1454.

Fayers, P.M., and Machin, D. (2000). *Quality of Life: Assessment, Analysis and Interpretation*. Wiley, Chichester.

Fisher, R.A. (1935). The logic of inductive inference. *Journal of the Royal Statistical Society, Series A* **98**:109–114.

Fleiss, J.L. (1981). *Statistical Methods for Rates and Proportions*, 2nd ed. Wiley, London.

Food and Drug Administration (FDA). (1992). *Points to Consider. Clinical Evaluation of Anti-infective Drug Products*.

Food and Drug Administration (FDA). (1997). *Draft Guidance for Industry. Food-Effect Bioavailability and Bioequivalence Studies*.

Food and Drug Administration (FDA). (1998). *Guidance for Industry. Pharmacokinetics in Patients with Impaired Renal Function–Study Design, Data Analysis and Impact on Dosing and Labelling.*

Food and Drug Administration (FDA). (1999a). *Draft Guidance for Industry. Pharmacokinetics in Patients with Impaired Hepatic Function: Study Design, Data Analysis and Impact on Dosing and Labelling.*

Food and Drug Administration (FDA). (1999b). *Guidance for Industry. In Vivo Drug Metabolism/Drug Interaction Studies—Study Design, Data Analysis, and Recommendations for Dosing and Labelling.*

Food and Drug Administration (FDA). (2000). *Guidance for Industry. Bioavailability and Bioequivalence Studies for Orally Administered Drug Products—General Considerations.*

Food and Drug Administration (FDA). (2001). *Statistical Approaches to Establishing Bioequivalence.*

Friendly, M. (1991). *SAS System for Statistical Graphics.* SAS, Cary, NC.

Frison, L.J., and Pocock, S.J. (1992). Repeated measures in clinical trials: analysis using mean summary statistics and its implication for design. *Statistics in Medicine* **11**:1685–1704.

Garrett, A.D. (2003). Therapeutic equivalence: fallacies and falsification. *Statistics in Medicine* **22**:741–762.

Grieve, A.P. (1989). Confidence intervals and trial sizes. *Lancet* February 11:337.

Grieve, A.P. (1990). Sample sizes and confidence intervals. *The American Statistician* **44**(2):190.

Grieve, A.P. (1991). Confidence intervals and sample sizes. *Biometrics* **47**:1597–1603.

Guenther, W.C. (1981). Sample size formulas for Normal theory t tests. *The American Statistician* **35**:243–244.

Hamilton, M. (1960). Hamilton Depression Scale. *Journal of Neurology, Neurosurgery and Psychiatry* **23**:56–62.

Hasselblad, V., and Kong, D.F. (2001). Statistical methods for comparison to placebo in active-control trials. *Drug Information Journal* **25**:435–449.

Hauck, W.W., and Anderson, S. (1992). Types of bioequivalence and related statistical considerations. *International Journal of Clinical Pharmacology, Therapy and Toxicology* **30**:181–187.

Hung, H.M.J., Wang, S.J., Lawrence, J., and O'Neil, R.T. (2003). Some fundamental issues with non-inferiority testing in active controlled trials. *Statistics in Medicine* **22**:213–225.

Hutton, J.L. (2000). Number needed to treat: properties and problems (with comments). *Journal of the Royal Statistical Society, Series A* **63**(3):403–419.

International Conference on Harmonisation of Technical Requirements for Registration of Pharmaceuticals for Human Use (ICH) E3. (1996). *Structure and Content of Clinical Study Reports.*

International Conference on Harmonisation of Technical Requirements for Registration of Pharmaceuticals for Human Use (ICH) E9. (1998). *Statistical Principles for Clinical Trials.*

International Conference on Harmonisation of Technical Requirements for Registration of Pharmaceuticals for Human Use (ICH) E10. (2000). *Choice of Control Group in Clinical Trials.*

Johnson, W.O., Su, C.L., Gardner, I.A., and Christensen, R. (2004). Sample size calculations for surveys to substantiate freedom of populations from infectious agents. *Biometrics* **60**:165–171.

Jones, B., Jarvis, P., Lewis, J.A., and Ebbutt, A.F. (1996). Trials to assess equivalence: the importance of rigorous methods. *British Medical Journal* **313**:36–39.

Jones, B., and Kenward, M.J. (2003). *Design and Analysis of Cross-Over Trials*, 2nd ed. Wiley, Chichester.

Jones, D., and Whitehead, J. (1979). Sequential forms of the log rank and modified Wilcoxon tests for censored data. *Biometrika* **66**:105–113.

Julious, S.A. (2000). Repeated measures in clinical trials: analysis using means summary statistics and its implications for design. *Statistics in Medicine* **19**:3133–3135.

Julious, S.A. (2002a). Designing early phase trials with uncertain estimates of variability. Paper presented at International Society for Clinical Biostatisticians Conference, Dijon.

Julious, S.A. (2004a). Designing clinical trials with uncertain estimates of variability. *The Journal of Pharmaceutical Statistics* **3**:261–268.

Julious, S.A. (2004c). Sample sizes for non-inferiority studies with binary data. Paper presented at International Society for Clinical Biostatisticians, Leiden.

Julious, S.A. (2004d). Tutorial in biostatistics: sample sizes for clinical trials with Normal data. *Statistics in Medicine* **23**:1921–1986.

Julious, S.A. (2005b). Sample size of twelve per group rule of thumb for a pilot study. *Journal of Pharmaceutical Statistics* **4**:287–291.

Julious, S.A. (2005d). Why do we use pooled variance analysis of variance? *Journal of Pharmaceutical Statistics* **4**:3–5.

Julious, S.A., and Campbell, M.J. (1996). Sample size calculations for ordered categorical data. *Statistics in Medicine* **15**:1065–1066.

Julious, S.A., and Campbell, M.J. (1998). Sample sizes for paired or matched ordinal data. *Statistics in Medicine* **17**:1635–1642.

Julious, S.A., Campbell, M.J., and Altman, D.G. (1999). Estimating sample sizes for continuous, binary and ordinal outcomes in paired comparisons: practical hints. *Journal of Biopharmaceutical Statistics* **9**(2):241–251.

Julious, S.A., and Debarnot, C.A.M. (2000). Why are pharmacokinetic data summarised as arithmetic means. *Journal of Biopharmaceutical Statistics* **10**(1): 55–71.

Julious, S.A., George, S., and Campbell, M.J. (1995). Sample size for studies using the Short Form 36 (SF-36). *Journal of Epidemiology and Community Health* **49**: 642–644.

Julious, S.A., George, S., Machin, D., and Stephens, R.J. (1997). Sample sizes for randomized trials measuring quality of life in cancer patients. *Quality of Life Research* **6**:109–117.

Julious, S.A., and Owen, R.J. (2006). Sample size calculations for clinical studies allowing for uncertainty about the variance. *Pharmaceutical Statistics* **6**(1): 29–37.

Julious, S.A., and Patterson, S.D. (2004). Sample sizes for estimation in clinical research. *Journal of Pharmaceutical Statistics* **3**:213–215.

Julious, S.A., Walker, S., Campbell, M., George, S.L., and Machin, D. (2000). Determining sample sizes for cancer trials involving quality of life instruments. *British Journal of Cancer* **83**(7):959–963.

Julious, S.A., and Zariffa, N. (2002). The ABC of pharmaceutical trial design: some basic principles. *The Journal of Pharmaceutical Statistics* **1**:45–53.

Keene, O. (2002). Alternatives to the hazard ratio in summarising efficacy in time to event studies: an example from influenza trials. *Statistics in Medicine* **21**: 3687–3700.

Kintz, J. (2007). NCSS, PASS and GESS. NCSS, Kaysville, UT.

Koch, G.G., and Gansky, S.A. (1996). Statistical considerations for multiplicity in confirmatory trials. *Drug Information Journal* **30**:523–534.

Koopman, P.A.R. (1984). Confidence intervals for the ratio of two binomial proportions. *Biometrics* **40**:513–517.

Kupper, L.L., and Hafner, K.B. (1989). How appropriate are popular sample size formulas? *The American Statistician* **43**:101–105.

Lacey, J.M., Keene, O.N., and Pritchard, J.F., and Bye, A. (1997). Common non-compartmental pharmacokinetic variables: are they Normally or log-Normally distributed? *Journal of Biopharmaceutical Statistics* **7**(1):171–178.

Lachin, J.M., and Foulkes, M.A. (1986). Evaluation of sample size and power for analyses of survival with allowance for non-uniform patient entry, losses to follow-up, non-compliance and stratification. *Biometrics* **42**:507–519.

Lemeshow, S., Hosmer, D.W., Klar, J., and Lwanga, S.K. (1990). *Adequacy of Sample Size in Health Studies*. Wiley, Chichester.

Liu, J.P. (1995). Use of the repeated cross-over designs in assessing bioequivalence. *Statistics in Medicine* **14**:1067–1078.

Lu, Y., and Bean, J.A. (1995). On the sample size for one-sided equivalence of sensitivities based upon the McNenar's test. *Statistics in Medicine* **14**:1831–1839.

Machin, D., Campbell, M.J., Fayers, P., and Pinol, A. (1997). *Statistical Tables for the Design of Clinical Studies*, 2nd ed. Blackwell Scientific, Oxford.

McCullagh, P. (1980). Regression models for ordinal data. *Journal of the Royal Statistical Society, Series B* **43**:109–142.

McIntyre, J. et al. (2005). Safety and efficacy of buccal midozolan versus rectal diazepam for emergency treatment of seizures in children: A randomised controlled trial. *The Lancet* **366**(9481): 205–210.

Medical Research Council. (1948). Streptomycin treatment of pulmonary tuberculosis. *British Medical Journal* **2**:769–782.

Medical Research Council Lung Cancer Working Party. (1996). Randomised trial of four-drug vs. less intensive two-drug chemotherapy in the palliative treatment of patients with small-cell lung cancer (SCLC) and poor prognosis. *British Journal of Cancer* **73**:406–413.

Miettinen, O., and Nurminen, M. (1985). Comparative analysis of two rates. *Statistics in Medicine* **4**:213–226.

Mood, A.M., and Snedecor, G.W. (1946). Query. *Biometrics Bulletin* **2**(6):120–122.

Morikawa, T., and Yoshida, M. (1995). A useful testing strategy in phase III trials: combined test of superiority and test of equivalence. *Journal of Biopharmaceutical Statistics* **5**(3):297–306.

Nam, J. (1997). Establishing equivalence of two treatments and sample size requirements in matched pairs design. *Biometrics* **50**:1422–1430.

Newcombe, R.G. (1998b). Interval estimation for the difference between independent proportions: comparison of eleven methods. *Statistics in Medicine* **17**:873–890.

Neyman, J., and Pearson, E.S. (1928). On the use and interpretation of test criteria. *Biometrika* **20**(A):175–294.

Neyman, J., and Pearson, E.S. (1933a). On the problem of the most efficient tests of statistical hypotheses. *Philosophical Transitions Royal Society (London)* **231**: 289–337.

Neyman, J., and Pearson, E.S. (1933b). The testing of statistical hypotheses in relation to the probabilities a priori. *Proceeds of the Cambridge Philosophical Society* **29**:492–510.

Neyman, J., and Pearson, E.S. (1936a). Contributions to the theory of testing hypotheses. *Journal Statistical Research Memoirs (University of London)* **1**:1–37.

Neyman, J., and Pearson, E.S. (1936b). Sufficient statistics and uniformly most powerful test of statistical hypothesis. *Journal Statistical Research Memoirs (University of London)* **1**:113–137.

Neyman, J., and Pearson, E.S. (1938). Contributions to the theory of testing statistical hypotheses. *Journal Statistical Research Memoirs (University of London)* **2**:25–57.

Noether, G.E. (1987). Sample size determination for some common nonparametric tests. *Journal of the American Statistical Association* **82**:645–647.

O'Brien, P.C., and Fleming, T.R. (1979). A multiple testing procedure for clinical trials. *Biometrics* **35**:549–546.

Olkin, I. (1998). Odds ratios revisited. *Evidence Based Medicine* **3**:71.

Owen, D.B. (1965). A special case of a bivariate non-central t-distribution. *Biometrika* **52**:437–446.

Patel, K., Kay, R., and Rowell, L. (2006). Comparing proportional hazards and accelerated failure time models: and application in influenza. *Pharmaceutical Statistics* **5**:213–224.

Pollock, M.A., Sturrock, A., Marshall, K., Davidson, K.M., Kelly, C.J.G., McMahaan, A.D., et al. (2005). Thyroxine treatment in patients with symptoms of hypothyroidism but thyroid function tests within the reference range: randomized double blind placebo controlled cross-over trial. *British Medical Journal* **323**:891–895.

Royston, P. (1993). Exact conditional and unconditional sample size for pair-matched studies with binary outcome: a practical guide. *Statistics in Medicine* **12**:699–712.

Schall, R., and Williams, R.L., for the Food and Drug Administration Individual Bioequivalence Working Group. (1996). Towards a practical strategy for assessing individual bioequivalence. *Journal of Pharmacokinetics and Biopharmaceutics* **24**:133–149.

Schesselman, J.J. (1982). *Case-Control Studies*. Oxford University Press, New York.

Schouten, H.J.A. (1999). Sample size formula with a continuous outcome for unequal group sizes and unequal variances. *Statistics in Medicine* **18**:87–91.

Senn, S. (1993). *Cross-over Trials in Clinical Research*. Wiley, Chichester.

Senn, S. (1997). *Statistical Issues in Drug Development*. Wiley, Chichester.

Senn, S. (1998). In the blood: proposed new requirements for the registering of generic drugs. *The Lancet* **352**:85–86.

Senn, S. (2001a). Guest editorial. The misunderstood placebo. *Applied Clinical Trials* **5**:40–46.

Senn, S. (2001b). Statistical issues in bioequivelance. *Statistics in Medicine* **20**:2787–2799.

Senn, S., Stevens, L., and Chaturvedi, N. (2000). Tutorial in biostatistics: repeated measures in clinical trials: simple measures for analysis using summary measures. *Statistics in Medicine* **19**:861–877.

Sheiner, L.B. (1997). Learning versus confirming in clinical drug development. *Clinical Pharmacology and Therapeutics* **61**:275–291.

Singer, J. (2001). A simple procedure to compute sample size needed to compared two independent groups when the population variances are unknown. *Statistics in Medicine* **20**:1089–1095.

Tang, M.L. (2003). Matched-pair non-inferiority using rate ratio: a comparison of current methods and sample size refinement. *Controlled Clinical Trials* **24**:364–377.

Tang, N.S., Tang, M.L., and Chan, S.F. (2003). On tests of equivalence via non-unity relative risk for matched pairs design. *Statistics in Medicine* **22**:1217–1233.

Tango, T. (1998). Equivalence test and confidence interval for the difference in proportions for the paired sample design. *Statistics in Medicine* **17**:891–908.

Tango, T. (1999). Improved confidence intervals for the difference between binomial proportions based on paired data. *Statistics in Medicine* **18**:3511–3513.

Troendle, J.F., and Frank, J. (2001). Unbiased confidence intervals for the odds ratio of two independent samples with applications to case control data. *Biometrics* **57**:484–489.

Tu, D. (1998). On the use of the ratio or the odds ratio of cure rates in therapeutic equivalence clinical trials with binary endpoints. *Journal of Biopharmaceutical Statistics* **8**:135–176.

Walker, S. (1998). Odds ratios revisited. *Evidence Based Medicine* **3**:71.

Whitehead, A., and Whitehead, J. (1991). A general parametric approach to the meta-analysis of randomised trials. *Statistics in Medicine* **10**:1665–1677.

Whitehead, J. (1993). Sample size calculations for ordered categorical data. *Statistics in Medicine* **12**:2257–2272.

Wiens, B.L. (2002). Choosing an equivalence limit for noninferiority and or equivalence studies. *Controlled Clinical Trials* **23**:2–14.

Wood, J., and Lambert, M. (1999). Sample-size calculations for trials in health services research. *Journal of Health Service Research and Policy* **4**:226–229.

Yardly, L., Donovan-Hall, M., Smith, H.E., Walsh, B.M, Mullee, M., and Bronstein, A.M. (2004). Effectiveness of primary care-based vestibular rehabilitation for chronic dizziness. *Annals of Internal Medicine* **141**:598–605.

Zigmond, A.S., and Snaith, R.P. (1983). The Hospital Anxiety and Depression Scale. *Acta Psychiatric Scandinavia* **67**:361–370.

Bibliography

Agresti, A. (2003). Dealing with discreteness: making 'exact' confidence intervals for proportions, differences of proportions and odds-ratios more exact. *Statistical Methods in Medical Research* **12**:3–21.

Altman, D.G. (1996). Better reporting of randomised trials: the CONSORT statement. *British Medical Journal* **313**:570–571.

Altman, D.G. (1998). Confidence intervals for the number needed to treat. *British Medical Journal* **317**:1309–1312.

Altman, D.G., and Bland, J.M. (1999). Treatment allocation in controlled trials: why randomise? *British Medical Journal* **318**:1209.

Altman, D.G., Deeks, J.L., and Sackett D. (1998). Odds-ratios should be avoided when events are common. *British Medical Journal* **317**:1318.

Anderson, T.W., and Burnstein, H. (1967). Approximating the upper binomial confidence limit. *Journal of the American Statistical Association* **63**:857–861.

Anderson, T.W., and Burnstein, H. (1968). Approximating the lower binomial confidence limit. *Journal of the American Statistical Association* **63**:1413–1415.

Angus, J.E., and Shafer, R.E. (1934). Improved confidence statements for the binomial parameter. *The American Statistician* **38**:189–191.

Beale, S.L. (1989). Sample size determination for confidence intervals on the population mean and on the difference between two population means. *Biometrics* **45**:969–977.

Begg, C., Cho, M., Eastwood, S., Horton, R., Moher, R., Olkin, I., et al. (1996). Improving the quality of reporting of randomised controlled trials: the CONSORT statement. *Journal of the American Medical Association* **276**:637–639.

Bender, R. (2001). Calculating confidence intervals for the number needed to treat. *Controlled Clinical Trials* **22**:102–110.

Birkett, M.A., and Day, S.J. (1994). Internal pilot studies for estimating sample size. *Statistics in Medicine* **13**:2455–2463.

Biswas, A. (2001). Adaptive designs for binary treatment responses in phase III clinical trials: controversies and progress. *Statistical Methods in Medical Research* **10**:353–364.

Blyth, C.R., and Still, H.A. (1983). Binomial confidence intervals. *Journal of the American Statistical Association* **78**:108–116.

Bradburn, M.J., Clark, T.G., Love, S.B., and Altman, D.G. (2003a). Survival analysis part II: multivariate data analysis—an introduction to concepts and methods. *British Journal of Cancer* 2003; **89**:431–436.

Bradburn, M.J., Clark, T.G., Love, S.B., and Altman, D.G. (2003b). Survival analysis part III: multivariate data analysis—choosing a model and assessing its adequacy and fit. *British Journal of Cancer* **89**:605–611.

Bradford Hill, A. (1990). Memories of the British streptomycin trial: the first randomized clinical trial. *Controlled Clinical Trials* **11**:77–79.

Browne, R.H. (1995). On the use of a pilot sample for sample size determination. *Statistics in Medicine* **14**:1933–1940.

Bunke, O., and Droge, B. (1984). Bootstrap and cross-validation estimates of the prediction error for linear regression models. *The Annals of Statistics* **12**: 1400–1424.

Burman, C.F., and Senn, S. (2003). Examples of options in drug development. *Pharmaceutical Statistics* **2**:113–125.

Campbell, M., Grimshaw, J., and Steen, N. (2000). Sample size calculations for cluster randomised trials. *Journal of Health Services Research and Policy* **5**:12–16.

Campbell, M.J. (2000). Cluster randomised trials in general (family) practice research. *Statistical Methods in Medical Research* **9**:81–94.

Campbell, M.K., and Grimshaw, J.M. (1998). Cluster randomised trials: time for improvement. The implications of adopting a cluster design are still largely ignored. *British Medical Journal* **317**:1171–1172.

Casella, G. (1986). Refining binomial confidence intervals. *The Canadian Journal of Statistics* **14**:113–129.

Chalmers, T.C., Celano, P., Sacks, H.S., and Smith, H. (1983). Bias in treatment assignment in controlled clinical trials. *New England Journal of Medicine* **309**: 1358–1361.

Charig, C.R., Webb, D.R., Payne, S.R., and Wickham, O.E. (1986). Comparison of treatment of renal calculi by operative surgery, percutaneous nephrolithotomy and extracoporeal shock wave lithotripsy. *British Medical Journal* **292**: 879–892.

Clark, T.G., Bradburn, M.J., Love, S.B., and Altman, D.G. (2003). Survival analysis part I: basic concepts and first analyses. *British Journal of Cancer* 2003; **89**:232–238.

Clayton, D., and Hills, M. (1993). *Statistical Models in Epidemiology*. Oxford University Press, Oxford.

Clopper, C.J., and Pearson, E.S. (1934). The use of confidence or fiducial limits illustrated in the case of the binomial. *Biometrika* **26**:404–413.

Committee for Proprietary Medicinal Products (CPMP). (2004a). *Notes for Guidance on the Evaluation of Medicinal Products Indicated for the Treatment of Bacterial Infections*. Doc. CPMP/EWP/558/95.

Committee for Proprietary Medicinal Products (CPMP). (2004b). *Points to Consider on the Choice of Non-Inferiority Margin (Draft)*. Doc. CPMP/EWP/2158/99 draft.

Conner, R.J. (1987). Sample size for testing differences in proportions for the paired-sample design. *Biometrics* **43**:207–211.

Cook, R.A., and Sackett, D.L. (1995). The number needed to treat: clinically useful measure of treatment effect. *British Medical Journal* **310**:452–454.

Cowell, R.G., Dawid, A.P., Hutchinson, T.A., Roden, S., and Spiegelhalter, D.J. (1993). Bayesian networks for the analysis of drug safety. *The Statistician* **42**(4): 369–384.

Crow, E.L. (1956). Confidence intervals for a proportion. *Biometrika* **43**:423–435.

Daly, L. (1992). Simple SAS macros for the calculation of exact binomial and Poisson confidence limits. *Computational and Biological Medicine* **22**:351–361.

Dark, R., Bolland, K., and Whitehead, J. (2003). Statistical methods for ordered data based on a constrained odds model. *Biometrical Journal* **45**(4):453–470.

Davies, H.T.O., Crombie, I.K., and Tavakoli, M. (1998). When can odds-ratios mislead? *British Medical Journal* **316**:989–991.

Day, S. (2000). Operational difficulties with internal pilot studies to update sample size. *Drug Information Journal* **34**:461–468.

Day, S.J., and Altman, D.G. (2000). Blinding in clinical trials and other studies. *British Medical Journal* **321**:504.

Deeks, J. (1998). Odds-ratios should be used only in case-control studies and logistic regression studies. *British Medical Journal* **317**:1155–1156.

de Haes, J.C.J.M., and van Knippenberg, F.C.E. (1985). The quality of life of cancer patients—a review of the literature. *Social Science and Medicine* **20**: 809–817.

de Haes, J.C.J.M., van Knippenberg, F.C.E., and Neijt, J.P. (1990). Measuring psychological and physical distress in cancer patients: structure and application of the Rotterdam Symptom Checklist. *British Journal of Cancer* **62**:1034–1038.

Desu, M.M., and Raghavarao, D. (1990). *Sample Size Methodology*. Academic Press, London.

Diggle, P.J., Liang, K.Y., and Zeger, S.L. (1996). *Analysis of Longitudinal Data*. Oxford University Press, Oxford.

Donner, A. (1983). Approaches to sample size estimation in the design of clinical trials—a review. *Statistics in Medicine* **3**:199–214.

Donner, A., and Wells, G. (1986). A comparison of confidence interval methods for the intra-class correlation coefficient. *Biometrics* **42**(2):401–412.

Ederer, F., and Mantel, N. (1974). Confidence limits on the ratio of two Poisson variables. *American Journal of Epidemiology* **100**(3):165–167.

Edwardes, M.D. (1998). The evaluation of confidence sets with application to binomial intervals. *Statistica Sinica* **8**:393–409.

Efron, B., and Gong, G. (1983). A leisurely look at the bootstrap, the jacknife and the cross-validation. *American Statistician*, **37**:36–48.

Efron, B., and Tibshirani, R.J. (1993). An introduction to the bootstrap. Chapman and Hall: New York.

Eldridge, S.M. (2005). Assessing, understanding an improving the efficiency of cluster randomized trials in primary care. Unpublished PhD dissertation, University of London.

Ellenberg, S.S., and Temple, R. (2000). Placebo-controlled trials and active control trials in the evaluation of new treatments. Part 2: practical issues and specific cases. *Annals of Internal Medicine* **133**:464–470.

Ellison, B.E. (1964). Two theorems for inferences about the Normal distribution with applications in acceptance sampling. *Journal of the American Statistical Association* **59**:89–95.

Enas, G., and Andersen, J.S. (2001). Enhancing the value delivered by the statistician throughout drug discovery and development: putting statistical science into regulated pharmaceutical innovation. *Statistics in Medicine* **20**:2697–2708.

Escobar, M.D. (1994). Estimating means with dirichlet process priors. *Journal of the American Statistical Association* **89**:268–277.

Escobar, M.D., and West, M. (1995). Bayesian density estimation and inference using mixtures. *Journal of the American Statistical Association* **90**:570–588.

Fayers, P., Ashby, D., and Parmar, M. (1997). Tutorial in biostatistics: Bayesian data monitoring in clinical trials. *Statistics in Medicine* **16**:1413–1430.

Fayers, P., and Machin, D. (1995). Sample size: how many patients are necessary? *British Journal of Cancer* **72**:1–9.

Feng, Z., and Grizzle, J.E. (1992). Correlated binomial variates: properties of estimator of intraclass correlation and its effect on sample size calculation. *Statistics in Medicine* **11**:1607–1614.

Ferguson, T.S. (1973). A Bayesian analysis of some nonparamatric problems. *The Annals of Statistics* **1**:209–230.

Ferguson, T.S. (1974). Prior distributions on spaces of probability measures. *The Annals of Statistics* **2**:615–629.

Fisher, R.A. (1925). *Statistical Methods for Research Workers*. Oliver and Boyd, Edinburgh.

Fleiss, J.L., and Levin, B. (1988). Sample size determination in studies with matched pairs. *Journal of Clinical Epidemiology* **41**:727–730.

Friede, T., and Kieser, M. (2001). A comparison of methods for adaptive sample size adjustment. *Statistics in Medicine* **20**:3861–3873.

Ghosh, B.K. (1979). A comparison of some approximate confidence limits for the binomial parameter. *Journal of the American Statistical Association* **74**: 894–900.

Gould, A.L. (1992). Interim analyses for monitoring clinical trials that do not materially affect the Type I error rate. *Statistics in Medicine* **11**:55–66.

Gould, A.L. (1995a). Group sequential extensions of a standard bioequivalence testing procedure. *Journal of Pharmacokinetics and Biopharmaceutics* **23**:5–86.

Gould, A.L. (1995b). Planning and revising the sample size for a trial. *Statistics in Medicine* **14**:1039–1051.

Gould, A.L. (2001). Sample size re-estimation: recent developments and practical considerations. *Statistics in Medicine* **20**:2625–2643.

Gould, A.L., and Shih, W.J. (1992). Sample size re-estimation without unblinding for Normally distributed data with unknown variance. *Communications in Statistics—Theory and Methods* **21**:2833–2853.

Gould, A.L., and Shih, W.J. (1998). Modifying the design of ongoing trials without unblinding. *Statistics in Medicine* **17**:89–100.

Graham, P.L., Mengersen, K., and Morton, A.P. (2003). Confidence limits for the ratio of two rates based on likelihood scores: noniterative method. *Statistics in Medicine* **22**:2071–2083.

Greenberg, R.P., and Fisher, S. (1994). Suspended judgement—seeing through the double masked design: a commentary. *Controlled Clinical Trials* **15**:244–246.

Greenland, S. (1988). On sample-size and power calculations for studies using confidence intervals. *American Journal of Epidemiology* **128**(1):231–237.

Grieve, A.P. (2003). The number needed to treat: a useful clinical measure or a case of the emperor's new clothes? *Journal of Pharmaceutical Statistics* **2**:87–102.

Guyatt, G.H., Juniper, E.F., Walter, S.D., Griffith, L.E., and Goldstein, R.S. (1998). Interpreting treatment effects in randomised trials. *British Medical Journal* **316**:690–693.

Hall, P. (1992). *Bootstrap and Edgeworth Expansion*. Springer-Verlag, New York.

Hilton, J.F., and Mehta. C.R. (1993). Power and sample size calculations for exact conditional tests with ordered data. *Biometrics* **49**:609–616.

Hinkley, D.V. (1988). Bootstrap methods. *Journal of the Royal Statistical Society, Series B* **50**:321–337.

Hinkley, D.V., and Schechtman, E. (1987). Conditional bootstrap methods in the mean shift model. *Biometrika* **74**:85–94.

Johnson, N.L., and Kotz, S. (1994a). *Distributions in Statistics: Continuous Univariate Distributions—1*. Wiley, Chichester.

Johnson, N.L., and Kotz, S. (1994b). *Distributions in Statistics: Continuous Univariate Distributions—2*. Wiley, Chichester.

Johnson, N.L., and Kotz, S. (1994c). *Distributions in Statistics: Discrete Distributions.* Wiley, Chichester.

Joseph, L., du Berger, R., and B'elisle, P. (1997). Bayesian and mixed Bayesian/ likelihood criteria for sample size determination. *Statistics in Medicine* **16**(7): 769–781.

Julious, S.A. (2004b). Sample size re-determination for repeated measures studies. *Biometrics* **60**:284–285.

Julious, S.A. (2004e). Using confidence intervals around individual means to assess statistical significance between two means. *The Journal of Pharmaceutical Statistics* **3**:217–222.

Julious, S.A. (2005a). Issues with number needed to treat [letter]. *Statistics in Medicine* **24**:3233–3235.

Julious, S.A. (2005c). Two-sided confidence intervals for the single proportion: comparison of seven methods [letter]. *Statistics in Medicine* **24**:3383–3384.

Julious, S.A., and Mullee, M.A. (1994). Confounding and Simpon's paradox. *British Medical Journal* **308**:1480–1481.

Julious, S.A., and Mullee, M.A. (2000). Crude rates of outcome. *British Journal of Surgery* **87**:8–9.

Julious, S.A., and Swank, D. (2005). Moving statistics beyond the individual clinical trial—applying decision science to optimise a clinical development plan. *Journal of Pharmaceutical Statistics* **4**:37–46.

Kendall, M., and Stuart, A. (1977). *Distribution Theory.* Vol. 1 of *The Advanced Theory of Statistics,* 4th ed. Griffin, London.

Kieser, M., and Friede, T. (2000). Re-calculating the sample size in internal pilot study designs with control of the Type I error rate. *Statistics in Medicine* **19**:901–911.

Korn, E.L. (1986) Sample size tables for bounding small proportions. *Biometrics* **42**:213–216.

Kunz, R., and Oxman, A.D. (1998). The unpredictability paradox: review of empirical comparisons of randomised trials and non-randomised clinical trials. *British Medical Journal* **317**:1185–1190.

Kwang, G.P.S., and Hutton, J.L. (2003). Choice of parametric models in survival analysis: applications to monotherapy for epilepsy and cerebral palsy. *Applied Statistics* **52**(2):153–168.

Lachin, J.M. (1977). Sample size determination for r x c comparative trials. *Biometrics* **33**:315–324.

Lake, S., Kammann, E., Klar, N., and Betensky, R. (2002). Samples size re-estimation in cluster randomisation trials. *Statistics in Medicine* **21**:1337–1350.

Laster, L.L., and Johnson, M.F. (2003). Non-inferiority trials: the 'at least as good as' criterion. *Statistics in Medicine* **22**:187–200.

Lee, M.K., Song, H.H., Kang, S.H., and Ahn, C.W. (2002). The determination of sample sizes in the comparison of two multinomial proportions from ordered categories. *Biometrical Journal* **44**(4):395–409.

Lesaffre, E., and Pledger, G. (1999). A note on the number needed to treat. *Controlled Clinical Trials* **20**:439–447.

Liu, K.J. (1991). Sample sizes for repeated measurements in dichotomous data. *Statistics in Medicine* **10**:463–472.

Liu, Q., Proschan, M.A., and Pledger, G.W. (2002). A unified theory of two-stage adaptive designs. *Journal of the American Statistical Association* **97**:1034–1041.

Lui, K.J. (2001). Interval estimation of simple difference with dichotomous data with repeated measurements. *Biometrical Journal* **43**:845–861.

Lunn, D.J., Wakefield, J., and Racine-Poon, R. (2001). Cumulative logic models for ordinal data: a case study involving allergic rhinitis severity scores. *Statistics in Medicine* **20**:2261–2285.

Matthews, J.N.S. (2000). *An Introduction to Randomised Controlled Trials*. Arnold, London.

May, W.L., and Johnson, W.D. (1997). The validity and power for tests of two correlation proportions. *Statistics in Medicine* **16**:1081–1096.

Miettinen, O.S. (1968). The matched pairs design in the case of all-or-none responses. *Biometrics* **24**:339–353.

Mood, A.M., Graybill, F.A., and Boes, D.C. (1974). *Introduction to the Theory of Statistics*. McGraw-Hill, London.

Moorey, S., Greer, S., Watsonm, M., Gormann, C., Rowdenn, L., Tunmore, R., et al. (1991). The factor structure and factor stability of the Hospital Anxiety and Depression Scale in patients with cancer. *British Journal of Psychiatry* **158**: 255–259.

Newcombe, R.G. (1998a). Improved confidence intervals for the difference between binomial proportions based on paired data. *Statistics in Medicine* **17**: 2633–2650.

Newcombe, R.G. (1998c). Two-sided confidence intervals for the single proportion: comparison of seven methods. *Statistics in Medicine* **17**:857–872.

Nixon, R.M., and Thompson, S.G. (2003). Baseline adjustments for binary data in repeated cross-sectional cluster randomised trials. *Statistics in Medicine* **22**: 2673–2692.

O'Brien, R.G., and Lohr, V.I. (1984). Power analysis for linear models: the time has come. SUGI Conference Proceedings.

O'Quigley, J., Pepe, M., and Fisher, L. (1990). Continual reassessment method: a practical guide for phase I clinical trials in cancer. *Biometrics* **46**:33–48.

O'Quigley, J., and Shen, L.Z. (1996). Continuous reassessment methods: a likelihood approach. *Biometrics* **52**:673–684.

Pham-Gia, T., and Turkkan, N. (1992). Sample size determination in Bayesian analysis. *The Statistician* **41**:389–392.

Pocock, S.J. (1983). *Clinical Trials: A Practical Approach*. Wiley, Chichester.

Posch, M., and Bauer, P. (2000). Interim analysis and sample size reassessment. *Biometrics* **56**:1170–1176.

Proschan, M.A., Liu, Q., and Hunsberger, S. (2003). Practical midcourse sample modification in clinical trials. *Controlled Clinical Trials* **23**:4–15.

Rabbee, N., Mehta, C., Patel, N., and Senchaudhuri, P. (2003). Power and sample for ordered data. *Statistical Methods in Medical Research* **12**:73–84.

Rao, C.R. (1965). *Linear Statistical Inference and Its Applications*. Wiley, Chichester.

Rasch, D., and Horrendorfer, G. (1986). *Experimental Design: Sample Size Determination and Block Designs*. Reidel, Lancaster.

Reiczigel, J. (2003). Confidence intervals for the binomial parameter: some new considerations. *Statistics in Medicine* **22**:611–621.

Robinson, L.D., and Jewell, N.P. (1991). Some surprising results about covariate adjustment in logistic regression models. *International Statistical Review* **58**(2): 227–240.

Sackett, D.L., Deeks, J.J., and Altman, D.G. (1996). Down with odds-ratios! *Evidence-Based Medicine* **1**(6):164–166.

Santer, T.J., and Snell, M.K. (1980). Small sample confidence intervals for p1-p2 and p1/p2 in 2x2 contingency tables. *Journal of the American Statistical Association* **75**:386–394.

Schulzer, M., and Mancini, G.B. (1996). 'Unqualified success' and 'unmitigated failure': number-needed-to-treat-related concepts for assessing treatment efficacy in the presence of treatment-induced adverse events. *International Journal of Epidemiology* **25**(4):704–712.

Seber, G.A.F. (1977) *Linear Regression Analysis*. Wiley, Chichester.

Senn, S. (2000). Consensus and controversy in pharmaceutical statistics (with discussion). *Journal of the Royal Statistical Society, Series D* **49**:135–176.

Shaban, S.A. (1980). Change-point problem and two-phase regression: an annotated bibliography. *International Statistical Review* **48**:83–93.

Simpson, E.H. (1951). The interpretation of interaction in contingency tables. *Journal of the Royal Statistical Society, Series B* **2**:238–241.

Smeeth, L., Haines, A., and Ebrahim, S. (1999). Numbers needed to treat derived from meta analyses—sometimes informative, usually misleading. *British Medical Journal* **318**:1548–1551.

Spiegelhalter, D., Abrams, K.R., and Myles, J.P. (2004). *Bayesian Approaches to Clinical Trials and Health-Care Evaluation*. Wiley, Chichester.

Spiegelhalter, D., Freedman, L., and Parmer, M. (1995). Bayesian approaches to randomized trials. *Journal of the Royal Statistical Society, Series A* **157**:387–416.

Spiegelhalter, D.J. (2001). Bayesian methods for cluster randomised trials with continuous responses. *Statistical in Medicine* **20**:435–452.

Spiegelhalter, D.J., Myles, J.P., Jones, D.R., and Abrams, K.R. (1999). Methods in health service research: an introduction to Bayesian methods in health service research. *British Medical Journal* **319**:508–512.

Sterne, T.E. (1945). Some remarks on confidence or fiducial limits. *Biometrika* **41**: 275–278.

Swiger, L.A., Harvey, W.R., Everson, D.O., and Gregory, K.E. (1964). The variance of intraclass correlation involving groups with one observation. *Biometrics* **20**:818–826.

Thompson, S.G., Warn, D.E., and Turner, R.M. (2004). Bayesian methods for analysis of binary data in cluster randomised trials on the absolute risk scale. *Statistics in Medicine* **23**:389–410.

Turner, R.M., Omar, R.Z., and Thompson, S.G. (2001). Bayesian methods of analysis for cluster randomised trials with binary outcome data. *Statistics in Medicine* **20**:453–471.

Turner, R.M., Omar, R.Z., and Thompson, S.G. (2006). Constructing intervals for the intra-cluster correlation coefficient using Bayesian modelling and application in cluster randomised trials. *Statistics in Medicine* **25**:1443–1456.

Turner, R.M., Prevost, A.T., and Thompson, S.G. (2004). Allowing for imprecision of the intracluster correlation coefficient in the design of cluster randomised trials. *Statistics in Medicine* **23**:1195–1214.

Ukoummunne, O.C. (2003a). A comparison of confidence intervals methods for the intraclass correlation coefficient in cluster randomised trials. *Statistics in Medicine* **21**:3757–3774.

Ukoummunne, O.C., Davison, A.C., Gulliford, M.C., and Chinn, C. (2003b). Non-parametric bootstrap confidence intervals for the intraclass correlation coefficient. *Statistics in Medicine* **22**:3805–3821.

Vollset, S.E. (1993). Confidence intervals for a binomial proportion. *Statistics in Medicine* **12**:809–824.

Whitehead, A., and Jones, N.M.B. (1994). A meta analysis of clinical trials involving different classifications of response into ordered categories. *Statistics in Medicine* **13**:2503–2515.

Whitehead, J., Zhou, Y., Patterson, S., Webber, D., and Francis, S. (2001). Easy to implement Bayesian methods for dose escalation studies in healthy volunteers. *Biostatistics* **2**:47–61.

Wilson, E.B. (1927). Probably inference, the law of succession and statistical inference. *Journal of the American Statistical Association* **22**:202–212.

Wittes, J., and Brittain, E. (1990). The role of internal pilot studies in increasing the efficacy of clinical trials. *Statistics in Medicine* **9**:65–72.

Wu, C.F.J. (1986). Jackknife, bootstrap and other re-sampling methods in regression analysis. *Annals of Statistics* **14**:1261–1295.

Yoshioka, A. (1998). Use of randomisation in the Medical Research Council's clinical trials of streptomycin in pulmonary tuberculosis in the 1940s. *British Medical Journal* **317**:1220–1223.

Zucker, D.M. (2004). Sample size re-determination for repeated measures studies. *Biometrics* **60**:284–285.

Zucker, D.M., and Denne, J. (2002). Sample size re-determination for repeated measures studies. *Biometrics* **48**(3):548–559.

Zucker, D.M., Wittes, J.T., Schabenberger, O., and Brittain E. (1999). Internal pilot studies II. Comparison of various procedures. *Statistics in Medicine* **18**: 3493–3509.

Appendix

All tables were created using Microsoft Excel®.

TABLE A.1

One-Sided Normal Probability Values

z	0.00	0.01	0.02	0.03	0.04	0.05	0.06	0.07	0.08	0.09
0.00	0.50000	0.49601	0.49202	0.48803	0.48405	0.48006	0.47608	0.47210	0.46812	0.46414
0.10	0.46017	0.45620	0.45224	0.44828	0.44433	0.44038	0.43644	0.43251	0.42858	0.42465
0.20	0.42074	0.41683	0.41294	0.40905	0.40517	0.40129	0.39743	0.39358	0.38974	0.38591
0.30	0.38209	0.37828	0.37448	0.37070	0.36693	0.36317	0.35942	0.35569	0.35197	0.34827
0.40	0.34458	0.34090	0.33724	0.33360	0.32997	0.32636	0.32276	0.31918	0.31561	0.31207
0.50	0.30854	0.30503	0.30153	0.29806	0.29460	0.29116	0.28774	0.28434	0.28096	0.27760
0.60	0.27425	0.27093	0.26763	0.26435	0.26109	0.25785	0.25463	0.25143	0.24825	0.24510
0.70	0.24196	0.23885	0.23576	0.23270	0.22965	0.22663	0.22363	0.22065	0.21770	0.21476
0.80	0.21186	0.20897	0.20611	0.20327	0.20045	0.19766	0.19489	0.19215	0.18943	0.18673
0.90	0.18406	0.18141	0.17879	0.17619	0.17361	0.17106	0.16853	0.16602	0.16354	0.16109
1.00	0.15866	0.15625	0.15386	0.15151	0.14917	0.14686	0.14457	0.14231	0.14007	0.13786
1.10	0.13567	0.13350	0.13136	0.12924	0.12714	0.12507	0.12302	0.12100	0.11900	0.11702
1.20	0.11507	0.11314	0.11123	0.10935	0.10749	0.10565	0.10383	0.10204	0.10027	0.09853
1.30	0.09680	0.09510	0.09342	0.09176	0.09012	0.08851	0.08691	0.08534	0.08379	0.08226
1.40	0.08076	0.07927	0.07780	0.07636	0.07493	0.07353	0.07215	0.07078	0.06944	0.06811
1.50	0.06681	0.06552	0.06426	0.06301	0.06178	0.06057	0.05938	0.05821	0.05705	0.05592
1.60	0.05480	0.05370	0.05262	0.05155	0.05050	0.04947	0.04846	0.04746	0.04648	0.04551
1.70	0.04457	0.04363	0.04272	0.04182	0.04093	0.04006	0.03920	0.03836	0.03754	0.03673
1.80	0.03593	0.03515	0.03438	0.03362	0.03288	0.03216	0.03144	0.03074	0.03005	0.02938
1.90	0.02872	0.02807	0.02743	0.02680	0.02619	0.02559	0.02500	0.02442	0.02385	0.02330
2.00	0.02275	0.02222	0.02169	0.02118	0.02068	0.02018	0.01970	0.01923	0.01876	0.01831
2.10	0.01786	0.01743	0.01700	0.01659	0.01618	0.01578	0.01539	0.01500	0.01463	0.01426
2.20	0.01390	0.01355	0.01321	0.01287	0.01255	0.01222	0.01191	0.01160	0.01130	0.01101
2.30	0.01072	0.01044	0.01017	0.00990	0.00964	0.00939	0.00914	0.00889	0.00866	0.00842
2.40	0.00820	0.00798	0.00776	0.00755	0.00734	0.00714	0.00695	0.00676	0.00657	0.00639
2.50	0.00621	0.00604	0.00587	0.00570	0.00554	0.00539	0.00523	0.00508	0.00494	0.00480
2.60	0.00466	0.00453	0.00440	0.00427	0.00415	0.00402	0.00391	0.00379	0.00368	0.00357
2.70	0.00347	0.00336	0.00326	0.00317	0.00307	0.00298	0.00289	0.00280	0.00272	0.00264
2.80	0.00256	0.00248	0.00240	0.00233	0.00226	0.00219	0.00212	0.00205	0.00199	0.00193
2.90	0.00187	0.00181	0.00175	0.00169	0.00164	0.00159	0.00154	0.00149	0.00144	0.00139
3.00	0.00135	0.00131	0.00126	0.00122	0.00118	0.00114	0.00111	0.00107	0.00104	0.00100
3.10	0.00097	0.00094	0.00090	0.00087	0.00084	0.00082	0.00079	0.00076	0.00074	0.00071
3.20	0.00069	0.00066	0.00064	0.00062	0.00060	0.00058	0.00056	0.00054	0.00052	0.00050
3.30	0.00048	0.00047	0.00045	0.00043	0.00042	0.00040	0.00039	0.00038	0.00036	0.00035
3.40	0.00034	0.00032	0.00031	0.00030	0.00029	0.00028	0.00027	0.00026	0.00025	0.00024
3.50	0.00023	0.00022	0.00022	0.00021	0.00020	0.00019	0.00019	0.00018	0.00017	0.00017
3.60	0.00016	0.00015	0.00015	0.00014	0.00014	0.00013	0.00013	0.00012	0.00012	0.00011
3.70	0.00011	0.00010	0.00010	0.00010	0.00009	0.00009	0.00008	0.00008	0.00008	0.00008
3.80	0.00007	0.00007	0.00007	0.00006	0.00006	0.00006	0.00006	0.00005	0.00005	0.00005
3.90	0.00005	0.00005	0.00004	0.00004	0.00004	0.00004	0.00004	0.00004	0.00003	0.00003
4.00	0.00003	0.00003	0.00003	0.00003	0.00003	0.00003	0.00002	0.00002	0.00002	0.00002

TABLE A.2

Two-Sided Normal Quantities

z	0.00	0.01	0.02	0.03	0.04	0.05	0.06	0.07	0.08	0.09
0.00	1.00000	0.99202	0.98404	0.97607	0.96809	0.96012	0.95216	0.94419	0.93624	0.92829
0.10	0.92034	0.91241	0.90448	0.89657	0.88866	0.88076	0.87288	0.86501	0.85715	0.84931
0.20	0.84148	0.83367	0.82587	0.81809	0.81033	0.80259	0.79486	0.78716	0.77948	0.77182
0.30	0.76418	0.75656	0.74897	0.74140	0.73386	0.72634	0.71885	0.71138	0.70395	0.69654
0.40	0.68916	0.68181	0.67449	0.66720	0.65994	0.65271	0.64552	0.63836	0.63123	0.62413
0.50	0.61708	0.61005	0.60306	0.59611	0.58920	0.58232	0.57548	0.56868	0.56191	0.55519
0.60	0.54851	0.54186	0.53526	0.52869	0.52217	0.51569	0.50925	0.50286	0.49650	0.49019
0.70	0.48393	0.47770	0.47152	0.46539	0.45930	0.45325	0.44725	0.44130	0.43539	0.42953
0.80	0.42371	0.41794	0.41222	0.40654	0.40091	0.39533	0.38979	0.38430	0.37886	0.37347
0.90	0.36812	0.36282	0.35757	0.35237	0.34722	0.34211	0.33706	0.33205	0.32709	0.32217
1.00	0.31731	0.31250	0.30773	0.30301	0.29834	0.29372	0.28914	0.28462	0.28014	0.27571
1.10	0.27133	0.26700	0.26271	0.25848	0.25429	0.25014	0.24605	0.24200	0.23800	0.23405
1.20	0.23014	0.22628	0.22246	0.21870	0.21498	0.21130	0.20767	0.20408	0.20055	0.19705
1.30	0.19360	0.19020	0.18684	0.18352	0.18025	0.17702	0.17383	0.17069	0.16759	0.16453
1.40	0.16151	0.15854	0.15561	0.15272	0.14987	0.14706	0.14429	0.14156	0.13887	0.13622
1.50	0.13361	0.13104	0.12851	0.12602	0.12356	0.12114	0.11876	0.11642	0.11411	0.11183
1.60	0.10960	0.10740	0.10523	0.10310	0.10101	0.09894	0.09691	0.09492	0.09296	0.09103
1.70	0.08913	0.08727	0.08543	0.08363	0.08186	0.08012	0.07841	0.07673	0.07508	0.07345
1.80	0.07186	0.07030	0.06876	0.06725	0.06577	0.06431	0.06289	0.06148	0.06011	0.05876
1.90	0.05743	0.05613	0.05486	0.05361	0.05238	0.05118	0.05000	0.04884	0.04770	0.04659
2.00	0.04550	0.04443	0.04338	0.04236	0.04135	0.04036	0.03940	0.03845	0.03753	0.03662
2.10	0.03573	0.03486	0.03401	0.03317	0.03235	0.03156	0.03077	0.03001	0.02926	0.02852
2.20	0.02781	0.02711	0.02642	0.02575	0.02509	0.02445	0.02382	0.02321	0.02261	0.02202
2.30	0.02145	0.02089	0.02034	0.01981	0.01928	0.01877	0.01827	0.01779	0.01731	0.01685
2.40	0.01640	0.01595	0.01552	0.01510	0.01469	0.01429	0.01389	0.01351	0.01314	0.01277
2.50	0.01242	0.01207	0.01174	0.01141	0.01109	0.01077	0.01047	0.01017	0.00988	0.00960
2.60	0.00932	0.00905	0.00879	0.00854	0.00829	0.00805	0.00781	0.00759	0.00736	0.00715
2.70	0.00693	0.00673	0.00653	0.00633	0.00614	0.00596	0.00578	0.00561	0.00544	0.00527
2.80	0.00511	0.00495	0.00480	0.00465	0.00451	0.00437	0.00424	0.00410	0.00398	0.00385
2.90	0.00373	0.00361	0.00350	0.00339	0.00328	0.00318	0.00308	0.00298	0.00288	0.00279
3.00	0.00270	0.00261	0.00253	0.00245	0.00237	0.00229	0.00221	0.00214	0.00207	0.00200
3.10	0.00194	0.00187	0.00181	0.00175	0.00169	0.00163	0.00158	0.00152	0.00147	0.00142
3.20	0.00137	0.00133	0.00128	0.00124	0.00120	0.00115	0.00111	0.00108	0.00104	0.00100
3.30	0.00097	0.00093	0.00090	0.00087	0.00084	0.00081	0.00078	0.00075	0.00072	0.00070
3.40	0.00067	0.00065	0.00063	0.00060	0.00058	0.00056	0.00054	0.00052	0.00050	0.00048
3.50	0.00047	0.00045	0.00043	0.00042	0.00040	0.00039	0.00037	0.00036	0.00034	0.00033
3.60	0.00032	0.00031	0.00029	0.00028	0.00027	0.00026	0.00025	0.00024	0.00023	0.00022
3.70	0.00022	0.00021	0.00020	0.00019	0.00018	0.00018	0.00017	0.00016	0.00016	0.00015
3.80	0.00014	0.00014	0.00013	0.00013	0.00012	0.00012	0.00011	0.00011	0.00010	0.00010
3.90	0.00010	0.00009	0.00009	0.00008	0.00008	0.00008	0.00007	0.00007	0.00007	0.00007
4.00	0.00006	0.00006	0.00006	0.00006	0.00005	0.00005	0.00005	0.00005	0.00005	0.00004

TABLE A.3

One-Sided Critical Values for a *t*-distribution

	Significance Level									
df	0.400	0.300	0.250	0.200	0.150	0.100	0.050	0.025	0.010	0.001
1	0.325	0.727	1.000	1.376	1.963	3.078	6.314	12.706	31.821	318.309
2	0.289	0.617	0.816	1.061	1.386	1.886	2.920	4.303	6.965	22.327
3	0.277	0.584	0.765	0.978	1.250	1.638	2.353	3.182	4.541	10.215
4	0.271	0.569	0.741	0.941	1.190	1.533	2.132	2.776	3.747	7.173
5	0.267	0.559	0.727	0.920	1.156	1.476	2.015	2.571	3.365	5.893
6	0.265	0.553	0.718	0.906	1.134	1.440	1.943	2.447	3.143	5.208
7	0.263	0.549	0.711	0.896	1.119	1.415	1.895	2.365	2.998	4.785
8	0.262	0.546	0.706	0.889	1.108	1.397	1.860	2.306	2.896	4.501
9	0.261	0.543	0.703	0.883	1.100	1.383	1.833	2.262	2.821	4.297
10	0.260	0.542	0.700	0.879	1.093	1.372	1.812	2.228	2.764	4.144
11	0.260	0.540	0.697	0.876	1.088	1.363	1.796	2.201	2.718	4.025
12	0.259	0.539	0.695	0.873	1.083	1.356	1.782	2.179	2.681	3.930
13	0.259	0.538	0.694	0.870	1.079	1.350	1.771	2.160	2.650	3.852
14	0.258	0.537	0.692	0.868	1.076	1.345	1.761	2.145	2.624	3.787
15	0.258	0.536	0.691	0.866	1.074	1.341	1.753	2.131	2.602	3.733
16	0.258	0.535	0.690	0.865	1.071	1.337	1.746	2.120	2.583	3.686
17	0.257	0.534	0.689	0.863	1.069	1.333	1.740	2.110	2.567	3.646
18	0.257	0.534	0.688	0.862	1.067	1.330	1.734	2.101	2.552	3.610
19	0.257	0.533	0.688	0.861	1.066	1.328	1.729	2.093	2.539	3.579
20	0.257	0.533	0.687	0.860	1.064	1.325	1.725	2.086	2.528	3.552
21	0.257	0.532	0.686	0.859	1.063	1.323	1.721	2.080	2.518	3.527
22	0.256	0.532	0.686	0.858	1.061	1.321	1.717	2.074	2.508	3.505
23	0.256	0.532	0.685	0.858	1.060	1.319	1.714	2.069	2.500	3.485
24	0.256	0.531	0.685	0.857	1.059	1.318	1.711	2.064	2.492	3.467
25	0.256	0.531	0.684	0.856	1.058	1.316	1.708	2.060	2.485	3.450
26	0.256	0.531	0.684	0.856	1.058	1.315	1.706	2.056	2.479	3.435
27	0.256	0.531	0.684	0.855	1.057	1.314	1.703	2.052	2.473	3.421
28	0.256	0.530	0.683	0.855	1.056	1.313	1.701	2.048	2.467	3.408
29	0.256	0.530	0.683	0.854	1.055	1.311	1.699	2.045	2.462	3.396
30	0.256	0.530	0.683	0.854	1.055	1.310	1.697	2.042	2.457	3.385
35	0.255	0.529	0.682	0.852	1.052	1.306	1.690	2.030	2.438	3.340
40	0.255	0.529	0.681	0.851	1.050	1.303	1.684	2.021	2.423	3.307
45	0.255	0.528	0.680	0.850	1.049	1.301	1.679	2.014	2.412	3.281
50	0.255	0.528	0.679	0.849	1.047	1.299	1.676	2.009	2.403	3.261
60	0.254	0.527	0.679	0.848	1.045	1.296	1.671	2.000	2.390	3.232
70	0.254	0.527	0.678	0.847	1.044	1.294	1.667	1.994	2.381	3.211
80	0.254	0.526	0.678	0.846	1.043	1.292	1.664	1.990	2.374	3.195
90	0.254	0.526	0.677	0.846	1.042	1.291	1.662	1.987	2.368	3.183
100	0.254	0.526	0.677	0.845	1.042	1.290	1.660	1.984	2.364	3.174
125	0.254	0.526	0.676	0.845	1.041	1.288	1.657	1.979	2.357	3.157
150	0.254	0.526	0.676	0.844	1.040	1.287	1.655	1.976	2.351	3.145
175	0.254	0.525	0.676	0.844	1.040	1.286	1.654	1.974	2.348	3.137
200	0.254	0.525	0.676	0.843	1.039	1.286	1.653	1.972	2.345	3.131
225	0.254	0.525	0.676	0.843	1.039	1.285	1.652	1.971	2.343	3.127
250	0.254	0.525	0.675	0.843	1.039	1.285	1.651	1.969	2.341	3.123
300	0.254	0.525	0.675	0.843	1.038	1.284	1.650	1.968	2.339	3.118
350	0.254	0.525	0.675	0.843	1.038	1.284	1.649	1.967	2.337	3.114
400	0.254	0.525	0.675	0.843	1.038	1.284	1.649	1.966	2.336	3.111
450	0.253	0.525	0.675	0.842	1.038	1.283	1.648	1.965	2.335	3.108
500	0.253	0.525	0.675	0.842	1.038	1.283	1.648	1.965	2.334	3.107
750	0.253	0.525	0.675	0.842	1.037	1.283	1.647	1.963	2.331	3.101
1,000	0.253	0.525	0.675	0.843	1.037	1.282	1.646	1.962	2.330	3.098

TABLE A.4

Two-Sided Critical Values for a *t*-distribution

	Significance Level										
df	0.500	0.400	0.300	0.250	0.200	0.150	0.100	0.050	0.025	0.010	0.001
1	1.000	1.376	1.963	2.414	3.078	4.165	6.314	12.706	25.452	63.657	636.619
2	0.816	1.061	1.386	1.604	1.886	2.282	2.920	4.303	6.205	9.925	31.599
3	0.765	0.978	1.250	1.423	1.638	1.924	2.353	3.182	4.177	5.841	12.924
4	0.741	0.941	1.190	1.344	1.533	1.778	2.132	2.776	3.495	4.604	8.610
5	0.727	0.920	1.156	1.301	1.476	1.699	2.015	2.571	3.163	4.032	6.869
6	0.718	0.906	1.134	1.273	1.440	1.650	1.943	2.447	2.969	3.707	5.959
7	0.711	0.896	1.119	1.254	1.415	1.617	1.895	2.365	2.841	3.499	5.408
8	0.706	0.889	1.108	1.240	1.397	1.592	1.860	2.306	2.752	3.355	5.041
9	0.703	0.883	1.100	1.230	1.383	1.574	1.833	2.262	2.685	3.250	4.781
10	0.700	0.879	1.093	1.221	1.372	1.559	1.812	2.228	2.634	3.169	4.587
11	0.697	0.876	1.088	1.214	1.363	1.548	1.796	2.201	2.593	3.106	4.437
12	0.695	0.873	1.083	1.209	1.356	1.538	1.782	2.179	2.560	3.055	4.318
13	0.694	0.870	1.079	1.204	1.350	1.530	1.771	2.160	2.533	3.012	4.221
14	0.692	0.868	1.076	1.200	1.345	1.523	1.761	2.145	2.510	2.977	4.140
15	0.691	0.866	1.074	1.197	1.341	1.517	1.753	2.131	2.490	2.947	4.073
16	0.690	0.865	1.071	1.194	1.337	1.512	1.746	2.120	2.473	2.921	4.015
17	0.689	0.863	1.069	1.191	1.333	1.508	1.740	2.110	2.458	2.898	3.965
18	0.688	0.862	1.067	1.189	1.330	1.504	1.734	2.101	2.445	2.878	3.922
19	0.688	0.861	1.066	1.187	1.328	1.500	1.729	2.093	2.433	2.861	3.883
20	0.687	0.860	1.064	1.185	1.325	1.497	1.725	2.086	2.423	2.845	3.850
21	0.686	0.859	1.063	1.183	1.323	1.494	1.721	2.080	2.414	2.831	3.819
22	0.686	0.858	1.061	1.182	1.321	1.492	1.717	2.074	2.405	2.819	3.792
23	0.685	0.858	1.060	1.180	1.319	1.489	1.714	2.069	2.398	2.807	3.768
24	0.685	0.857	1.059	1.179	1.318	1.487	1.711	2.064	2.391	2.797	3.745
25	0.684	0.856	1.058	1.178	1.316	1.485	1.708	2.060	2.385	2.787	3.725
26	0.684	0.856	1.058	1.177	1.315	1.483	1.706	2.056	2.379	2.779	3.707
27	0.684	0.855	1.057	1.176	1.314	1.482	1.703	2.052	2.373	2.771	3.690
28	0.683	0.855	1.056	1.175	1.313	1.480	1.701	2.048	2.368	2.763	3.674
29	0.683	0.854	1.055	1.174	1.311	1.479	1.699	2.045	2.364	2.756	3.659
30	0.683	0.854	1.055	1.173	1.310	1.477	1.697	2.042	2.360	2.750	3.646
35	0.682	0.852	1.052	1.170	1.306	1.472	1.690	2.030	2.342	2.724	3.591
40	0.681	0.851	1.050	1.167	1.303	1.468	1.684	2.021	2.329	2.704	3.551
45	0.680	0.850	1.049	1.165	1.301	1.465	1.679	2.014	2.319	2.690	3.520
50	0.679	0.849	1.047	1.164	1.299	1.462	1.676	2.009	2.311	2.678	3.496
60	0.679	0.848	1.045	1.162	1.296	1.458	1.671	2.000	2.299	2.660	3.460
70	0.678	0.847	1.044	1.160	1.294	1.456	1.667	1.994	2.291	2.648	3.435
80	0.678	0.846	1.043	1.159	1.292	1.453	1.664	1.990	2.284	2.639	3.416
90	0.677	0.846	1.042	1.158	1.291	1.452	1.662	1.987	2.280	2.632	3.402
100	0.677	0.845	1.042	1.157	1.290	1.451	1.660	1.984	2.276	2.626	3.390
125	0.676	0.845	1.041	1.156	1.288	1.448	1.657	1.979	2.269	2.616	3.370
150	0.676	0.844	1.040	1.155	1.287	1.447	1.655	1.976	2.264	2.609	3.357
175	0.676	0.844	1.040	1.154	1.286	1.446	1.654	1.974	2.261	2.604	3.347
200	0.676	0.843	1.039	1.154	1.286	1.445	1.653	1.972	2.258	2.601	3.340
225	0.676	0.843	1.039	1.153	1.285	1.444	1.652	1.971	2.257	2.598	3.334
250	0.675	0.843	1.039	1.153	1.285	1.444	1.651	1.969	2.255	2.596	3.330
300	0.675	0.843	1.038	1.153	1.284	1.443	1.650	1.968	2.253	2.592	3.323
350	0.675	0.843	1.038	1.152	1.284	1.443	1.649	1.967	2.251	2.590	3.319
400	0.675	0.843	1.038	1.152	1.284	1.442	1.649	1.966	2.250	2.588	3.315
450	0.675	0.842	1.038	1.152	1.283	1.442	1.648	1.965	2.249	2.587	3.312
500	0.675	0.842	1.038	1.152	1.283	1.442	1.648	1.965	2.248	2.586	3.310
750	0.675	0.842	1.037	1.151	1.283	1.441	1.647	1.963	2.246	2.582	3.304
1,000	0.675	0.842	1.037	1.151	1.282	1.441	1.646	1.962	2.245	2.581	3.300

TABLE A.5

Chi-Squared Critical Values

	Significance Level												
df	0.999	0.990	0.975	0.950	0.900	0.750	0.500	0.250	0.100	0.050	0.025	0.010	0.001
1	0.000002	0.0002	0.001	0.004	0.02	0.10	0.45	1.32	2.71	3.84	5.02	6.63	10.83
2	0.002	0.020	0.05	0.10	0.21	0.58	1.39	2.77	4.61	5.99	7.38	9.21	13.82
3	0.02	0.11	0.22	0.35	0.58	1.21	2.37	4.11	6.25	7.81	9.35	11.34	16.27
4	0.09	0.30	0.48	0.71	1.06	1.92	3.36	5.39	7.78	9.49	11.14	13.28	18.47
5	0.21	0.55	0.83	1.15	1.61	2.67	4.35	6.63	9.24	11.07	12.83	15.09	20.52
6	0.38	0.87	1.24	1.64	2.20	3.45	5.35	7.84	10.64	12.59	14.45	16.81	22.46
7	0.60	1.24	1.69	2.17	2.83	4.25	6.35	9.04	12.02	14.07	16.01	18.48	24.32
8	0.86	1.65	2.18	2.73	3.49	5.07	7.34	10.22	13.36	15.51	17.53	20.09	26.12
9	1.15	2.09	2.70	3.33	4.17	5.90	8.34	11.39	14.68	16.92	19.02	21.67	27.88
10	1.48	2.56	3.25	3.94	4.87	6.74	9.34	12.55	15.99	18.31	20.48	23.21	29.59
11	1.83	3.05	3.82	4.57	5.58	7.58	10.34	13.70	17.28	19.68	21.92	24.72	31.26
12	2.21	3.57	4.40	5.23	6.30	8.44	11.34	14.85	18.55	21.03	23.34	26.22	32.91
13	2.62	4.11	5.01	5.89	7.04	9.30	12.34	15.98	19.81	22.36	24.74	27.69	34.53
14	3.04	4.66	5.63	6.57	7.79	10.17	13.34	17.12	21.06	23.68	26.12	29.14	36.12
15	3.48	5.23	6.26	7.26	8.55	11.04	14.34	18.25	22.31	25.00	27.49	30.58	37.70
16	3.94	5.81	6.91	7.96	9.31	11.91	15.34	19.37	23.54	26.30	28.85	32.00	39.25
17	4.42	6.41	7.56	8.67	10.09	12.79	16.34	20.49	24.77	27.59	30.19	33.41	40.79
18	4.90	7.01	8.23	9.39	10.86	13.68	17.34	21.60	25.99	28.87	31.53	34.81	42.31
19	5.41	7.63	8.91	10.12	11.65	14.56	18.34	22.72	27.20	30.14	32.85	36.19	43.82
20	5.92	8.26	9.59	10.85	12.44	15.45	19.34	23.83	28.41	31.41	34.17	37.57	45.31
21	6.45	8.90	10.28	11.59	13.24	16.34	20.34	24.93	29.62	32.67	35.48	38.93	46.80
22	6.98	9.54	10.98	12.34	14.04	17.24	21.34	26.04	30.81	33.92	36.78	40.29	48.27
23	7.53	10.20	11.69	13.09	14.85	18.14	22.34	27.14	32.01	35.17	38.08	41.64	49.73
24	8.08	10.86	12.40	13.85	15.66	19.04	23.34	28.24	33.20	36.42	39.36	42.98	51.18
25	8.65	11.52	13.12	14.61	16.47	19.94	24.34	29.34	34.38	37.65	40.65	44.31	52.62
26	9.22	12.20	13.84	15.38	17.29	20.84	25.34	30.43	35.56	38.89	41.92	45.64	54.05
27	9.80	12.88	14.57	16.15	18.11	21.75	26.34	31.53	36.74	40.11	43.19	46.96	55.48
28	10.39	13.56	15.31	16.93	18.94	22.66	27.34	32.62	37.92	41.34	44.46	48.28	56.89
29	10.99	14.26	16.05	17.71	19.77	23.57	28.34	33.71	39.09	42.56	45.72	49.59	58.30
30	11.59	14.95	16.79	18.49	20.60	24.48	29.34	34.80	40.26	43.77	46.98	50.89	59.70
35	14.69	18.51	20.57	22.47	24.80	29.05	34.34	40.22	46.06	49.80	53.20	57.34	66.62
40	17.92	22.16	24.43	26.51	29.05	33.66	39.34	45.62	51.81	55.76	59.34	63.69	73.40
45	21.25	25.90	28.37	30.61	33.35	38.29	44.34	50.98	57.51	61.66	65.41	69.96	80.08
50	24.67	29.71	32.36	34.76	37.69	42.94	49.33	56.33	63.17	67.50	71.42	76.15	86.66
60	31.74	37.48	40.48	43.19	46.46	52.29	59.33	66.98	74.40	79.08	83.30	88.38	99.61
70	39.04	45.44	48.76	51.74	55.33	61.70	69.33	77.58	85.53	90.53	95.02	100.43	112.32
80	46.52	53.54	57.15	60.39	64.28	71.14	79.33	88.13	96.58	101.88	106.63	112.33	124.84
90	54.16	61.75	65.65	69.13	73.29	80.62	89.33	98.65	107.57	113.15	118.14	124.12	137.21
100	61.92	70.06	74.22	77.93	82.36	90.13	99.33	109.14	118.50	124.34	129.56	135.81	149.45
125	81.77	91.18	95.95	100.18	105.21	114.00	124.33	135.27	145.64	152.09	157.84	164.69	179.60
150	102.11	112.67	117.98	122.69	128.28	137.98	149.33	161.29	172.58	179.58	185.80	193.21	209.26
175	122.83	134.44	140.26	145.41	151.49	162.04	174.33	187.23	199.36	206.87	213.52	221.44	238.55
200	143.84	156.43	162.73	168.28	174.84	186.17	199.33	213.10	226.02	233.99	241.06	249.45	267.54
225	165.10	178.61	185.35	191.28	198.28	210.35	224.33	238.92	252.58	260.99	268.44	277.27	296.29
250	186.55	200.94	208.10	214.39	221.81	234.58	249.33	264.70	279.05	287.88	295.69	304.94	324.83
300	229.96	245.97	253.91	260.88	269.07	283.14	299.33	316.14	331.79	341.40	349.87	359.91	381.43
350	273.90	291.41	300.06	307.65	316.55	331.81	349.33	367.46	384.31	394.63	403.72	414.47	437.49
400	318.26	337.16	346.48	354.64	364.21	380.58	399.33	418.70	436.65	447.63	457.31	468.72	493.13
450	362.96	383.16	393.12	401.82	412.01	429.42	449.33	469.86	488.85	500.46	510.67	522.72	548.43
500	407.95	429.39	439.94	449.15	459.93	478.32	499.33	520.95	540.93	553.13	563.85	576.49	603.45

Index

CPSIA information can be obtained at www.ICGtesting.com
Printed in the USA
LVOW04*1001151214

418617LV00009B/35/P